Adolescent Substance Use Disorders

Guest Editor

YIFRAH KAMINER, MD, MBA

CHILD AND ADOLESCENT PSYCHIATRIC CLINICS OF NORTH AMERICA

www.childpsych.theclinics.com

Consulting Editor
HARSH K. TRIVEDI, MD

July 2010 • Volume 19 • Number 3

SAUNDERS an imprint of ELSEVIER, Inc.

W.B. SAUNDERS COMPANY
A Division of Elsevier Inc.

Elsevier Inc. • 1600 John F. Kennedy Boulevard • Suite 1800 • Philadelphia, Pennsylvania 19103-2899

http://www.childpsych.theclinics.com

CHILD AND ADOLESCENT PSYCHIATRIC CLINICS OF NORTH AMERICA Volume 19, Number 3
July 2010 ISSN 1056–4993, ISBN-13: 978-1-4377-2432-5

Editor: Sarah E. Barth
Developmental Editor: Theresa Collier

Child and Adolescent Psychiatric Clinics of North America (ISSN 1056-4993) is published quarterly by Elsevier Inc., 360 Park Avenue South, New York, NY 10010-1710. Months of issue are January, April, July, and October. Business and Editorial Offices: 1600 John F. Kennedy Boulevard, Suite 1800, Philadelphia, PA 19103-2899. Periodicals postage paid at New York, NY and additional mailing offices. Subscription prices are $257.00 per year (US individuals), $386.00 per year (US institutions), $132.00 per year (US students), $292.00 per year (Canadian individuals), $466.00 per year (Canadian institutions), $168.00 per year (Canadian students), $347.00 per year (international individuals), $466.00 per year (international institutions), and $168.00 per year (international students). International air speed delivery is included in all Clinics subscription prices. All prices are subject to change without notice. **POSTMASTER:** Send address changes to Child and Adolescent Psychiatric Clinics of North America, Elsevier Health Sciences Division, Subscription Customer Service, 3251 Riverport Lane, Maryland Heights, MO 63043. **Customer Service: 1-800-654-2452 (U.S. and Canada); 314-447-8871 (outside U.S. and Canada). Fax: 314-447-8029. E-mail: JournalsCustomerService-usa@ elsevier.com (for print support) or journalsonlinesupport-usa@elsevier.com (for online support).**

Reprints. For copies of 100 or more of articles in this publication, please contact the Commercial Reprints Department, Elsevier Inc., 360 Park Avenue South, New York, New York 10010-1710 Tel.: (212) 633-3812; Fax: (212) 462-1935, e-mail: reprints@elsevier.com.

Child and Adolescent Psychiatric Clinics of North America is covered in *MEDLINE/PubMed (Index Medicus), ISI, SSCI, Research Alert, Social Search, Current Contents,* and *EMBASE/Excerpta Medica.*

Printed in the United States of America.

Contributors

CONSULTING EDITOR

HARSH K. TRIVEDI, MD
Executive Medical Director and Chief-of-Staff, Vanderbilt Psychiatric Hospital;
Associate Professor of Psychiatry, Vanderbilt Medical School, Nashville, Tennessee

CONSULTING EDITOR EMERITUS

ANDRÉS MARTIN, MD, MPH

FOUNDING CONSULTING EDITOR

MELVIN LEWIS, MBBS, FRCPSYCH, DCH

GUEST EDITOR

YIFRAH KAMINER, MD, MBA
Professor of Psychiatry and Pediatrics, Alcohol Research Center, University of
Connecticut Health Center, Farmington, Connecticut

AUTHORS

GILBERT J. BOTVIN, PhD
Professor of Public Health and Psychiatry, Director of Cornell's Institute for Prevention
Research; Chief, Division of Prevention and Health Behavior, Department of Public Health,
Weill Cornell Medical College, Cornell University, New York, New York

CHRISTINA BREZING, MD
University of Florida College of Medicine, Gainesville, Florida

ALAN J. BUDNEY, PhD
Professor, Center for Addiction Research, Department of Psychiatry, University of
Arkansas for Medical Sciences, Little Rock, Arkansas

OSCAR G. BUKSTEIN, MD, MPH
Professor of Psychiatry, Western Psychiatric Institute and Clinic, University of Pittsburgh
School of Medicine, Pittsburgh, Pennsylvania

KAREN G. CHARTIER, PhD
Faculty Associate, University of Texas School of Public Health, Dallas, Texas

JEFFREY L. DEREVENSKY, PhD
International Centre for Youth Gambling, Problems and High Risk Behaviors, McGill
University, Montreal, Quebec, Canada

DANIELLE M. DICK, PhD
Assistant Professor of Psychiatry, Psychology and Human and Molecular Genetics, Virginia Institute of Psychiatric and Behavioral Genetics, Virginia Commonwealth University, Richmond, Virginia

BRETTON ENGLE, PhD, LCSW
Assistant Professor, School of Social Work, Barry University, Miami Shores, Florida

MARK GODLEY, PhD
Director of Research and Development, Chestnut Health Systems, Normal, Illinois

SEVERIN GRENOBLE, MD
Resident, Department of Psychiatry, University of South Alabama College of Medicine, Mobile, Alabama

KENNETH W. GRIFFIN, PhD, MPH
Professor of Public Health, Division of Prevention and Health Behavior, Department of Public Health, Weill Cornell Medical College, Cornell University, New York, New York

MICHIE N. HESSELBROCK, PhD
Professor, Department of Psychiatry, University of Connecticut School of Medicine, Farmington, Connecticut

VICTOR M. HESSELBROCK, PhD
Professor and Interim Chairman, Department of Psychiatry, University of Connecticut School of Medicine, Farmington, Connecticut

MICHELLE S. HORNER, DO
Postdoctoral Research Scholar, Western Psychiatric Institute and Clinic, University of Pittsburgh School of Medicine, Pittsburgh, Pennsylvania

YIFRAH KAMINER MD, MBA
Professor of Psychiatry and Pediatrics, Alcohol Research Center, University of Connecticut Health Center, Farmington, Connecticut

WILLIAM LATIMER, PhD, MPH
Associate Professor, Department of Mental Health, Johns Hopkins Bloomberg School of Public Health, Baltimore, Maryland

MARK J. MACGOWAN, PhD, LCSW
Associate Professor, School of Social Work, College of Public Health and Social Work; Associate Director, Community-Based Intervention Research Group, Florida International University, Miami, Florida

LINDA C. MAYES, MD
Arnold Gesell Professor, Child Psychiatry, Pediatrics, Psychology, Yale Child Study Center, Yale University School of Medicine, New Haven, Connecticut

JACQUELYN L. MEYERS, BS
Doctoral Candidate, Department of Human and Molecular Genetics, Virginia Institute of Psychiatric and Behavioral Genetics, Virginia Commonwealth University, Richmond, Virginia

MARC N. POTENZA, MD, PhD
Professor of Psychiatry and Child Study, Yale Child Study Center; Department
of Psychiatry, Connecticut Mental Health Center, Yale University School of Medicine,
New Haven, Connecticut

CYNTHIA L. ROWE, PhD
Associate Professor, Department of Epidemiology and Public Health, Center for
Treatment Research on Adolescent Drug Abuse, University of Miami Miller School
of Medicine, Miami, Florida

HELENA J.V. RUTHERFORD, PhD
Postdoctoral Associate, Yale Child Study Center, Yale University School of Medicine,
New Haven, Connecticut

DEBORAH R. SIMKIN, MD
Associate Professor; Residency Director; Head, Division of Child and Adolescent
Psychiatry, Department of Psychiatry, University South Alabama College of Medicine,
Mobile, Alabama

CATHERINE STANGER, PhD
Associate Professor, Center for Addiction Research, Department of Psychiatry, University
of Arkansas for Medical Sciences, Little Rock, Arkansas

JULIA ZUR, BS
Doctoral Candidate, Department of Mental Health, Johns Hopkins Bloomberg School
of Public Health, Baltimore, Maryland

Contents

This article provides an overview of drug and alcohol use and risk factors among American adolescents. Current trends indicate that tobacco, alcohol, and marijuana are the most frequently used substances among this age group. Further, the greatest risk factors for using these substances are being male, being White, being an older adolescent, engaging in sexual risk behaviors, having a family history of substance abuse, associating with peers who abuse substances, and lacking a sense of school commitment and connectedness. These findings underscore the need to involve communities, families, schools, and peer groups to effectively prevent and treat this problem.

Substance dependence disorders are chronic relapsing disorders with immense societal consequences. Twin and family studies have found that there are critical genetic and environmental components in the inheritance of substance use disorders, and modern advances in genetics are making it possible to identify specific variants that may predispose an individual to these disorders. Adolescence is a crucial period for initiation, experimentation, and the establishment of more regular patterns of use of alcohol and other drugs. Adolescent substance use is a known risk factor for the development of later alcohol and substance use problems, as well as related externalizing disorders such as antisocial personality disorder. Understanding the early risk factors and processes that make these youths vulnerable to substance use disorders is crucial to the development of effective strategies for prevention. This article reviews the genetic origins of adolescent substance use problems and the potential this field of research offers for prevention.

Adolescence represents a unique period of development with neuronal maturation accompanied by increases in behavioral risk taking. Although risky behavior is a likely marker of normative adolescent development, there is an early emergence of substance use disorders in this population. Adolescence represents a distinct period of vulnerability to substance use initiation and transitions to substance abuse and dependence. Of recent interest is understanding the neurobiology of adolescent substance use disorders, with adult studies being limited in their applicability to this developmentally sensitive maturation period and providing restricted insight into potential treatment and intervention. First, the authors review the neurobiology of adolescent substance use disorders and, second, the authors consider the implications of these findings for prevention and treatment.

This article provides an overview of the characteristics of adolescent alcohol use, normative and subgroup variations in drinking behavior, and the important factors associated with an increased risk for developing alcohol problems in later adolescence and young adulthood. Parental or family histories of alcoholism, temperament traits, conduct problems, cognitive functioning, alcohol expectancies, and peer and other social relations are identified as factors influencing an adolescent's susceptibility for initiating a variety of alcohol use behaviors. The deviance prone model, proposed by Sher in 1991, is presented as an important tool for testing possible relationships among the various risk factors and their sequencing that leads to early adolescent alcohol use and drug initiation. It is also possible to extend the model to allow for an examination of the complex interplay of risk factors that lead to the development of alcohol use problems in late adolescence and young adults.

Substantial progress has been made in developing prevention programs for adolescent drug abuse. The most effective interventions target salient risk and protective factors at the individual, family, and community levels and are guided by relevant psychosocial theories regarding the etiology of substance use and abuse. This article reviews the epidemiology, etiologic risk and protective factors, and evidence-based approaches that have been found to be most effective in preventing adolescent substance use and abuse. Exemplary school- and family-based prevention programs for universal (everyone in population), selected (members of at-risk groups), and indicated (at-risk individuals) target populations are reviewed, along with model community-based prevention approaches. Challenges remain in widely disseminating evidence-based prevention programs into schools, families, and communities.

This article reviews behavior therapies, motivational interviewing interventions, and combined behavioral-psychosocial therapies across 34 peer-reviewed publications. Studies were included if they involved youth with alcohol and other drug (AOD) use, included measures of AOD outcomes, and used controlled research designs with a control or comparison condition. The level of empirical support of the interventions was evaluated using established guidelines. The article determined that behavior therapies were "probably efficacious," and motivational interviewing interventions easily met the criteria for "promising." Because of small sample sizes, combined behavioral-psychosocial therapies marginally met the criteria for "promising." The findings from this article underscore the value of individual and group behavior therapies and motivational interviewing in helping reduce mild to serious AOD use among adolescents.

Catherine Stanger and Alan J. Budney

The addition of contingency management (CM) to the menu of effective treatments for adolescent substance abuse has generated excitement in the research and treatment communities. CM interventions are based on extensive basic science and clinical research evidence demonstrating that drug use is sensitive to systematically applied consequences. This article provides (a) a review of basic CM principles, (b) implementation guidelines, (c) a review of the clinical CM research targeting adolescent substance abuse, and (d) a discussion of implementation successes and challenges. Although the research base for CM with adolescents is in its infancy, there are multiple reasons for high expectations.

Cynthia L. Rowe

Adolescent substance abuse rarely occurs without other psychiatric and developmental problems, but it is often treated and researched as if it can be isolated from comorbid conditions. Few comprehensive interventions are available that effectively address the range of co-occurring problems associated with adolescent substance abuse. This article reviews the clinical interventions and research evidence supporting the use of Multidimensional Family Therapy (MDFT) for adolescents with substance abuse and co-occurring problems. MDFT is uniquely suited to address adolescent substance abuse and related disorders given its comprehensive interventions that systematically target the multiple interacting risk factors underlying many developmental disruptions of adolescence.

Yifrah Kaminer and Mark Godley

This article addresses less developed areas of clinical research that are of great importance for better understanding the therapeutic process along the continuum of care in youth with alcohol and other substance use disorders (AOSUD). These include the rationale, design, mechanisms of behavior change (MBCs), implementation, monitoring, and outcome-based modification of treatment continuum for youth with AOSUD. The specific objectives are: (1) present current knowledge pertaining to the pretreatment phase including the effect of baseline assessment on treatment outcome; (2) address potential MBCs in treatment; (3) discuss the importance of aftercare, also known as continued care, to prevent postintervention relapse; (4) consider how reconceptualization of therapeutic paradigms might advance the field, in particular treatment algorithm or adaptive treatment strategies addressing poor response to treatment.

Deborah R. Simkin and Severin Grenoble

There is a paucity of research on pharmacotherapies in adolescents with substance use disorders. This paucity is partly because of the fact that most people with substance dependence do not get diagnosed until early adulthood, that is, after 18 years of age. This article reviews pharmacotherapies used for aversion, substitution, anti-craving, and detoxification of alcohol, nicotine, cocaine, and opioids dependence. Adult research is referenced when applicable and generalized to adolescents with caution. Continued evaluation and development of pharmacotherapy for youth in controlled studies are needed to examine medication effectiveness, safety, potential for abuse, compliance, and potential interactions with other medications or substances of abuse.

Oscar G. Bukstein and Michelle S. Horner

Substance use disorders are common in youth, and co-occurring psychiatric disorders are present in the majority of cases. This article reviews clinical considerations unique to the population, including intricacies of assessment and special treatment considerations. Several psychotherapeutic intervention models are discussed, including cognitive-behavioral therapy, dialectic behavior therapy, motivational enhancement therapy/motivational interviewing, family behavior therapy, multidimensional family therapy, and multisystemic therapy. Research on psychopharmacologic treatment is limited, and primarily focuses on mood disorders and attention deficit/hyperactivity disorder. To maximize outcome, recommendations based on practice parameters promote integration of treatment modalities versus serial or concurrent treatment of co-occurring substance use and psychiatric disorders.

Christina Brezing, Jeffrey L. Derevensky, and Marc N. Potenza

Adolescence is characterized by participation in multiple novel and potentially risky behaviors. Amongst these behaviors are gambling and use of the Internet, and excessive engagement in these activities (as seen in pathological gambling and problematic Internet use) may be accompanied by serious impairments in school, mental health, and social functioning. This article reviews the potential impact of pathological gambling and problematic Internet use in youth, the relevance of subsyndromal levels of participation, and how prevention and treatment strategies may be considered and tested within a developmental framework.

Yifrah Kaminer

Energy drinks (EDs) are caffeine-based beverages that commonly contain large doses of sugar, carbohydrates, and a variety of legal stimulants and supplements, such as guarana, taurine, ginseng, and vitamin B complex. These drinks are marketed for young people as natural alternatives that increase fun and improve physical and cognitive performance such as concentration, attention, and alertness. There are commonly held false perceptions that the consumption of EDs can reverse alcohol-related impairment, including motor coordination and visual reaction time, which are crucial for driving safety. This article reviews the literature on EDs and examines problematic use and potential negative consequences in young people. Special emphasis is devoted to safety concerns following combination of EDs with alcohol, which gives the user a false sense of control.

THE CLINICS ARE NOW AVAILABLE ONLINE!

Access your subscription at:
www.theclinics.com

Foreword

The Elephant in the Room

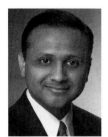

Harsh K. Trivedi, MD
Consulting Editor

The National Institute on Drug Abuse has found that 46.7% of 12th graders have already used an illicit substance and 72.3% have used alcohol. Unfortunately, we are not talking exclusively about kids "testing the waters" or "getting high on some dope" or "experimenting with alcohol." When asked about the nonmedical use of prescription pain-killers, nearly 1 in 10 high school seniors reported using Vicodin and 1 in 20 reported abuse of OxyContin within the past year. Add to that nearly 45% of 12th graders having used cigarettes, 10% having used inhalants, 9% having used tranquilizers, 7% having used ecstasy, 7% having used hallucinogens, 6% having used nonprescription cough medicine, and 6% having used crack cocaine...and the numbers seem quite staggering.[1]

What is most amazing about the issue of substance abuse in kids is how little is done, at the level of training programs as well as in treatment programs, to help diagnose and treat this population. Most training programs (pediatrics, child and adolescent psychiatry, psychology, social work, nursing, and others) gloss over this topic by providing a few reference articles to their respective students or muddling through it in a few lectures over the course of an entire training program. Where this starts to get scary is when there is an identified youth who needs help. The remarkable lack of appropriate treatment programs (across the board in most parts of the country) is shocking. For the ones that do exist, finding ones that provide high-quality and competent care with pediatric-trained providers (ie, not using adult providers to treat youth) can prove even more difficult. Even inpatient adolescent psychiatric units that admit patients with comorbid substance abuse problems often choose to treat the psychiatric condition and refer out for the substance abuse treatment.

I thank Yifrah Kaminer for taking on this extremely important topic. Anyone treating youth likely encounters patients who have substance abuse problems. Due to the paucity of services, the responsibility of identifying (and often treating) these youth

Child Adolesc Psychiatric Clin N Am 19 (2010) xiii–xiv
doi:10.1016/j.chc.2010.04.001   **childpsych.theclinics.com**
1056-4993/10/$ – see front matter © 2010 Elsevier Inc. All rights reserved.

also falls to these same providers. I thank Dr Kaminer for being a leader in this field and contributing substantially to our understanding of this issue. Likewise, I thank him for being able to produce an excellent volume that brings forth practical knowledge to help each of us do a better job in caring for these youth. I am also grateful to all of the respected contributors, who have each shared their expertise on this topic. Let us hope that, through the efforts of our youth, concerned loved ones, researchers, clinical treatment providers, the media, scientific publications, and advocacy efforts; that we can begin talking more comprehensively about the elephant in room (and potentially have an intervention to get him some necessary help).

Harsh K. Trivedi, MD
Vanderbilt Psychiatric Hospital
1601 23rd Avenue South, Suite 1157
Nashville, TN 37212, USA

E-mail address:
harsh.k.trivedi@vanderbilt.edu

REFERENCE

1. National Institute on Drug Abuse (NIDA) InfoFacts. High school and youth trends. Available at: http://www.drugabuse.gov/infofacts/HSYouthtrends.html. Accessed April 17, 2010.

Preface

Been There, Done That, and Now What? Adolescent Addictive Behaviors from Etiology to Postvention

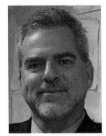

Yifrah Kaminer, MD, MBA
Guest Editor

Childhood and adolescence are not only critical phases for normal development but also periods when various pathological behaviors or disorders, including substance use disorders (SUD), are first recognized. Substance use and SUD among American youth continues to present a challenging public health problem because of concerns regarding the short- and long-term physical and mental health outcomes of adolescents who use psychoactive drugs. The use of alcohol and other drugs is a leading cause of morbidity and mortality among adolescents from motor vehicle accidents, suicidal behavior, violence, drowning, and unprotected sexual activity, including unplanned pregnancy and sexually transmitted diseases.[1] Lifetime diagnoses of alcohol and drug abuse among adolescents in the United States range from 3% to 10%. Six percent and 5.4% of youths ages 12 to 17 were classified as needing treatment for alcohol use and illicit drug use, respectively.[2] Only a small segment of adolescents in need of treatment (10% –15%) end up receiving services because of lack of motivation for treatment among youth, poor screening and assessment skills of providers, limited resources, inadequate age-appropriate quality programs, and lack of a broad consensus on preferred treatment strategies. Nevertheless, the number of published treatment studies has grown dramatically during the last decade.[3]

The main objective of this compilation of thirteen articles is to provide updated contributions on important topics pertaining to better understanding the development of SUD in youth and responding to their treatment needs. Additional information is provided on new emerging issues in the study of newer addictive behaviors in youth.

One article reviews the epidemiologic trends of adolescent substance use. Another two articles look at risk factors for the development of substance use disorders and the interphase between genetic[4] and environmental influences. The authors address the

Child Adolesc Psychiatric Clin N Am 19 (2010) xv–xvi
doi:10.1016/j.chc.2010.03.014
1056-4993/10/$ – see front matter © 2010 Elsevier Inc. All rights reserved.

childpsych.theclinics.com

implications for prevention and treatment. Two other articles address the development and transitions of substance abuse from adolescence into early adulthood and prevention approaches.

Six articles examine treatment approaches. The four psychotherapy articles address motivational interviewing and cognitive behavioral therapy with special attention to the difference between individual and group interventions. Also included are two articles on contingency reinforcement approaches and on multidimensional family therapy. The psychotherapy section is concluded with a synthesis on the process of treatment from the assessment phase through treatment and aftercare (known also as continued care). Two articles address pharmacotherapy and the management of youth substance abuse with psychiatric comorbidity.

Finally, there is still an ongoing debate whether nonsubstance-related addictions are actually addictions.[5] A clever article on the use of butterbeer by Harry Potter and his friends indirectly addresses the question of youth habit formation and exposure to addictive drinks even though it occurs in a fantasy world.[6] Internet addiction and the availability of gambling online are relatively new developments in the study of addictive behaviors in youth. Associations with predictive psychiatric symptoms that might serve as markers for the identification of adolescents at high-risk for these behaviors are intriguing.[7] Unique and relevant contributions are two articles addressing emerging addictive disorders, which include gambling, Internet preoccupation, the use of "energy" drinks, and, perhaps, the next vogue of "antienergy drinks."

I am grateful to the experts who have contributed scholarly articles for this special issue.

Yifrah Kaminer, MD, MBA
Alcohol Research Center
University of Connecticut Health Center
263 Farmington Avenue
Farmington, CT 06030-2103, USA

E-mail address:
Kaminer@uchc.edu

REFERENCES

1. Kaminer Y, Bukstein O, editors. Adolescent substance abuse: dual diagnosis and high risk behaviors. NewYork: Routledge/Taylor & Francis; 2008.
2. Kaminer Y, Winters K, editors. Clinical manual of adolescent substance abuse treatment. Washington, DC: American Psychiatric Publishing Inc; 2010.
3. Dennis ML, Kaminer Y. Introduction to special issue on advances in the assessment and treatment of adolescent substance use disorders. Am J Addict 2008; 15(Suppl 1):1–3.
4. Sartor C, Grant JD, Bucholz KK, et al. Common genetic contributions to alcohol and cannabis use and dependence symptomatology. Alcohol Clin Exp Res 2010;34(3):545–54.
5. Martin PR, Petry NM. Are non-substance-related addictions really addictions? Am J Addictions 2005;14(1):1–7.
6. Welsh CJ. Harry Potter and butterbeer. J Am Acad Child Adolesc Psychiatry 2004; 43(1):9–10.
7. Ko CH, Yen JY, Chen CS, et al. Predictive values of psychiatric symptoms for internet addiction in adolescents:a 2-year prospective study. Arch Pesiatr Adolesc Med 2009;163(10):937–43.

Epidemiologic Trends of Adolescent Use of Alcohol, Tobacco, and Other Drugs

William Latimer, PhD, MPH*, Julia Zur, BS

KEYWORDS

- Adolescence • Youth • Drug • Alcohol epidemiologic trends
- Risk factors

This article provides an overview of adolescent substance abuse, including rates of use, risk and protective factors, and demographic trends for various licit and illicit drugs. Most of this article focuses on adolescent tobacco, alcohol, and marijuana use, because these 3 substances are most commonly used among this age group. Significantly less research has been conducted on the use of other substances among adolescents, because these areas are substantially less problematic. For this reason, a basic overview of rates of use of these substances is included in the article to provide a general sense of patterns of use, whereas the remainder of the article focuses on the most commonly used substances. **Table 1** provides an overview of all of the information sources used to compile this article.

TOBACCO
Rates of Use

In the Monitoring the Future survey of 2008, it was found that cigarette use among 12th grade students reached its lowest rates in over 30 years.[1] Although this finding presents promising information about the success of the efforts taken to minimize the use of cigarettes, the problem is certainly not resolved. In fact, it was also found that by eighth grade, 21% of students have experimented with cigarettes, and 7% of eighth grade students were reported being current smokers. By 12th grade, this number is a great deal higher, with 45% of students reporting having tried cigarettes in the past and 20% of students reporting that they are current smokers. The Monitoring the Future survey also examined rates of adolescent cigarette use during the past 30-day period and found that 7% of 8th graders, 12% of 10th graders, and 20% of

Department of Mental Health, Johns Hopkins Bloomberg School of Public Health, 2213 McElderry Street, 4th Floor, Baltimore, MD 21205, USA
* Corresponding author.
E-mail address: wlatimer@jhsph.edu

Child Adolesc Psychiatric Clin N Am 19 (2010) 451–464
doi:10.1016/j.chc.2010.03.002
1056-4993/10/$ – see front matter © 2010 Elsevier Inc. All rights reserved.
childpsych.theclinics.com

Table 1
Overview of information sources

Year	Authors	Sample	Findings
2008	Johnston et al[1]	More than 46,000 8th, 10th, and 12th grade students from 386 high schools	Rates of use and risk factors for most licit and illicit drugs among American high school students
2004	Beyers et al[2]	32,403 adolescents; 48% male; 85% White	Risk factors for substance use include perceived availability, low school commitment, poor family management, family history of substance use, interaction with antisocial peers, sensation seeking. Protective factors include social skills and a belief in the moral order
2007	Bond et al[3]	2678 eighth grade students in 26 secondary schools; 47% male	School connectedness and social connectedness associated with a decreased likelihood for initiating smoking
1998	Flay et al[4]	6695 seventh grade students; 50% male; 32.5% White; 35.5% Hispanic; 15.5% African American	Family and peer use of cigarettes, alcohol use, and marijuana use are all risk factors for cigarette use
2007	Xue et al[5]	824 9th graders; 50% male; 83% African American; 17% White	Participation in prosocial activities is protective against cigarette smoking
1995	Aaron et al[6]	1211 adolescents aged 12–16 y; 51% boys; 73% White	Physical activity is protective against smoking in girls but increases risk of alcohol consumption in boys
1994	Kelder et al[7]	2376 6th–12th grade students	Students who experimented with smoking were more likely to become regular smokers
2000	Blum et al[8]	10,803 7th–12th high school students; 71% White, 9% Hispanic, and 16% African American	For younger students, highest rates of smoking and drinking were among White
1975	Jessor and Jessor[9]	432 junior high school students	Alcohol use is associated with onset of sexual intercourse and onset of marijuana use
2009	Nelson et al[10]	Biennial 1993–2005 data from state school–based Youth Risk Behavior Survey for 9th–12th grade students	Within particular geographic locations, rates of adolescent alcohol use is correlated with rates of adult alcohol use and rates of adult drunk driving
2008	Beebe et al[11]	134 Native Americans, aged 13–19 y	Nonparental role models, strong family communication, and religious involvement are protective against use of alcohol and other drugs

2007	Leaver-Dunn[12]	1690 10th–12th grade students; 81% White	Participation in recreational activities is protective against alcohol abuse
2007	Watt and Rogers[13]	11,413 adolescents aged 12–17 y; 81% White; 19% African American	White adolescents are more likely to drink alcohol than African American adolescents, but the difference is almost entirely explained by influence of peers and family members
2007	Lonczak et al[14]	97 youth aged 13–19 y; 100% Native American; 44% male	Youth are more likely to begin using alcohol if they live in a single-parent home
2007	Walls et al[15]	603 Native American families with female caretakers of youths aged 10–13 y	Caregiver substance abuse influences adolescent substance abuse
1991	Wallace and Bachman[16]	77,500 adolescents; 77.5% White; 11.9% African American	Native American and White adolescents use alcohol more frequently than other racial group, largely because of lifestyle differences
2004	Brook et al[17]	1332 7th–10th grade students from East Harlem; primarily African American and Puerto Rican	Early illicit drug use is associated with risky sexual behavior later in young adulthood
1994	Lowry et al[18]	11,631 adolescents from 124 high schools	Students who do not use illegal substances are least likely to report high-risk sexual behaviors
2004	Patton et al[19]	5769 students aged 10–15 y	Early-onset puberty increases risk for substance use
2008	Cleveland et al[20]	91,778 students from grades 6, 8, 10, and 12; 90% White	Boys exhibit higher levels of substance use than girls
2005	van den Bree and Pickworth[21]	13,718 high school students aged 11–21 y	Peer involvement with substances, delinquency, and school problems increase the risk for marijuana use
2006	Herman-Stahl et al[22]	17,709 adolescents aged 12–17 y; 51.1% male; 62.8% White; 14.6% African American; 15.9% Hispanic	Low religiosity, binge drinking, and selling drugs increase risk of methamphetamine use
1997	Shrier et al[23]	3054 9th–12th grade students	Marijuana and cocaine use associated with high-risk sexual behavior
2007	Guxens et al[24]	1056 seventh grade students; 52.2% male	Single-parent household increases risk for adolescent marijuana use
2001	Brook et al[25]	3 samples: 739 predominately white adolescents from the Northeast (50% male), 1900 adolescents from East Harlem (55% male), and 1374 adolescents from Colombia (51% male)	Risk factors for marijuana use: rebelliousness, sensation seeking, depression, and delinquency. Protective factors: intolerance for deviance, church attendance, and careful reasoning
2004	Brown et al[26]	1354 sixth grade students; 49.7% male; 77.4% White; 22.6% African American	Developmental patterns of adolescent marijuana use differ between White and African Americans

(continued on next page)

Table 1
(continued)

Year	Authors	Sample	Findings
1992	Beauvais[27]	NA, literature review	Native American adolescents are more likely to use marijuana than adolescents from other racial or ethnic groups
1988	Binion et al[28]	13- to 17-year-old Native American youth from the Add Health survey	Native Americans are more likely to use marijuana in response to feelings of boredom
2008	Terry-McElrath et al[29]	82,106 high school seniors from 1977–2005; split evenly by gender; 80% White	Girls are more likely than boys to plan to abstain from marijuana
2007	Springer et al[30]	15,240 adolescents; 51.4% male; 61.4% White; 14.1% Hispanic; 13.9% African American	Methamphetamine use associated with low religiosity, high binge drinking, selling drugs, sexual risk behaviors; rates are higher among boys, White, and Hispanics
2008	Johnston et al[31]	Nationally representative sample of secondary school students followed longitudinally beginning in 1977	Trends of use for most licit and illicit drugs among American high school students
2006	Teter et al[32]	4580 college students; 50% male; 65% White	Lifetime and past-year rates of prescription stimulant use were 8.3% and 5.9%, respectively; rates highest among White
2007	McCabe et al[33]	1086 secondary school students; 46% male; 52% White; 45% African American	Combined medical/nonmedical use of prescription drugs is more common than nonmedical use alone
2009	Ford[34]	17,875 adolescents aged 12–17 y; 51.18% male; 60.02% White	Rates of over-the-counter drug abuse are increasing; more common among older, female, and low-income adolescents
2006	Arria and Wish[35]	NA, literature review	College students more likely to use prescription stimulants than noncollege students due to lifestyle differences

Abbreviation: NA, not available.

12th graders reported using cigarettes during the past month. Moreover, perceived availability of cigarettes is quite high, with 58% of 8th graders and 77% of 10th graders reporting that cigarettes are easy for them to access.

Risk Factors

Several risk factors for the onset of cigarette smoking among adolescents have been identified. The following factors have been specifically cited as increasing an adolescent's risk for initiating cigarette smoking:

Community-level factors
    Perceived availability of cigarettes[2]
    Community norms that favor cigarette use[2]
    Low school commitment[2]
    Low level of school connectedness[3]
Family factors
    Poor family management[2]
    Family history of cigarette use[2,4]
    Parental attitudes that favor cigarette use[2]
    Family conflicts[4]
Peer influence
    Friends' cigarette use[4]
    Friends' approval of smoking[4]
    Interaction with antisocial peers[2]
Individual-level factors
    Antisocial behavior[2]
    Sensation seeking[2]
    Alcohol use[4]
    Marijuana use.[4]

Protective Factors

Some researchers have suggested that social skills and a belief in the moral order are protective factors against cigarette smoking among this age group.[2] Other researchers have reported that participating in prosocial neighborhood activity serves as a protective factor against cigarette smoking during adolescence. This protective effect was specifically apparent in response to participation in school and community activities in neighborhoods with primarily White residents. In contrast, participation in church activities had a stronger protective effect on adolescents from neighborhoods with primarily African American residents.[5] A protective effect due to participation in competitive athletics has also been identified, such that adolescents who participated in such sports were significantly less likely to initiate cigarette smoking.[6] Finally, some research has suggested that high levels of both school connectedness and social connectedness are associated with a decreased likelihood of initiating smoking during adolescence.[3]

Cessation Efforts

The findings on adolescent cigarette use thus far suggest that despite recent successes at decreasing the rates of cigarette use among adolescents, much work is needed to continue this trend. One study found that students who began experimenting with cigarette smoking reported significant difficulties associated with quitting.[7] This finding necessitates further smoking-cessation programs for adolescents, as well as additional preventative efforts.

Demographic Factors

Cigarette smoking is usually initiated during adolescence. In comparison to African American and Hispanic adolescents, White adolescents have higher rates of cigarette use.[8]

With regard to gender, during early adolescence, girls typically have higher rates of cigarette use. This trend levels out during midadolescence, such that 10th grade boys and girls have comparable rates of cigarette use. By later adolescence, however, boys generally report higher rates of cigarette use than girls.[1]

In terms of geographic trends, when compared with other areas of the country, adolescent cigarette use has been found to be significantly lower on the West Coast.[1] Finally, cigarette smoking is also associated with being college-bound, such that college-bound adolescents have a lower likelihood of using cigarettes than adolescents who are not.[1]

Smokeless Tobacco

Smokeless tobacco is used almost exclusively among boys. When adolescent boys in the Monitoring the Future survey were asked about their use of smokeless tobacco during the past month, approximately 5.5% of 8th graders, 8.2% of 10th graders, and 11.8% of 12th graders reported using it. In comparison, among girls, only 1.5% of 8th graders, 2% of 10th graders, and 11.8% of 12th graders reported the use of smokeless tobacco during the past month.[1]

ALCOHOL
Rates of Use

Approximately 39% of eighth grade students report having consumed more than a few sips of alcohol, and nearly half of these students report having been drunk at least once in their lives. By 12th grade, 72% of adolescents report having consumed more than a few sips of alcohol in the past, and 55% of 12th grade students report having been drunk at least once in the past.[1]

When asked about alcohol use during the last month, approximately 16% of 8th graders, 29% of 10th graders, and 43% of 12th graders reported having had at least 1 alcohol drink. Moreover, approximately 9% of 8th graders, 16% of 10th graders, and 25% of 12th graders reported having 5 or more drinks in 1 sitting during the past 2 weeks.[1] In terms of availability, 63% of 8th graders, 81% of 10th graders, and 92% of 12th graders reported that alcohol is easily accessible to them.[1]

Risk Factors

As is the case for initiation of cigarette smoking, several community, family, peer, and individual factors that are associated with adolescent alcohol use have been identified as risk factors for adolescent alcohol use. Specific factors include perceived availability of alcohol, community norms that favor alcohol use; poor family management, a family history of substance use, and parental attitudes that favor substance use; friends' drug use; and antisocial behavior and sensation seeking.[2] Moreover, it has been found that adolescent alcohol use is associated with the onset of sexual intercourse as well as with the onset of marijuana use.[9] Another study has demonstrated that within particular geographic locations rates of adolescent alcohol use is correlated with both the rates of adult alcohol use and adult drunk driving, suggesting that the environmental norms likely have a strong influence on adolescent behavior.[10] Finally, adolescents who are involved with competitive athletics have been shown to be more likely to begin using alcohol than adolescents who are not involved with such activities.[6]

Protective Factors

Social skills and a belief in the moral order have also been cited as primary protective factors against adolescent alcohol use.[2] Another research has also suggested that the presence of nonparental adult role models and religious involvement are protective factors against the use of alcohol during adolescence.[11] Finally, participation in organized recreational activities has been shown to be protective against both the abuse of alcohol and the intent to abuse it.[12]

Demographics

In terms of race, research has demonstrated that White adolescents were more likely to drink alcohol than both African American[13] and Hispanic[1,8] adolescents. However, in the case of African American youth, this difference was almost entirely explained by the influence of peers and family members, illustrating the role that cultural norms play in alcohol abuse among adolescents.[13] Further supporting the contribution of the cultural environment in shaping these behaviors is the finding that Native American youth are more likely to begin using alcohol if they live in a single-parent home than in a double-parent home[14] and that caregiver substance abuse influences adolescent substance abuse among this population.[15] Another study reported that in comparison to other racial or ethnic groups, Native American and White adolescents use alcohol more frequently and that this difference is largely explained by lifestyle differences between different cultural groups.[16]

Moreover, adolescents who are not college-bound are more likely to drink heavily than those who are college-bound.[1] In terms of geography, rates of adolescent alcohol use are significantly higher in the Northeast and in the Midwest than they are in the south and in the west.[1]

ILLICIT DRUGS—GENERAL INFORMATION

According to the 2008 Monitoring the Future survey, 28% of American adolescents have tried an illicit drug by the end of eighth grade, and 47% of adolescents have done so by the end of high school. Further, 25% of American adolescents report having used an illicit drug other than marijuana by the end of high school.[1]

Risk Factors

Early onset of illicit drug use is commonly associated with risky sexual activity later in life, necessitating the importance of fully examining and addressing this topic. Moreover, early risky sexual behavior, such as inconsistent condom use, has been associated with later drug use.[17] Similarly, students who do not use illegal substances are least likely to report sexual intercourse or high-risk sexual behaviors, such as having multiple partners.[18] Early-onset puberty has also been shown to be a risk factor for illegal drug use among adolescents.[19]

Protective Factors

Protective factors against the onset of adolescent illicit drug use include the presence of nonparental adult role models and strong family communication.[11]

Demographics

Among older adolescents, a gender difference in illicit drug use has been identified, such that boys typically exhibit higher levels of substance use than girls.[20] In addition, high school students who are not college-bound have a higher likelihood of abusing illicit drugs than college-bound students.[1] In terms of geography, the Northeast and the West Coast have been found to have the highest rates of adolescent illicit drug use, whereas the south has the lowest rates.[1]

Finally, the Monitoring the Future survey identified several racial differences with regard to illicit drug use. For instance, White adolescents reported the highest rates of overall use for any illicit drug when compared with other groups. When broken down into subcategories, however, the rates of use varied slightly by racial group. Specifically, among 12th grade students, Hispanic adolescents reported the highest rates of crack, heroin, and crystal methamphetamine use when compared with other racial groups. For other drugs, however, the rates of use in Hispanic adolescents were lower than that in White adolescents and higher than that in African American adolescents. Moreover, among eighth grade students, Hispanic youth reported the highest rates of use for nearly all drugs, with amphetamines being the exception. It has been hypothesized that the change in rates of use among Hispanic youth from 8th grade to 12th grade can be explained by the higher high school dropout rates among this population, because those who begin using drugs at an earlier age are more likely to drop out of school.[1]

MARIJUANA
Rates of Use

Marijuana is the most widely used illicit drug among adolescents, with 11% of 8th graders, 23% of 10th graders, and 33% of 12th graders reporting that they used marijuana during the last 12 months. This rate of use is likely related to the availability of the drug, because approximately 39% of 8th graders, 67% of 10th graders, and 84% of 12th graders reported that marijuana is an easily accessible drug.[1]

Risk Factors

The risk factors commonly associated with adolescent marijuana use are similar to those for cigarette and alcohol use. Similar community, family, peer, and individual-level factors have been cited as increasing the risk of adolescent marijuana use. These factors include the perceived availability of drugs,[2] community norms favorable toward drug use,[2] poor family management,[2] family history of substance use,[2] parental attitudes favoring drug use,[2] low school commitment,[2] antisocial peers,[2] friends' and peers' drug use,[21] low school commitment,[2] problems at school,[21] interaction with antisocial peers,[2] antisocial behavior,[2] delinquency,[21] prior history of cigarette smoking,[2] alcohol consumption,[2] and other substance use.[21]

Prior use of both prescription stimulants and methamphetamine has also been shown to be associated with the onset of marijuana use.[22] Moreover, an increased number of sexual partners as well as a lower likelihood of condom use among adolescents are both commonly associated with use of marijuana.[23] Research has also shown that growing up in a single-parent home is a risk factor for the use of marijuana during adolescence.[24] Finally, several personality traits have been found to increase the odds of adolescent marijuana use, including rebelliousness, sensation seeking, delinquency, and depression.[25]

Protective Factors

As was the case for both cigarette use and alcohol use, social skills and a belief in the moral order have been cited as protective factors against the onset of adolescent marijuana use.[2] Other research has suggested that an intolerance of deviance,[25] church attendance,[25] a tendency to rely on careful reasoning,[25] positive emotions,[21] and relations with a father figure[21] are all traits that are also protective against adolescent marijuana use.

Demographics

Research on marijuana use among different racial or ethnic groups has been somewhat inconsistent. For example, one study reported that developmental patterns and outcomes of marijuana use differ significantly between African American and White adolescents.[26] Another research has suggested that the risk and protective factors for marijuana use are quite similar among adolescents from different racial or ethnic groups.[25] Finally, some research has suggested that Native American adolescents are more likely to use this drug than adolescents from other racial or ethnic groups,[27] and the documented explanation for this difference is a response to feelings of boredom,[28] demonstrating that lifestyle and cultural norms likely play a large role in the onset of marijuana use.

Several gender differences with regard to marijuana use have been identified as well. Specifically, boys were significantly more likely to report having used marijuana than girls, and among adolescents who have used marijuana in the past, boys were more likely to continue using in the future than girls. Similarly, boys were more likely to report that their marijuana use was problematic than girls. In contrast, when asked whether they planned to use marijuana during the following 12 months, female respondents were more likely than males to report that they probably or definitely would be abstaining from use.[29]

METHAMPHETAMINES
Rates of Use

The Monitoring the Future survey of 2008 found that about 1% of 12th graders reported using crystal methamphetamine in the past 12 months, and 12% of 8th graders, 16% of 10th graders, and 24% of 12th graders reported that crystal methamphetamine is easily available.[1] Moreover, among a group of US high school students, rates of lifetime methamphetamine use were comparable to those of lifetime cocaine use but were more than double the rate of lifetime heroin use.[30]

Risk Factors

Previous research has indicated that adolescent methamphetamine use is associated with low levels of religiosity,[22] high rates of binge drinking,[22] selling drugs,[22] early onset of sexual intercourse,[30] having multiple sexual partners,[30] and having been pregnant or having gotten someone else pregnant in the past.[30]

Demographics

Several gender differences have been reported with regard to adolescent methamphetamine use, with boys generally demonstrating higher rates of methamphetamine use than girls.[30] Racial differences have been observed as well, such that rates of lifetime methamphetamine use among white and Hispanic adolescents have been found to be almost twice as high as the rates for black adolescents.[30]

COCAINE
Rates of Use

During the past 12 months, approximately 5% of 12th graders, 3% of 10th graders, and 2% of 8th graders reported having used cocaine. Moreover, less than 2% of those surveyed reported any crack use during the past 12 months. However, 42% of 12th grade adolescents reported that cocaine is easily accessible to them.[1]

Risk Factors

Both early-onset cocaine use and lifetime frequency of cocaine use were found to be associated with increased number of sexual partners and a lower likelihood of using condoms during sexual activity. This finding demonstrates that high-risk behaviors among adolescents often occur simultaneously.[23]

INHALANTS
Rates of Use

In comparison to the substances described previously, the rate of inhalant use among adolescents is relatively low. Moreover, the trends in use with regard to age are the reverse of what is typically expected with substance use. According to the Monitoring the Future survey of 2008, only 9% of 8th graders, 6% of 10th graders, and 4% of 12th graders reported inhalant use during the past 12 months. It is believed that the drug is common among younger adolescents because it is one of the few drugs that they can access due to its cheapness, availability, and legality to purchase and possess.[1]

LYSERGIC ACID DIETHYLAMIDE
Rates of Use

Approximately 3% of 12th graders, 2% of 10th graders, and 1% of 8th graders reported using lysergic acid diethylamide during the last 12 months. Although these rates are quite low in comparison to the rates of use for other drugs, it is worth noting that the reported availability of these drugs are somewhat higher, with 30% of 12th graders, 19% of 10th graders, and 11% of 8th graders reporting that the drug is easily accessible to them.[1]

AMPHETAMINES
Rates of Use

When asked about amphetamine use during the past 12 months, approximately 5% of 8th graders, 7% of 10th graders, and 7% of 12th graders reported using amphetamines. These rates are among the lowest-reported rates of use among adolescents since the 1970s. However, the accessibility of the drug is a bit higher, with approximately 21% of 8th graders, 33% of 10th graders, and 48% of 12th graders reporting that these drugs are easily available.[1]

HEROIN
Rates of Use

The rate of heroin use among adolescents is low, with less than 1% of respondents reporting any heroin use during the past 12 months. In terms of accessibility, approximately 15% of 8th graders, 18% of 10th graders, and 25% of 12th graders reported that heroin is easily available.[1]

PRESCRIPTION AND OVER-THE-COUNTER DRUGS
Rates of Use

The rates of nonmedical use of prescription drugs among adolescents are relatively low in comparison to other substances. Specifically, in 2007, 2.1% of 8th grade students, 2.8% of 10th grade students, and 3.9% of 12th grade students reported using methylphenidate in a nonmedical manner during the past year.[31] Research has suggested somewhat higher rates among undergraduate college students, with lifetime and past-year estimates of use at 8.1% and 5.4%, respectively.[32] Although the rates of use are somewhat lower than other drugs, one study examining both medical and nonmedical use of prescription stimulants found that whereas only 3.3% of adolescent respondents reported nonmedical use only, 17.5% reported using these drugs both medically and nonmedically in the past. This finding suggests that this problem is significantly larger among adolescents who are supposed to be taking these drugs to treat medical problems than among those who do receive a prescription for the drugs.[33] In terms of over-the-counter drugs, the 2006 National Survey on Drug Use and Health found that the rates of lifetime, past-year, and past-month misuse among adolescents aged 12 to 17 years were 4%, 2%, and 1%, respectively.[34]

Demographics

Research has indicated that white adolescents are more likely to abuse both prescription and over-the-counter medications than other adolescent groups.[22,32,34] Moreover, boys are significantly more likely to report nonmedical use of prescription drugs than girls, whereas girls are more likely to report misuse of over-the-counter drugs than boys.[34,35]

Risk Factors

High levels of both family conflict and sensation-seeking behavior have been associated with using these drugs in a nonprescribed manner.[22] Moreover, adolescents who are not college-bound and come from families of lower socioeconomic groups have a higher likelihood of abusing prescription and over-the-counter drugs.[32,34,35]

NARCOTICS
Rates of Use

When asked about use of narcotics other than heroin, such as oxycodone (OxyContin) and hydrocodone (Vicodin), approximately 9% of 12th graders reported abusing these drugs during the past 12 months. Moreover, approximately 13% of 8th graders, 20% of 10th graders, and 36% of 12th graders reported that these drugs would be easy for them to access.[1]

TRANQUILIZERS
Rates of Use

Among all available tranquilizers, diazepam (Valium) and alprazolam (Xanax) are the most commonly abused among adolescents. However, relative to other abused drugs, the rates of use remain low, with only 2% of 8th graders, 4% of 10th graders, and 6% of 12th graders reporting use during the past 12 months. When asked about availability of these drugs, 17% of 8th graders, 25% of 10th graders, and 24% of 12th graders reported that they could access them easily.[1]

SEDATIVES
Rates of Use

During the past year, approximately 5% of 12th graders reported abusing sedatives. Moreover, approximately 19% of 8th graders, 24% of 10th graders, and 39% of 12th graders reported that these drugs are easy for them to access.[1]

CLUB DRUGS
Rates of Use

3,4-Methylenedioxymethamphetamine (Ecstasy) is among the most common club drugs used by adolescents, with approximately 5% of 12th graders, 3% of 10th graders, and 2% of 8th graders reporting use during the past 12 months. Perceived availability of this drug is fairly high, and when surveyed, 15% of 8th graders, 25% of 10th graders, and 42% of 12th graders reported that Ecstasy is easily accessible for them. Lower–rates of use were identified for gamma hydroxybutyric acid (Xyrem) and ketamine, with rates of use during the past year being close to 1% for 8th, 10th, and 12th graders.[1]

SUMMARY

From the literature, it is apparent that tobacco, alcohol, and marijuana represent the greatest problematic areas for adolescents and that use of other illicit drugs is rare in comparison, although it is certainly not absent. Further, research suggests that older adolescents typically struggle the most with substance abuse. The highest risk groups are generally White males, although significant problems are observable among females and among adolescents of other racial or ethnic groups. Other risk factors commonly associated with substance abuse among adolescents are family and peer substance use, low levels of school commitment and connectedness, and early-onset sexual risk behaviors.

The fact that substance abuse affects adolescents from a variety of demographic groups demonstrates the importance of developing culturally sensitive interventions that target the many different risk factors affecting the various adolescent groups. Moreover, because factors at many levels contribute to the onset of adolescent substance abuse, it is essential that prevention and treatment interventions target this issue from a variety of areas. Researchers and treatment providers must reach out to adolescents by targeting their communities, families, schools, and peer groups as well as the adolescents themselves who are at risk for developing problems with licit and illicit drug use.

REFERENCES

1. Johnston LD, O'Malley PM, Bachman JG, et al. Monitoring the Future national results on adolescent drug use. Bethesda (MD): NIDA; 2008. Available at: http://www.drugabuse.gov/PDF/overview2008.pdf. Accessed August, 2009.
2. Beyers JM, Toumbourou JW, Catalano R, et al. A cross-national comparison of risk and protective factors for adolescent substance use: the United States and Australia. J Adolesc Health 2004;35:3–16.
3. Bond L, Butler H, Thomas L, et al. Social and school connectedness in early secondary school as predictors of late teenage substance use, mental health, and academic outcomes. J Adolesc Health 2007;40:e9–18.
4. Flay BR, Hu FB, Richardson J. Psychosocial predictors of different stages of cigarette smoking among high school students. Prev Med 1998;27:9–18.
5. Xue Y, Zimmerman MA, Caldwell CH. Neighborhood residence and cigarette smoking among urban youths: the protective role of prosocial activities. Am J Public Health 2007;97:1865–72.
6. Aaron DJ, Dearwater SR, Anderson R, et al. Physical activity and the initiation of high-risk health behaviors in adolescents. Med Sci Sports Exerc 1995;27:1639–45.
7. Kelder SH, Perry CL, Klepp KI, et al. Longitudinal tracking of adolescent smoking, physical activity, and food choice behaviors. Am J Public Health 1994;84:1121–6.

8. Blum RW, Beuhring T, Shew ML, et al. The effects of race/ethnicity, income, and family structure on adolescent risk behaviors. Am J Public Health 2000;90: 1879–84.

9. Jessor R, Jessor SL. Adolescent development and the onset of drinking. A longitudinal study. J Stud Alcohol 1975;36:27–51.

10. Nelson DE, Naimi TS, Brewer RD, et al. State alcohol-use estimates among youth and adults, 1993–2005. Am J Prev Med 2009;36:218–24.

11. Beebe LA, Vesely SK, Oman RF, et al. Protective assets for non-use of alcohol, tobacco and other drugs among urban American Indian youth in Oklahoma. Matern Child Health J 2008;12:82–90.

12. Leaver-Dunn D. Influence of sports' programs and club activities on alcohol use intentions and behaviors among adolescent males. J Alcohol Drug Educ 2007;51: 57–72.

13. Watt TT, Rogers JM. Factors contributing to differences in substance use among Black and White adolescents. Youth Soc 2007;39:54–74.

14. Lonczak HS, Fernandez A, Austin L, et al. Family structure and substance use among American Indian youth: a preliminary study. Fam Syst Health 2007;25: 10–22.

15. Walls ML, Whitbeck LB, Hoyt DR, et al. Early-onset alcohol use among Native American youth: examining female caretaker influence. J Marriage Fam 2007; 69:451–64.

16. Wallace JM, Bachman JG. Explaining racial/ethnic differences in adolescent drug use: the impact of background and lifestyle. Soc Probl 1991;38:333–57.

17. Brook JS, Adams RE, Balka EB, et al. Illicit drug use and risky sexual behavior among African American and Puerto Rican urban adolescents: the longitudinal links. J Genet Psychol 2004;165:203–20.

18. Lowry R, Holtzman D, Truman BI, et al. Substance use and HIV-related sexual behaviors among US high school students: are they related? Am J Public Health 1994;84:1116–20.

19. Patton GC, McMorris BJ, Toumbourou JW, et al. Puberty and the onset of substance use and abuse. Pediatrics 2004;114:300–6.

20. Cleveland MJ, Feinberg ME, Bontempo DE, et al. The role of risk and protective factors in substance use across adolescence. J Adolesc Health 2008;43:157–64.

21. van den Bree M, Pickworth WB. Risk factors predicting changes in marijuana involvement in teenagers. Arch Gen Psychiatry 2005;62:311–9.

22. Herman-Stahl MA, Krebs CP, Kroutil LA, et al. Risk and protective factors for nonmedical use of prescription stimulants and methamphetamine among adolescents. J Adolesc Health 2006;39:374–80.

23. Shrier LA, Emans SJ, Woods ER, et al. The association of sexual risk behaviors and problem drug behaviors in high school students. J Adolesc Health 1997; 20:377–83.

24. Guxens M, Nebot M, Ariza C. Age and sex differences in factors associated with the onset of cannabis use: a cohort study. Drug Alcohol Depend 2007; 88:234–43.

25. Brook JS, Brook DW, Arencibia-Mireles O, et al. Risk factors for adolescent marijuana use across cultures and across time. J Genet Psychol 2001;162:357–74.

26. Brown TL, Flory K, Lynam DR, et al. Comparing the developmental trajectories of marijuana use of African American and Caucasian adolescents: patterns, antecedents, and consequences. Exp Clin Psychopharmacol 2004;12:47–56.

27. Beauvais F. Trends in Indian adolescent drug and alcohol use. Am Indian Alsk Native Ment Health Res 1992;5:1–12.

28. Binion A, Miller CD, Beauvais F, et al. Rationales for the use of alcohol, marijuana, and other drugs by eighth-grade Native American and Anglo youth. Int J Addict 1988;23:47–64.
29. Terry-McElrath YM, O'Malley PM, Johnston LD. Saying no to marijuana: why American youth report quitting or abstaining. J Stud Alcohol Drugs 2008;69: 796–805.
30. Springer AE, Peters RJ, Shegog R, et al. Methamphetamine use and sexual risk behaviors in U.S. high school students: findings from a national risk behavior survey. Prev Sci 2007;8:103–13.
31. Johnston LD, O'Malley PM, Bachman JG, et al. Monitoring the Future national survey results on drug use, 1975–2007; I: Secondary school students. Bethesda (MD): US Department of Health and Human Services, National Institutes of Health, National Institute on Drug Abuse; 2008.
32. Teter CJ, McCabe SE, LaGrange K, et al. Illicit use of specific prescription stimulants among college students: prevalence, motives, and routes of administration. Pharmacotherapy 2006;26:1501–10.
33. McCabe SE, Boyd CJ, Young A. Medical and nonmedical use of prescription drugs among secondary school students. J Adolesc Health 2007;40:76–83.
34. Ford JA. Misuse of over-the-counter cough or cold medications among adolescents: prevalence and correlates in a national sample. J Adolesc Health 2009; 44:505–7.
35. Arria AM, Wish ED. Nonmedical use of prescription stimulants among students. Pediatr Ann 2006;35:565–71.

Genetic and Environmental Risk Factors for Adolescent-Onset Substance Use Disorders

Jacquelyn L. Meyers, BS[a], Danielle M. Dick, PhD[a,b,*]

KEYWORDS

• Alcohol use • Substance use • Drug use • Adolescence
• Genetics • Gene-environment interaction

Substance dependence disorders are chronic relapsing disorders with immense societal consequences. Twin and family studies have found that there are critical genetic and environmental components in the inheritance of substance use disorders, and modern advances in genetics are making it possible to identify specific variants that may predispose an individual to these disorders. There is no "gene for alcoholism"; rather there are a multitude of genes, each with small effects, that interact with each other (epitasis) as well as with their biologic and external environments (gene-environment interaction) to make an individual more or less susceptible to the development of these complex disorders. The onset of substance dependence is rarely sudden; it is usually preceded by a trajectory of risk-related behavior, with its origins in childhood. Adolescence is a crucial period for the initiation of, and experimentation with, alcohol and other drugs. This experimentation, as well as a degree of other conduct-disordered behavior, is normative; however, adolescent substance use is a known risk factor for the development of later alcohol and substance use problems as well as related externalizing disorders such as antisocial personality disorder. Understanding the early risk factors and trajectories that make these youths vulnerable to substance use

a Department of Human & Molecular Genetics, Virginia Institute of Psychiatric and Behavioral Genetics, Virginia Commonwealth University, PO Box 980126, Richmond, VA 23298-0126, USA
b Department of Psychiatry, Virginia Institute of Psychiatric and Behavioral Genetics, Virginia Commonwealth University, PO Box 980126, Richmond, VA 23298-0126, USA
* Corresponding author. Departments of Psychiatry and Human and Molecular Genetics, Virginia Institute for Psychiatric and Behavioral Genetics, Virginia Commonwealth University, PO Box 980126, Richmond, VA 23298-0126.
E-mail address: ddick@vcu.edu

Child Adolesc Psychiatric Clin N Am 19 (2010) 465–477
doi:10.1016/j.chc.2010.03.013
1056-4993/10/$ – see front matter © 2010 Elsevier Inc. All rights reserved.

childpsych.theclinics.com

disorders is crucial to the development of effective strategies for prevention. This article reviews the genetic origins of adolescent substance use problems, which create one of the largest public health concerns in the United States, and the potential this field of research offers for prevention.

ADOLESCENT DRUG AND ALCOHOL USE

Adolescent alcohol use is a major public health problem. Youths who drink alcohol are more likely to experience many negative outcomes including academic, social, and legal problems, in addition to unwanted, unplanned, and unprotected sexual activity.[1,2] Biologically, adolescence is characterized by strong neuronal plasticity, with sprouting and pruning of synapses, myelinization of nerve fibers, and changes in neurotransmitter concentrations and their receptor levels in brain areas essential for behavioral and cognitive functions.[3] Adolescent drinkers are at higher risk for changes in brain development that may have life-long effects.[3] Long-term alcohol misuse is associated with liver disease, cancer, cardiovascular disease, and neurologic damage, as well as psychiatric problems such as depression, anxiety, and antisocial personality disorder.[4]

In addition to the personal risks to the adolescent, the societal and economic costs of alcohol and other substance use disorders in the United States also are substantial. Alcohol is used by more young people in the United States than tobacco or illicit drugs.[1] Although it is illegal to drink alcohol before the age of 21 years in all states, in 2007, 26% of high-school students reported episodic heavy or binge drinking and 11% of high-school students reported driving a car or other vehicle during the past 30 days when they had been drinking alcohol. In addition, 29% of students reported riding in a car or other vehicle during the past 30 days driven by someone who had been drinking alcohol.[5] In 2005, there were more than 145,000 emergency rooms visits by youths aged 12 to 20 years for injuries and other conditions linked to alcohol.[6]

COMORBIDITY AND ILLICIT DRUG USE

Cannabis is the most commonly used illicit substance among adolescents and young adults in the United States.[7] In 2004, 46% of high-school seniors reported having tried cannabis at some time, 34% reported having used within the past month, and 5.6% reported having smoked cannabis daily.[8] Initiation into cannabis use typically begins in adolescence, as youths aged 12 to 17 years constitute about two-thirds of the new cannabis users.[9] Approximately 14% of adolescent-onset cannabis users develop cannabis dependence, a rate roughly twice that reported for adult-onset users.[10] Further work has focused on the biologic mechanisms involved in the development of cannabis dependence, and this has elucidated some of the underlying pathways from cannabis use to behavior and the potential for the development of problems. For example, the receptor for cannabinoids (CB1) belongs to the Gi/Go protein-coupled receptor family, and, in the mammalian brain, is densely diffused in regions involved in the processing of emotional inputs, rewarding stimuli, habit formation, and higher cognitive functions.[11]

In recent years there have been reductions in the rates of illicit drug use among adolescents. Current marijuana use decreased from 27% in 1999 to 20% in 2007. Lifetime use of ecstasy among high-school students decreased from 11% in 2003 to 6% in 2007. Hallucinogenic drug use decreased from 13% in 2001 to 8% in 2007.[12] Although illicit drug use has declined among youths, rates of nonmedical use of prescription and over-the-counter (OTC) medications, including pain relievers, tranquilizers, stimulants, and depressants, remain high. These easily accessible drugs are falsely believed to be safer than illicit drugs; however, misuse of prescription and OTC medications can cause serious health effects, addiction, and death.[7,13,14]

EARLY INITIATION

One of the most robust findings in the alcohol literature came out of an influential study by Grant and Dawson[15] reporting that individuals who reported that they had first tried alcohol before the age of 15 years were 4 times more likely to have a lifetime diagnosis of alcohol dependence than individuals who reported that they had first tried alcohol after the age of 20 years. This finding has been replicated in many independent samples, using retrospective[16–19] and prospective[20] data. Alcohol use before 15 years of age is also found to predict other forms of adult disinhibitory psychopathology, including substance use disorders and antisocial personality disorder. Many mechanisms for this association have been proposed.

One theory suggests that early use of alcohol may increase alcoholism risk by altering the course of adolescent development.[16] Adolescent alcohol use could alter the course of development by increasing the likelihood that an adolescent is affiliated with deviant peers, thus decreasing the likelihood that an adolescent is affiliated with individuals who reinforce and model prosocial behaviors. A second theory hypothesizes that early use of alcohol may influence biologic development directly, through its effects in the developing adolescent brain.[21] Research with rodents[22] and humans[23] suggests that heavy use of alcohol during adolescence can result in neurocognitive changes that increase the likelihood of subsequent abuse of alcohol in adulthood.

A third hypothesis is that the association of early alcohol use with alcoholism risk arises because early use of alcohol in adolescence and alcoholism in adulthood are manifestations of a general inherited liability to disinhibitory psychopathology.[24,25] Support for this idea came initially from a study of nearly 9000 twins that showed that early use of alcohol was heritable and that its association with alcoholism risk was mediated entirely by genetic factors.[19] This model also predicts that early use of alcohol should be a nonspecific risk factor for a wide range of behavioral pathologies because it is an indicator of a general disposition toward disinhibited behavior. Consistent with this expectation, alcohol use before 15 years of age is associated with attention deficit/hyperactivity disorder, conduct disorder, personality measures of impulsivity, psychophysiological indicators of disinhibition, academic underachievement, and abuse of substances other than alcohol.[18] In their 2008 review of these mechanisms, McGue and Iacono[26] point out that none of these mechanisms are mutually exclusive, and that early use of alcohol may be an indicator of inherited risk and disrupt the course of adolescent development.

HERITABILITY

Alcoholism runs in families. This is likely a result of the transmission of genetics as well as the familial environment. Twin methodology has been used to study the measurable contribution of genetic and environmental influences on a particular trait or disease state. Twin studies provide an estimation of a trait's heritability in a population; that is, what proportion of phenotypic variation is produced by genetic variation underlying the trait. Twin studies accomplish this by comparing phenotypic similarity between monozygotic twins, who share all of their genetic variation, with dizygotic twins, who share (on average) half of their genetic variation. Measures of heritability are a function of the specific population. Heritability of substance use disorders varies among substances (and the measure of substance use), populations, age, and sex.

A 2006 meta-analysis of twin studies showed that the heritability of all addictive substances ranges from 40% to 60%.[27] Heritabilities in the range of 30% to 60% are also observed for illicit drug dependences.[28,29] Variability in the exact estimates is likely a function of the age of the participants (genetic influences often increase across development[30]), cohort differences, and the exact measure of the phenotype being studied. Current research on the heritability of youth drug and alcohol problems suggests that these disordered behaviors are manifestations of risk to a spectrum of externalizing disorders and that to consider each of these disorders separately may lead us to miss important etiologic clues.

HERITABILITY ACROSS DEVELOPMENT

The use of longitudinal studies of behavior across development has elucidated the dramatic changes that are evident in the importance of genetic and environmental influences throughout the lifespan, observed across multiple behavioral domains including intellectual abilities[31] and depression.[32] Substance use is another area in which dramatic changes in the relative importance of genetic and environmental effects across development are apparent. This finding has been documented in data from our longitudinal Finnish Twin Studies, in which the authors have found that the importance of genetic effects on drinking patterns increases dramatically from adolescence to young adulthood. At the age of 14 years, genetic influences accounted for only 18% of the variance in drinking initiation, and this was significant only in girls, with no evidence of genetic influence on drinking patterns in boys at this early age.[33] However, by 16 years of age, genetic factors accounted for one-third of the variation in drinking patterns in both sexes, and by 18 years of age genetic factors accounted for half of the variation.[34] Thus, in a period of slightly more than 4 years, genetic influences changed from having virtually no detectable effect on drinking patterns to accounting for the majority of the variance. Conversely, the importance of common environmental effects decreased significantly from adolescence into adulthood, accounting for more than 70% of the variance at 14 years of age, but only approximately 15% of the variance by 18 years of age. Thus, as drinking patterns develop, differentiate, and stabilize across adolescence, genetic factors assume increasing importance to drinking patterns; however, alcohol use early in adolescence seems to be almost entirely influenced by family, school, and neighborhood.[35]

In 2008, Kendler and colleagues[30] examined these relative changes in the importance of genes and environment in substance use from early adolescence to middle adulthood. The study provides more support for an etiologic model in which initiation and early patterns of use are more strongly influenced by social and familial environmental factors, while later levels of use are more heavily influenced by genetic factors. The importance of environment has been theorized to reflect the important influence of social and familial structure that characterizes development across adolescence. Early on, there is usually less opportunity for adolescents to express their genetic predisposition, as more of their activities and decisions are influenced by figures of authority. As adolescents move into adulthood, and usually out of the social structure of their youth, emerging adults have more opportunity to express their genetic predispositions, choosing more freely their friends and activities. In some studies, it has been observed that some of the environmental influences are still evident after individuals moves out of their parents' homes. This is believed to reflect personal values that one's family or community has instilled in the individual, such as religious beliefs.

THE EXTERNALIZING SPECTRUM

Another consideration for understanding genetic influences on pathways of risk for alcohol problems is the robust finding that the overlap between childhood conduct problems and later alcohol problems is largely the result of shared genetic factors. This finding has been shown across multiple twin samples.[24,25,36,37] In addition, an offspring of twins study found increased rates of conduct disorder in alcohol-dependent fathers, with transmission patterns supporting the common-genes hypothesis.[38] Specific genes that have been associated with adult alcohol dependence have been associated with conduct problems in younger children and adolescents (rather than early adolescent alcohol dependence),[39] again suggesting that childhood behavior problems may be an early manifestation of an underlying predisposition to subsequent alcohol problems. The association with behavior problems may emerge earlier in development because genetic factors are apparent in behavior problems (showing up early in childhood) before their effects on patterns of alcohol use (for which genetic influences assume greater importance later in adolescence).

Epidemiologic studies find that individuals rarely abuse a single substance. Instead, polysubstance abuse/dependence is normative, with high rates of comorbidity across various drug classes. In addition, persons with substance use disorders also exhibit higher rates of other psychiatric disorders including mood disorders and antisocial personality disorder. Twin studies suggest that this comorbidity is due at least in part to a shared genetic cause underlying susceptibility to different types of substance use and other psychopathologies. Kendler and colleagues[36] used the Virginia Twin Registry sample to identify common genetic factors underlying the major class of psychiatric and substance use disorders, and found that a common genetic factor was shared across alcohol dependence, illicit drug dependence, adult antisocial behavior, and childhood conduct disorder. These results suggest a common genetic factor for substance dependence/abuse and general externalizing psychopathologies **(Fig. 1)**. Alcohol dependence and illicit drug dependence also showed some disorder-specific genetic influences. However, 69% of the total genetic variance on alcohol dependence, and 64% of the genetic variance on illicit drug dependence resulted from the genetic factor shared across externalizing psychopathology. This finding indicates that much of the genetic predisposition to alcohol and other drug dependence is not specific to that disorder. Using only male twins from the same population, Kendler and colleagues[40] found that a common genetic factor loaded strongly onto abuse/dependence of all classes of illicit drugs. There has now been much evidence

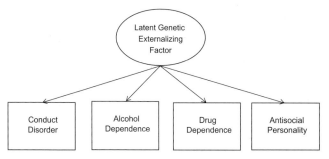

Several studies have found that a common genetic factor, broadly termed the externalizing factor, accounts for a significant portion of the variance in alcohol dependence, abuse/dependence on other drugs, adult antisocial behavior and childhood conduct disorder. Alcohol and other drug dependence also show some disorder specific genetic influences.

Fig. 1. The latent genetic externalizing factor.

to suggest that youth drug and alcohol problems are a manifestation of risk to a spectrum of externalizing disorders, and that to consider each of these disorders separately may lead us to miss important etiologic clues.

GENE-ENVIRONMENT INTERACTION

There is an emerging literature documenting how specific environmental factors moderate the importance of genetic effects. A growing number of variables have been shown to moderate the relative importance of genetic effects on substance use and dependence and externalizing behavior. Among the environmental moderators being studied are childhood stressors (emotional, physical, and sexual abuse), availability and access to drugs and alcohol, peer-group antisocial and prosocial behavior, religiosity, parental attitudes toward drugs and alcohol, parental monitoring, and socioregional factors. Religiosity has been shown to moderate genetic influences on alcohol use among females, with genetic factors playing a larger role among individuals without a religious upbringing.[41] Social contact and cotwin dependency[42] have also been shown to moderate twin similarity, with reduced genetic effects and enhanced environmental influences among more codependent pairs. Genetic influences on adolescent substance use are also enhanced in environments with lower parental monitoring.[43] These analyses suggest that when adolescents receive little parental monitoring, it creates an environment that allows for greater opportunity to express genetic predispositions. The moderating effects of peer alcohol use on adolescent drinking has been shown to operate in a similar fashion: among adolescents with a larger number of peers who used alcohol, there was greater expression of genetic predispositions.[44] These findings may reflect a situation in which environments characterized by low parental monitoring or high peer substance use create opportunity for adolescents to express genetic predispositions. These results support previous findings from the Finnish Twin Studies, which indicated that in neighborhoods in which there is less stability, presumably engendering less community monitoring, there was greater evidence of genetic influence.[45] Conversely, in more supervised and restricted environments, there was less opportunity to express genetic predispositions and greater influence of environmental effects.[34,45] Hicks and colleagues[46] examined the specificity of each of these environmental risk factors on externalizing spectrum disorders, including substance dependence/abuse. They concluded that, in the context of environmental adversity, broadly defined, genetic factors become more important in the etiology of externalizing disorders. In addition, their results suggest a general mechanism of environmental influence on externalizing disorders, regardless of the specific form of environmental risk.

These analyses illustrate the importance of incorporating measured aspects of the environment into genetically informative twin models to understand how specific environments act and interact with genetic predispositions. They may also have implications for studying the risk associated with specific genes. For example, a recent study[47] aimed to characterize the pathway of risk associated with GABRA2 (for each known human gene the Human Genome Organization [HUGO] Gene Nomenclature Committee approves a gene name and symbol [short-form abbreviation]. Details on this process can be found on the HUGO Web site at http://www.hugo-international.org/comm_genenomenclaturecommittee.php), a gene previously associated with adult alcohol dependence,[48] in a community sample of children followed longitudinally from childhood to young adulthood. Association between GABRA2 and trajectories of externalizing behavior was tested from adolescence to young adulthood and moderation of genetic effects by parental monitoring was also tested. Two classes of externalizing behavior emerged: a stable, high externalizing class and a moderate, decreasing externalizing-behavior class. The *GABRA2* gene was associated with class membership, with subjects who showed persistent increased trajectories of externalizing behavior more likely to carry the genotype previously associated with increased risk of adult alcohol dependence. A significant interaction with parental monitoring emerged; the association of *GABRA2* with externalizing trajectories diminished with high levels of parental monitoring.[43]

GENE IDENTIFICATION EFFORTS
Candidate Gene Approach

Evidence for significant heritability for all of the addictive disorders has led to considerable efforts to identify the specific genes involved. The gene search has been complicated by addictive behaviors being complex genetic traits that are phenotypically and genetically heterogeneous. It is expected that there are multiple genetic loci influencing manifestation and variation in these behaviors, and that these loci vary in the direction and magnitude of their effects. Beyond the multiple loci involved, it is likely that there are also many layers of intricate interactions between loci (epistasis), in addition to gene-environment interactions.

Because of the challenges associated with gene identification efforts for multifactorial traits (traits that are influenced by multiple genes and environments) such as substance dependence, several strategies have been used to identify genes involved in addictive disorders. One approach is the candidate gene approach. This strategy involves investigation of a gene that is believed to be involved in the cause of a specific disorder for known or hypothesized biologic reasons. A classic example of the candidate gene approach is the association of genes involved in alcohol metabolism with susceptibility to alcohol dependence. Multiple alcohol-metabolism genes have been repeatedly implicated in the development of alcohol addiction and susceptibility to dependence on other drugs. These genes were initially suspected as having a role in dependence, as they are known to be involved in the metabolism of ethanol. For example, alcohol dehydrogenase 1B (*ADH1B*) is involved in the conversion of ethanol to acetaldehyde; acetaldehyde is toxic and its accumulation leads to an unpleasant physiologic reaction involving headache, nausea, and heart palpitations. Polymorphisms in alcohol metabolism genes that affect acetaldehyde levels can have a profound effect on drinking behavior.[49,50] For example, the *ADH1B*2* allele rapidly oxidizes ethanol, and is protective against alcoholism; this effect is most evident among East Asian and Ashkenazi Jewish populations, in whom the frequency of this allele is high. Individuals carrying at least 1 of these alleles are far less likely to develop alcoholism. The advantage of the candidate gene approach is that it provides targeted hypothesis testing, but this approach is limited by knowledge of human biology.

Linkage and Association

With the increasing availability of genetic markers localized across the genome, more systematic approaches to gene identification have gained favor. Such studies are hypothesis free in their design, scanning large portions of the genome to identify regions that are significantly associated with the phenotype of interest. Linkage mapping was an early technique used to systematically scan the genome, in which approximately 400 to 1000 highly polymorphic markers were genotyped to test for genomic regions showing increased allele sharing among affected family members. Many large-scale alcohol-dependence gene identification projects have used genetic linkage mapping; the largest of these is the Collaborative Study of the Genetics of

Alcoholism (COGA). COGA is a family-based study that has collected detailed phenotypic data on individuals in families with multiple alcoholic members. The strongest linkage regions with alcohol dependence to emerge from this project were on chromosomes 4 and 7. Follow-up association studies of candidate genes in the linkage regions have identified association with several genes in each region, including GABRA2,[48] NFKB1,[51] ADH4, ADH1A, ADH1B,[49] CHRM2,[52] and TAS2R16.[53] Although these studies illustrate the potential of genome-wide linkage approaches (followed by targeted association tests in the linked regions) to identify novel genetic variants, linkage studies are largely underpowered to detect genes of small effect, such as those hypothesized to be involved in addiction. Although linkage was successful in the identification of genes involved in monogenic diseases, mapping polygenic disease genes requires a large number of family members to ensure sufficient power to detect genetic variants.[54] In addition, linkage mapping lacks the precision other methods provide, because the linkage peaks resulting from this strategy do not precisely localize the associated genes, and imprecise linkage peaks make it difficult to know the exact region to target for follow-up with association studies.

For these reasons, genome-wide association studies (GWAS) has gained favor. GWAS theoretically combines the advantages of linkage mapping (a systematic genome-wide scan that has the capability of identifying novel genetic variants) and the advantages of association (higher resolution that provides more power to detect genes of subtle effect). Currently, there is only 1 published GWAS for alcohol dependence.[55] Treutlein and colleagues[55] found 2 genome-wide significant results in closely linked intergenic single nucleotide polymorphisms (SNPs), located on chromosome region 2q35, and 9 SNPs located in genes (CDH13 and ADH1C), all of which have previously been implicated in the alcohol dependence literature. This study is the first published GWAS to identify a genome-wide significant association in alcohol dependence. In addition to this study, many GWAS are currently underway for alcohol-related phenotypes including efforts from large gene identification projects, the COGA, the Irish Affected Sib-Pair Substance and Alcohol Dependence (IASPSAD), and the Study of Addiction: Genetics and Environment (SAGE), with results expected imminently. Although GWAS provides several advantages, including the ability to more precisely localize associated variants, it also provides many challenges including the need for large samples to detect genes of small effect, many genetic markers, and multiple testing concerns.[56] There are strengths and weaknesses to all gene-finding techniques, and converging evidence of association across techniques will be key to validating specific genetic variants involved in complex traits.

GENE IDENTIFICATION IN ADOLESCENT POPULATIONS

Many of these gene identification efforts focus on adult alcohol and substance dependence. This focus is in part so that subjects will have passed through the age of onset for common addictive substance disorders and to ensure that there is no ambiguity associated with whether an unaffected individual simply has not yet manifested problems. However, some projects have focused specifically on adolescent samples. Many of these studies have come from the Colorado Center for the Genetics of Antisocial Drug Dependence (CADD), which is an ongoing multicomponent, collaborative study at the University of Colorado[57] consisting of more than 5000 youths. The CADD is using several research designs and strategies in its study of the genetic basis for antisocial drug dependence in adolescents. Stallings and colleagues[57] reported a genome-wide linkage study for the average number of substance dependence symptoms (a quantitative index of substance use liability) that implicated several genomic regions, including chromosomes 3q24-25 (near markers D3S1279 and D3S1614) and 9q34 (near markers D9S1826 and D9S1838). A 2008 study[58] reported SNP association results from a targeted gene assay designed to test 50 candidate genes with previous associations with substance use disorders and conduct disorder, in a sample of male probands in treatment of antisocial drug dependence and a matched set of community controls. After gene-based permutation tests, 2 genes probed with multiple SNPs (*OPRM1* and *CHRNA2*) emerged as plausible candidates for a role in antisocial drug dependence. Other studies have focused on candidate genes, such as the neuronal nicotinic acetylcholine receptors and tobacco and alcohol phenotypes. Ehringer and colleagues[59] examined 2 neuronal nicotinic receptor subunit candidate genes, and found that *CHRNA4* was associated with past 6-month use of alcohol in White, and *CHRNB2* was associated with the initial subjective response to alcohol and tobacco.

Another strategy that has been used to identify genes involved in adolescent substance dependence is to initially search for genetic variants associated with adult substance dependence, and then to study the risk associated with these variants in adolescent samples. One example of this strategy in use is the identification of the gene *GABRA2*, first found in association with alcohol dependence,[48,60] and subsequently with illicit drug dependence, antisocial personality disorder, and conduct disorder, suggesting that this gene may be involved in addictions through general externalizing pathways.[61] In 2006, Dick and colleagues[39] extended the work on *GABRA2* by using children and adolescents recruited from alcohol-dependent COGA families and control families obtained from community sources. Results suggested that individuals carrying at least 1 A allele of the SNP rs279871, which was significantly overtransmitted to alcohol-dependent subjects in the adult COGA sample, were twice as likely to meet the 3-symptom threshold of DSM-III-R conduct disorder. This effect has subsequently been replicated in an independent sample.[62] These findings suggest that this gene may be involved in addictions through general externalizing pathways that manifest first as conduct problems in adolescence, and later in adulthood as a spectrum of related disorders, including alcohol and drug dependence and antisocial personality disorder.

APPLICATIONS FOR PREVENTION

When disseminating this research to the public, it is crucial to convey how to appropriately interpret this information. Substance dependences are complex disorders, phenotypically and etiologically. There is no gene that makes an individual an alcoholic or a cocaine user; instead, there are multiple genes of subtle effects that interact to make the individual more vulnerable to a host of behaviors and disorders, many of which are characterized by behavioral disinhibition, including alcoholism and illicit drug use. These genetic vulnerabilities work in tandem with the individual's dynamic environment to protect or promote the development of externalizing spectrum problems. Although knowledge of the specific genes involved in addiction is not sufficiently advanced for this information to be used in clinical settings at the present time, the hope is that eventually information about specific genes that alter susceptibility for addictive disorders can be used to provide more individual-specific risk assessments. This information could be used to create more tailored programs for prevention and intervention. Recognizing this potential for genetic information will necessitate our understanding the pathways of risk and environmental factors that moderate risk associated with specific genetic profiles.

REFERENCES

1. US Department of Health and Human Services. The surgeon general's call to action to prevent and reduce underage drinking. Bethesda (MD): US Department of Health and Human Services, Office of the Surgeon General; 2007.
2. Hedlund JH, Ulmer RG, Preusser DF. Determine why there are fewer young alcohol impaired drivers. Washington, DC: National Highway Traffic Safety Administration; 2001. DOT HS 809 348.
3. Rice D, Barone S Jr. Critical periods of vulnerability for the developing nervous system: Evidence from humans and animal models. Environ Health Perspect 2000;108(3 Suppl):511–33.
4. Centers for Disease Control and Prevention (CDC). Alcohol-attributable deaths and years of potential life lost–United States, 2001. MMWR Morb Mortal Wkly Rep 2004;53(37):866–70.
5. Centers for Disease Control and Prevention (CDC). Youth Risk Behavior Surveillance—United States, 2007. MMWR Morb Mortal Wkly Rep 2008; 57(4 Suppl):S1–131.
6. Substance Abuse and Mental Health Services Administration. Drug Abuse Warning Network, 2005: national estimates of drug-related emergency department visits. Rockville (MD): Substance Abuse and Mental Health Services Administration; 2005. Available at: http://dawninfo.samhsa.gov/pubs/edpubs/default. asp. Accessed August 24, 2009.
7. Substance Abuse and Mental Health Services Administration. Results from the 2006 National Survey on Drug Use and Health: national findings. Rockville (MD): Substance Abuse and Mental Health Services Administration; 2006. Available at: http://dawninfo.samhsa.gov/pubs/edpubs/default.asp. Accessed August 24, 2009.
8. Merline AC, O'Malley PM, Schulenberg JE, et al. Substance use among adults 35 years of age: prevalence, adulthood predictors, and impact of adolescent substance use. Am J Public Health 2004;94(1):96–102.
9. Substance Abuse and Mental Health Services Administration. 2004 National Survey on Drug Use and Health: detailed tables. Rockville (MD): Substance Abuse and Mental Health Services Administration; 2004. Available at: http://www.oas.samhsa. gov/NSDUH/2k6NSDUH/tabs/LOTSect2pe.htm#AlcAge. Accessed August 24, 2009.
10. Chen K, Kandel DB, Davies M. Relationships between frequency and quantity of marijuana use and last year proxy dependence among adolescents and adults in the United States. Drug Alcohol Depend 1997;46(1):53–67.
11. Howlett AC, Bidaut-Russell M, Devane WA, et al. The cannabinoid receptor: biochemical, anatomical and behavioral characterization. Trends Neurosci 1990;13(10):420–3.
12. Johnston LD, O'Malley PM, Bachman JG, et al. Overall, illicit drug use by American teens continues gradual decline in 2007. Available at: www.monitoringthefuture. org. Accessed August 24, 2009.
13. Substance Abuse and Mental Health Services Administration. Misuse of over-the-counter cough and cold medications among persons aged 12 to 25. Rockville (MD): Substance Abuse and Mental Health Services Administration; 2008. Available at: http://dawninfo.samhsa.gov/pubs/edpubs/default.asp. Accessed August 24, 2009.
14. National Institute on Drug Abuse. Research report series: prescription drugs: abuse and addiction. NIH publication no. 01-4881. Bethesda (MD): US Department

of Health and Human Services, National Institutes of Health; 2001. Revised August 2005. Available at: http://www.cdc.gov/healthyYouth/alcoholdrug/index. htm. Accessed August 24, 2009.

15. Grant BF, Dawson DA. Age of onset of drug use and its association with DSM-IV drug abuse and dependence: results from the national longitudinal alcohol epidemiologic survey. J Subst Abuse 1998;10(2):163–73.

16. Dewit DJ, Adlaf EM, Offord DR, et al. Age at first alcohol use: a risk factor for the development of alcohol disorders. Am J Psychiatry 2000;157(7):45–50.

17. Hingson RW, Heeren T, Winter MR. Age at drinking onset and alcohol dependence: age at onset, duration, and severity. Arch Pediatr Adolesc Med 2006; 160(7):739–46.

18. McGue M, Iacono WG, Legrand LN, et al. Origins and consequences of age at first drink: associations with substance-use disorders, disinhibitory behavior and psychopathology, and P3 amplitude. Alcohol Clin Exp Res 2001;25(8):1156–65.

19. Prescott CA, Kendler KS. Age at first drink and risk for alcoholism: a noncausal association. Alcohol Clin Exp Res 1999;23(1):101–7.

20. Keyes MA, Iacono WG, McGue M. Early onset problem behavior, young adult psychopathology, and contextual risk. Twin Res Hum Genet 2007;10(1):45–53.

21. Tapert SF, Caldwell L, Burke C. Alcohol and the adolescent brain: human studies. Alcohol Res Health 2004;28(4):205–12.

22. Spear LP. The adolescent brain and the college drinker: biological basis of propensity to use and misuse alcohol. J Stud Alcohol 2002;14(Suppl):71–81.

23. Brown SA, Tapert SF. Adolescence and the trajectory of alcohol use: basic to clinical studies. Ann N Y Acad Sci 2004;10(21):234–44.

24. Krueger RF, Hicks BM, Patrick CJ, et al. Etiologic connections among substance dependence, antisocial behavior, and personality: modeling the externalizing spectrum. J Abnorm Psychol 2002;111(3):411–24.

25. Young SE, Stallings MC, Corley RP, et al. Genetic and environmental influences on behavioral disinhibition. Am J Med Genet 2000;96(5):684–95.

26. McGue M, Iacono WG. The adolescent origins of substance use disorders. Int J Methods Psychiatr Res 2008;17(Suppl 1):S30–8.

27. Goldman D, Oroszi G, Ducci F. The genetics of addictions: uncovering the genes. Nat Rev Genet 2005;6(7):521–32.

28. Kendler KS, Prescott CA. Cannabis use, abuse, and dependence in a population-based sample of female twins. Am J Psychiatry 1998;155(8):1016–22.

29. Tsuang MT, Lyons MJ, Meyer JM, et al. Co-occurrence of abuse of different drugs in men: the role of drug-specific and shared vulnerabilities. Arch Gen Psychiatry 1998;55(11):967–72.

30. Kendler KS, Schmitt E, Aggen SH, et al. Genetic and environmental influences on alcohol, caffeine, cannabis, and nicotine use from early adolescence to middle adulthood. Arch Gen Psychiatry 2008;65(6):674–82.

31. Bouchard TJ Jr, McGue M. Genetic and environmental influences on human psychological differences. J Neurobiol 2003;54(1):4–45.

32. Boomsma DI, van Beijsterveldt CE, Hudziak JJ. Genetic and environmental influences on Anxious/Depression during childhood: a study from the Netherlands twin register. Genes Brain Behav 2005;4(8):466–81.

33. Rose RJ, Dick DM, Viken RJ, et al. Drinking or abstaining at age 14? A genetic epidemiological study. Alcohol Clin Exp Res 2001;25(11):1594–604.

34. Rose RJ, Dick DM, Viken RJ, et al. Gene-environment interaction in patterns of adolescent drinking: regional residency moderates longitudinal influences on alcohol use. Alcohol Clin Exp Res 2001;25(5):637–43.

35. Rose RJ, Viken RJ, Dick DM, et al. It does take a village: nonfamilial environments and children's behavior. Psychol Sci 2003;14(3):273–7.
36. Kendler KS, Prescott C, Myers J, et al. The structure of genetic and environmental risk factors for common psychiatric and substance use disorders in men and women. Arch Gen Psychiatry 2003;60(9):929–37.
37. Slutske WS, Heath AC, Dinwiddie SH, et al. Common genetic risk factors for conduct disorder and alcohol dependence. J Abnorm Psychol 1998;107(3): 363–74.
38. Haber JR, Jacob T, Heath AC. Paternal alcoholism and offspring conduct disorder: evidence for the 'common genes' hypothesis. Twin Res Hum Genet 2005;8(2):120–31.
39. Dick DM, Bierut L, Hinrichs A, et al. The role of GABRA2 in risk for conduct disorder and alcohol and drug dependence across developmental stages. Behav Genet 2006;36(4):577–90.
40. Kendler KS, Jacobson KC, Prescott CA, et al. Specificity of genetic and environmental risk factors for use and abuse/dependence of cannabis, cocaine, hallucinogens, sedatives, stimulants, and opiates in male twins. Am J Psychiatry 2003; 160(4):687–95.
41. Koopmans JR, Slutske WS, Van Baal GC, et al. The influence of religion on alcohol use initiation: evidence for genotype X environment interaction. Behav Genet 1999;29(6):445–53.
42. Rose RJ, Kaprio J, Williams CJ, et al. Social contact and sibling similarity: facts, issues, and red herrings. Behav Genet 1990;20(6):763–78.
43. Dick DM, Viken R, Purcell S, et al. Parental monitoring moderates the importance of genetic and environmental influences on adolescent smoking. J Abnorm Psychol 2007;116(1):213–8.
44. Marshal MP, Chassin L. Peer influence on adolescent alcohol use: the moderating role of parental support and discipline. Appl Dev Sci 2000;4:80–8.
45. Dick DM, Rose RJ, Viken RJ, et al. Exploring gene-environment interactions: socioregional moderation of alcohol use. J Abnorm Psychol 2001;110(4):625–32.
46. Hicks BM, South SC, Dirago AC, et al. Environmental adversity and increasing genetic risk for externalizing disorders. Arch Gen Psychiatry 2009;66(6):640–8.
47. Dick DM, Latendresse SJ, Lansford JE, et al. Role of GABRA2 in trajectories of externalizing behavior across development and evidence of moderation by parental monitoring. Arch Gen Psychiatry 2009;66(6):649–57.
48. Edenberg HJ, Dick DM, Xuei X, et al. Variations in GABRA2, encoding the alpha 2 subunit of the GABA(A) receptor, are associated with alcohol dependence and with brain oscillations. Am J Hum Genet 2004;74(4):705–14.
49. Edenberg HJ, Xuei X, Chen HJ, et al. Association of alcohol dehydrogenase genes with alcohol dependence: a comprehensive analysis. Hum Mol Genet 2006;15(9):1539–49.
50. Kuo PH, Kalsi G, Prescott CA, et al. Association of ADH and ALDH genes with alcohol dependence in the Irish Affected Sib Pair Study of Alcohol Dependence (IASPSAD) sample. Alcohol Clin Exp Res 2008;32(5):785–95.
51. Edenberg HJ, Xuei X, Wetherill LF, et al. Association of NFKB1, which encodes a subunit of the transcription factor NF-kappaB, with alcohol dependence. Hum Mol Genet 2008;17(7):963–70.
52. Wang JC, Hinrichs AL, Stock H, et al. Evidence of common and specific genetic effects: association of the muscarinic acetylcholine receptor M2 (CHRM2) gene with alcohol dependence and major depressive syndrome. Hum Mol Genet 2004;13(17):1903–11.

53. Wang JC, Hinrichs AL, Bertelsen S, et al. Functional variants in TAS2R38 and TAS2R16 influence alcohol consumption in high-risk families of African-American origin. Alcohol Clin Exp Res 2007;31(2):209–15.
54. Risch N, Merikangas K. The future of genetic studies of complex human diseases. Science 1996;273(5281):1516–7.
55. Treutlein J, Cichon S, Ridinger M, et al. Genome-wide association study of alcohol dependence. Arch Gen Psychiatry 2009;66(7):773–84.
56. Sebastiani P, Timofeev N, Dworkis DA, et al. Genome-wide association studies and the genetic dissection of complex traits. Am J Hematol 2009;84(8):504–15.
57. Stallings MC, Corley RP, Hewitt JK, et al. A genome-wide search for quantitative trait loci influencing substance dependence vulnerability in adolescence. Drug Alcohol Depend 2003;70(3):295–307.
58. Corley RP, Zeiger JS, Crowley T, et al. Association of candidate genes with anti-social drug dependence in adolescents. Drug Alcohol Depend 2008;96(1-2): 90–8.
59. Ehringer MA, Clegg HV, Collins AC, et al. Association of the neuronal nicotinic receptor beta2 subunit gene (CHRNB2) with subjective responses to alcohol and nicotine. Am J Med Genet B Neuropsychiatr Genet 2007;144(5):596–604.
60. Dick DM, Plunkett J, Wetherill LF, et al. Association between GABRA1 and drinking behaviors in the collaborative study on the genetics of alcoholism sample. Alcohol Clin Exp Res 2006;30(7):1101–10.
61. Dick DM. Identification of genes influencing a spectrum of externalizing psycho-pathology. Curr Dir Psychol Sci 2007;16(6):331–5.
62. Sakai JT, Stallings MC, Crowley TJ, et al. Test of association between GABRA2 (SNP rs279871) and adolescent conduct/alcohol use disorders utilizing a sample of clinic referred youth with serious substance and conduct problems, controls and available first degree relatives. Drug Alcohol Depend 2010;106(2–3): 199–203.

Neurobiology of Adolescent Substance Use Disorders: Implications for Prevention and Treatment

Helena J.V. Rutherford, PhD[a],*, Linda C. Mayes, MD[a],
Marc N. Potenza, MD, PhD[a,b]

KEYWORDS

- Neurobiology • Adolescence • Substance use
- Treatment • Prevention

Adolescence marks an important developmental period of neurobiological change, with heightened vulnerability to substance use. Greater severity in progression of drug usage in adolescence has been observed, with higher dependency rates during this developmental period.[1] Adolescents also show greater experimental use and

Funding Sources and Disclosures: This work was supported by the National Institutes of Health (NIH) grants R01 DA019039, R01 DA020908, RL1 AA017539, R01 DA06025, R01 DA017863, R01 HD044796, R21 DA024232, P01 DA022446, P50 DA09241, P50 DA016556, UL1 DE19586, NIH Roadmap for Medical Research/Common Fund, the Office of Research on Women's Health, the Gustavus and Louise Pfeiffer Research Foundation, and the Anna Freud Centre (UK). This publication was also made possible by CTSA Grant Number UL1 RR024139 from the National Center for Research Resources (NCRR), a component of the NIH, and NIH roadmap for Medical Research. The contents of the manuscript are solely the responsibility of the authors and do not necessarily represent the official views of any of the funding agencies. Dr Potenza has received financial support or compensation for the following: Dr Potenza consults for and is an advisor to Boehringer Ingelheim; has consulted for and has financial interests in Somaxon; has received research support from NIH, Department of Veterans Affairs, Mohegan Sun Casino, the National Center for Responsible Gaming and its affiliated Institute for Research on Gambling Disorders, and Forest Laboratories, Ortho-McNeil, Oy-Control/Biotie, and Glaxo-SmithKline pharmaceuticals; has participated in surveys, mailings, or telephone consultations related to drug addiction, impulse control disorders, or other health topics; has consulted for law offices and the federal public defender's office in issues related to impulse control disorders; provides clinical care in the Connecticut Department of Mental Health and Addiction Services Problem Gambling Services Program; has performed grant reviews for NIH and other agencies; has given academic lectures in grand rounds, continuing medical education events and other clinical or scientific venues; and has generated books or book chapters for publishers of mental health texts.

[a] Yale Child Study Center, Yale University School of Medicine, 230 South Frontage Road, New Haven, CT 06520, USA
[b] Department of Psychiatry, Yale University School of Medicine, Connecticut Mental Health Center, 34 Park Street, New Haven, CT 06519, USA
* Corresponding author.
E-mail address: helena.rutherford@yale.edu

Child Adolesc Psychiatric Clin N Am 19 (2010) 479–492
doi:10.1016/j.chc.2010.03.003
1056-4993/10/$ – see front matter © 2010 Elsevier Inc. All rights reserved.

report higher rates of substance use disorders (SUDs),[2] suggesting potential neurobiological vulnerability to substance use or a critical period in adolescent development. Early substance use may influence later social and occupational functioning,[3] as well as physical and psychological health,[4,5] with earlier onset of substance use predicting greater addiction severity and morbidity with other clinical disorders in adulthood.[6] Consequently, an improved understanding of the neurobiology of adolescent substance use initiation and development of SUDs should facilitate advances in prevention and treatment during adolescence.

This article is organized into 3 sections. The first section discusses the neurobiology of adolescent decision making and how this contributes to initiation of substance use before maintained use and abuse or dependence. The second section presents the empirical research that has started to identify neurobiological differences in structural and functional neuroanatomy in adolescents with SUDs and healthy controls. The third section considers the implications of structural and functional differences for prevention and treatment of adolescent SUDs.

THE NEUROBIOLOGY OF ADOLESCENT DECISION MAKING

Behavioral tests have been used to investigate decision making in laboratory settings. One such paradigm, the Iowa Gambling Task (IGT), was developed to investigate why individuals with stroke lesions in specific brain areas (eg, the ventromedial prefrontal cortex) exhibited poor performance in real-life measures of functioning while not displaying impairment on standard neuropsychological tests.[7] Adults with drug addictions have been shown to perform disadvantageously on the IGT (that is, selecting larger immediate rewards despite longer-term losses and not learning to change this behavior over time), and performance has been associated with real-life measures of functioning (eg, disadvantageous performance has been positively associated with unemployment[8]). However, decision-making tasks like the IGT involve multiple components including risk/reward assessment, strategic learning, and cognitive flexibility. In making decisions, the valence, probability, and magnitude of potential outcomes should be considered.[9] Impaired consideration of any of these processes may lead to engagement in risky behavior such that immediate rewarding outcomes drive decision making regardless of future (potentially negative) outcomes. As such, it has been hypothesized that such dysfunctions in decision making serve to underscore the development of substance use disorders.[10] Thus, additional tasks that probe specific components of decision making can be used to fractionate the construct and better understand the relationships of the core components to adolescent substance use behaviors.

Risk/reward assessment as it contributes to decision making has been investigated from a behavioral neuroeconomic perspective. Specifically, temporal discounting (or delay discounting) paradigms have been used to investigate reward preferences as they relate to substance use behaviors.[11] Delay discounting refers to the selection of small immediate rewards over larger delayed rewards, with higher rates of discounting demonstrated by individuals scoring high on measures of impulsivity.[12] Adults with SUDs typically show a rapid discounting of rewards, tending to prefer smaller, immediate rewards over larger, delayed ones.[13] As compared with adults, adolescents have been found to discount rewards more rapidly,[14] with heavy alcohol-drinking adolescents discounting more than light alcohol-drinking adolescents.[15] Individual differences in the ability to delay gratification and select larger delayed rewards over smaller immediate ones have been demonstrated in youth as young as 3 to 4 years of age,[16] suggesting that the propensity to exhibit self-control in the setting of appetitive stimuli may manifest early in life. As related to adolescent SUDs, more rapid

characterized by increases in myelination and initial aborization and then pruning of gray matter.[46] Further, evidence suggests that the adolescent brain is more vulnerable to the effects of substance use,[47] with animal studies showing that substance use in adolescent rats disturbs neuroendocrine functioning.[48] Consequently, studies in adults with SUDs may not provide adequate insight into the neurobiology of adolescent SUDs, limiting treatment and prevention options and identifying the need for research during adolescence in this field. Advances in techniques such as magnetic resonance imaging (MRI) and diffusion tensor imaging (DTI) have provided a unique opportunity to probe structural differences that may exist in adolescent SUDs. Arguably, 3 brain regions have received the most attention in this regard: the hippocampus, corpus callosum, and frontal cortex.

Hippocampus

Hippocampal structure has been implicated in learning and memory,[49] and evidence from animal studies has shown sensitivity of the hippocampus to neurotoxicity.[48] Initial work[50] showed reduced left and right hippocampal volumes in adolescents with alcohol use disorders (AUDs) relative to controls, in the absence of any volumetric differences in corpus callosum, gray and white matter, amygdala, and cerebrum. Furthermore, these decreases in hippocampal volume were significantly correlated with the age of onset and duration of AUDs, suggesting a direct association between the development of AUDs and hippocampal volume reduction. In a subsequent study, when recruiting adolescents with no additional comorbid disorders, only left hippocampal volume reductions in adolescents with AUDs were observed.[51] In a separate study, increases (rather than decreases) in left hippocampal volume have been reported in adolescents using both marijuana and alcohol relative to adolescents using only alcohol.[52] However, these populations appear more reflective of regular substance users than individuals with formal SUDs; nonetheless, these findings suggest a complex influence of multiple substance use on adolescent hippocampal structure.

Corpus callosum

Increases in myelination occur during adolescent brain development,[46] and thus research has investigated the integrity of the corpus callosum in adolescents with SUDs, although with seemingly conflicting results. DTI research[53] has revealed that the integrity of white matter tracts in adolescents with AUDs, compared with controls, is reduced in the splenium and body (at statistical trend level) of the corpus callosum, with the integrity of the white matter tracts showing significant relationships with AUD characteristics such as duration of heavy drinking and withdrawal symptoms. However, group differences in callosal white matter between adolescents with AUDs and controls have not been reported elsewhere.[50,54] Furthermore, increases (vs decreases) in white matter integrity have been reported in the anterior corpus callosum in adolescents with AUDs, suggesting premature myelination rather than neurotoxicity.[54]

Frontal cortex

The importance of understanding structural abnormalities in frontal cortex in adolescent SUDs is evident from the executive dysfunction observed in substance dependent adults,[55] as well as the later maturation of this region in adolescence.[33] Recent DTI research has begun to investigate substance use in adolescents as related to white matter tract integrity, identifying frontal and parietal circuits.[56] PFC total volume and white matter volume has been reported as significantly smaller in adolescents with AUDs as compared with those without.[57] Furthermore, PFC volume and gray matter volume in the PFC in this sample were related to alcohol characteristics, specifically the average amount of alcohol consumed at a given time. In a similar study, structural MRI examined frontal regions with specific interest in gender effects in adolescents with AUDs.[58] Adolescent girls with AUDs were found to have smaller PFC and white matter PFC volume relative to control girls, whereas adolescent boys with AUDs were found to have larger PFC and white matter PFC volume relative to control boys. Such an effect was not found previously,[57] but important sample differences, including a younger cohort and comorbid psychiatric disorder exclusion criteria present in the former study,[58] may represent important differences.

Brain Function

Several studies using functional MRI (fMRI) have begun to elucidate differences in brain function during different tasks in adolescent substance dependence. Evidence to suggest functional abnormalities between adolescents with SUDs and adolescents without have been drawn from 3 task domains: executive functioning including working memory, cerebral perfusion at rest, and presentation of substance-related cues.

Working memory and executive functioning

Multiple studies have required participants to complete a spatial working memory task during fMRI. Distinct differences in functional brain activation emerged in adolescents with AUDs,[59] who show reduced functional activity compared with controls in multiple areas including the left precentral gyrus, left inferior temporal and fusiform gyri, and bilaterally in the cerebellum. Greater activity was also found in bilateral parietal regions relative to control participants. Interestingly, functional differences in this task between adolescents with AUDs and those without were heightened in girls (vs boys), suggesting increased neurobiological vulnerability to the effects of alcohol use in girls.[60] This result also converges with structural findings of the differential effects of alcohol use on PFC volume as a function of gender.[58] The differences in functional activity in both studies[59,60] are more compelling taking into consideration the absence of any behavioral difference in performance between the AUD and control adolescents in the spatial working memory task. This performance indifference suggests the involvement of compensatory neural mechanisms engaged during task performance. An earlier study[61] using the same task but completed by an older (aged 18–25 years) cohort of women with alcohol dependence observed poorer behavioral performance on the same spatial working memory task relative to controls, with reduced activity in parietal regions, accompanied by a reduction in activity in prefrontal regions (including right medial frontal gyrus and left superior frontal gyrus). These studies taken together suggest that alcohol dependence during adolescence manifests in subtle neurophysiological changes in the absence of specific behavioral impairments, although as this dependence continues through the course of development, increased brain dysfunction emerges that is accompanied by objective behavioral difficulties.

Recent research suggests that adolescents with marijuana and alcohol dependence (MAUD) show no behavioral differences relative to controls in spatial working memory; however, a wider network of dysfunction appears to emerge.[62] Specifically, relative to controls, adolescents with MAUD show increased activity in the dorsolateral prefrontal cortex, with reduced activity in the anterior cingulate, right inferior frontal, and bilateral temporal regions. These findings are consistent with the notion that functional activity observed in adolescents with MAUD may reflect compensatory networks of activation needed to maintain behavioral performance. Also noteworthy in this study were the comparisons between adolescents with MAUDs and AUDs that revealed similar functional patterns of activation in frontal regions, although functional activity in adolescents with AUDs did not statistically differ from controls. These findings suggest a gradation of substance use effects on neurophysiology, with additive effects of polysubstance use having more detrimental consequences on functional brain activity.

These studies investigating spatial working memory reveal dysfunction in regions typically associated with cognitive control, including frontal, temporal, and parietal cortex. Additional research using an auditory memory (n-back) task has revealed behavioral and neurobiological hippocampal dysfunction in adolescents frequently using both marijuana[63] and ecstasy.[64] Other studies have investigated the neurobiology of attentional control in adolescent substance users, particularly those with both SUDs and conduct problems (SCP[65]). Consistent with other studies described previously, activation differences were observed, often in the absence of behavioral deficits; for example, under conditions of attentional conflict, adolescents with SCP showed increased activation in multiple regions including bilateral hippocampal gyrus, superior frontal gyrus, thalamus, and the caudate.

Cerebral perfusion at rest

Important for understanding fMRI findings, which rely on blood flow measures during task performance, are the potential for existing differences in blood flow at rest. Resting cerebral perfusion in frontal regions have been examined in young women recruited from an existing adolescent substance abuse cohort and compared with control women.[66] Here it was found that although global differences in perfusion were absent, perfusion was less in prefrontal and parietal regions in the SUD cohort relative to the control group. Such resting state differences may contribute to differences observed in the functional studies outlined previously (those when engaged in spatial working memory tasks), although the contribution of age as a factor may need to be considered and this finding replicated in adolescents. Nevertheless, it is interesting to note that such resting state differences can exist and future research will benefit from determining how and whether changes in resting state manifest in functional and behavioral differences in adolescents with SUDs.

Substance-related cues

The neural correlates of substance cue reactivity has been examined in adolescents with and without SUDs.[67] On each trial, participants were presented a single picture drawn from a series of advertisements containing either alcohol- or non–alcohol-relevant cues, and these cues were personalized to suit the beverage preference of each individual participant. Responding was task-irrelevant, with participants making a discrimination response to the presence or absence of people in the advertisements. Adolescents with AUDs showed an overall increased activation in response to alcohol cues compared with controls. This functional increase was observed predominantly in frontal and limbic regions, areas that have previously been identified as important in processing emotionally and motivationally salient and rewarding stimuli.[68] This finding suggests that alcohol-related cues may be processed as rewarding by adolescents with AUDs. In studies that directly investigate reward processing, adolescents as compared with adults, including adolescents with a family history of alcoholism, have shown relatively diminished activation of the ventral striatum.[69,70] These findings resonate with studies of adults with AUDs in which relatively diminished ventral striatal activation is observed in the AUD group, and this diminished ventral striatal activation correlates with impulsivity measures.[71,72]

Thus far we have reviewed both structural and functional evidence that points to neurobiological differences present in adolescents with SUDs relative to controls. We now turn our attention to considering the implications of these studies for the prevention and treatment of adolescent SUDs.

IMPLICATIONS FOR PREVENTION AND TREATMENT

The evidence discussed previously suggests that identifiable structural and functional abnormalities emerge in adolescents with SUDs, indicating the potential for prevention and treatment during this period. However, it is important to consider whether these abnormalities emerge as a consequence of substance use, or reflect preexisting differences that serve to increase vulnerability to initial substance use and subsequent abuse and dependence. On the one hand, substances such as alcohol may be exerting neurotoxic effects in cortical and subcortical regions, disrupting normative trajectories of neural myelination in adolescence. The inhibitory effects of ethanol on N-methyl-D-aspartate (NMDA) receptors is such that it impairs excitatory glutamate neurotransmission[48] and the effects of alcohol on NDMA receptors has been hypothesized as a possible mechanism underlying reduced hippocampal volume in adolescent SUD (eg, DeBellis and colleagues[50]).

On the other hand, structural and functional abnormalities may represent preexisting morbidity and vulnerability to the development of SUDs. One approach to teasing this apart with existing data sets would be to correlate age of onset of substance use and dependency with structural and functional data; presumably if these abnormalities were a consequence, rather than a cause, of substance use then there should be a numerical relation between neurobiology and chronology. The absence of such a relationship may instead speak to a preexisting vulnerability to substance use. In the structural data for instance, PFC volume reduction was not related to age of onset,[57] suggesting an initial volume deficit before substance use. Relating structure to function, existing research has documented the importance of frontal regions in impulse control and decision making,[73] perhaps suggesting that these structural impairments may be a precursor to these behavioral and cognitive dysfunctions, and increase the likelihood of initial and maintained substance use.[57] As described in an earlier section, animal data suggest a role for both preexisting vulnerabilities for substance use in substance-naïve individuals and that substance use leads to changes in behavior, mediated by functional and structural brain-based changes. Thus, it will be the goal of future research to investigate developmental interactions between substance use and adolescent (and adult) neurobiology.

If preexisting structural and functional vulnerabilities can be considered risk factors to the development and maintenance of SUDs, then these neurobiological characteristics could potentially be used to identify those most at risk in adolescence and into adulthood. The pragmatics of neurobiological screening during adolescence though is limited, but brain-behavior relationships may be useful here. As detailed previously, certain constructs such as impulsivity and related factors may contribute significantly to decision-making processes and engagement in risky behaviors, and if a strong association can be demonstrated between such behavioral measures and brain findings, then this could prove fruitful in identifying those individuals at greatest risk. An important caveat in understanding neural substrates of adolescent substance use is that part and parcel of adolescence are biological changes that promote novelty seeking and risk taking, which are adaptive in promoting independence from caregivers.[2,31] It is when these normative changes lead to more negative outcomes, with initial substance use leading to repeated substance use and dependence, that intervention is crucial. Nevertheless, identification of those individuals who may show atypical responses in behavioral measures of risk may still prove beneficial. This could be greatly facilitated by establishing relations between risk factors identified in behavioral measures and neurobiological changes in adolescent populations with SUDs. Prevention programs could identify those most at risk, targeting behavioral characteristics associated with risk rather than a more general intervention approach, and this has proven successful in changing the attitudes of young adults who report high scores on sensation seeking.[74]

Relevant to findings in non-SUD adolescents, understanding the contribution of reward sensitivity may also prove important here. According to the neurobiological model of adolescent brain development,[35] the maturation of the limbic system with heightened reward sensitivity in conjunction with the protracted development of prefrontal cortex and immature cognitive control, suggests that an imbalance between the development of these 2 systems may be at the core of risk-taking behavior. Indeed, in healthy participants across development, activity in the ventral striatum positively correlated with an increased likelihood of self-reported engagement with risky behaviors.[75] Although this neurobiological approach speaks to a general increase in risk-taking behavior during this developmental period, intervention programs need to identify those adolescents more likely to engage in risky behaviors, potentially through reward sensitivity, who may be susceptible to the negative outcomes beyond the normative adolescent trajectory.

As described previously, substance-related cues are processed by the affective system similarly to motivationally rewarding cues in adolescents with SUDs, with increased responsiveness in frontal and limbic circuits to these cues.[67] Similarly in adult studies, substance use cues have been shown to influence neural activity in frontal and subcortical (eg, thalamic) regions,[76] thus converging with findings in adolescents. As such, the marketing and advertising of commonly used substances, such as alcohol and tobacco, warrant consideration, particularly as related to adolescents. Overlapping reward systems processing substances and nonsubstances also suggest the utility of treatment programs in replacing risk-taking behavior with other stimulating or novel behaviors that have rewarding outcomes but are not substance-based.[74] This could be completed in conjunction with interventions enhancing the rewarding value of naturally occurring reinforcers.[77] However, as these investigations are at very early stages and some prevention strategies with seemingly rational foundations have been shown not to be very helpful in adolescents,[78] additional research is needed to determine empirically the validity of such approaches.

It is worthwhile to consider the role of gender in the development of adolescent SUDs. Findings of differential PFC structural volumes in boys and girls with AUDs,[58] and functional differences during spatial working memory tasks,[60] suggest gender differences in the neurobiological substrates of adolescent SUDs may be a significant factor.[79,80] Indeed, the pathways to substance use and dependence may differ significantly by gender; for example, women with AUDs use alcohol more to facilitate regulation of negative affect than men with AUDs.[81] Gender differences in psychopathology (for instance, adolescent girls have higher rates of mood disorders[82]; boys have higher rates of conduct disorder[83]) may also serve to demonstrate the importance of gender more generally in the development of clinical disorders, especially considering these disorders typically onset in adolescence and are highly comorbid with substance use.[20] Consequently, structural and functional gender differences may reflect distinct mechanisms underlying substance use, and both screening and intervention programs should consider gender to optimize efforts.

Finally, identifying those at risk for the development of adolescent SUDs to target intervention will benefit greatly from consideration of whether the implications of these findings are in standing within the realms of genetic or environmental contributions. Family studies have found that there are high concordance rates between substance-using children and parents, suggesting a heritable component to illicit drug use, with increased rates of adolescent substance use when parents are perceived as substance users (see Mayes and Suchman[84] for a review). Although this may suggest a genetic component, the familial environment with exposure (and potentially access) to drugs may reinforce substance-using behaviors, specifically initiation of use. Genetic components are also important, with susceptibility and vulnerability to substance use and SUDs found to have substantial heritable contributions.[85] Furthermore, repeated substance use may alter the expression of specific genes involved in the pathophysiology of SUDs (eg, DeBellis and colleagues[50]). Thus, it may be that genetic and environmental factors modulate substance use experimentation, and the complex transition from initiation to repeated use and subsequent dependence with specific periods, like adolescence, of particular neurodevelopmental vulnerability.[84]

SUMMARY

Adolescence is characterized by distinct neurobehavioral changes with more rapid development of limbic systems and relatively immature prefrontal cognitive system that may promote risky behaviors and substance use. Research understanding the neurobiological substrates of SUDs has historically focused on adults, and findings from studies of adults may have limited applicability to adolescents. Recent studies are identifying distinct structural and functional differences in adolescents with SUDs, providing a biological basis for prevention and treatment programs. These data coupled with a better understanding of individual differences and their relation to brain structure and function will be important for the successful development and implementation of prevention and treatment before, during, and following adolescence.

ACKNOWLEDGMENTS

We are grateful to Naaila Panjwani for her assistance with the preparation of the manuscript.

REFERENCES

1. Wagner FA, Anthony JC. From first drug use to drug dependence—developmental periods of risk for dependence upon marijuana, cocaine, and alcohol. Neuropsychopharmacology 2002;26(4):479–88.
2. Kelley AE, Schochet T, Landry CF. Risk taking and novelty seeking in adolescence: introduction to part I. Ann N Y Acad Sci 2004;1021(1):27–32.
3. Friedman AS, Terras A, Zhu W. Early adolescent substance use/abuse as predictor to employment in adulthood: gender differences. J Child Adolesc Subst Abuse 2004;13(4):49–60.
4. Jones DR, Macias C, Barreira PJ, et al. Prevalence, severity, and co-occurrence of chronic physical health problems of persons with serious mental illness. Psychiatr Serv 2004;55(11):1250–7.
5. McGue M, Lacono WG. The association of early adolescent problem behavior with adult psychopathology. Am J Psychiatry 2005;162(6):1118–24.

6. Grant BF, Dawson DA. Age of onset of drug use and its association with DSM-IV drug abuse and dependence: results from the national longitudinal alcohol epidemiologic survey. J Subst Abuse 1998;10(2):163–73.
7. Damasio AR. Descartes' error: emotion, reason and the human brain. New York: Crosset/Putnam; 1994.
8. Bechara A. Risky business: emotion, decision-making, and addiction. J Gambl Stud 2003;19(1):23–51.
9. Montague PR, Berns GS. Neural economics and the biological substrates of valuation. Neuron 2002;36(2):265–84.
10. Paulus MP. Decision-making dysfunctions in psychiatry—altered homeostatic processing? Science 2007;318:602–6.
11. Bickel WK, Marsch LA. Toward a behavioral economic understanding of drug dependence: delay discounting processes. Addiction 2001;96(1):73–86.
12. Mitchell SH. Measures of impulsivity in cigarette smokers and non-smokers. Psychopharmacology (Berl) 1999;146(4):455–64.
13. Petry NM. Substance abuse, pathological gambling, and impulsiveness. Drug Alcohol Depend 2001;63(1):29–38.
14. Steinberg L, Graham S, O'Brien L, et al. Age differences in future orientation and delay discounting. Child Dev 2009;80(1):28–44.
15. Field M, Christiansen P, Cole J, et al. Delay discounting and the alcohol Stroop in heavy drinking adolescents. Addiction 2007;102(4):579–86.
16. Mischel W, Shoda Y, Rodriguez M. Delay of gratification in children. Science 1989;244:933–8.
17. Reynolds B, Karraker K, Horn K, et al. Delay and probability discounting as related to different stages of adolescent smoking and non-smoking. Behav Processes 2003;64(3):333–44.
18. Reynolds B. Do high rates of cigarette consumption increase delay discounting? A cross-sectional comparison of adolescent smokers and young-adult smokers and nonsmokers. Behav Processes 2004;67(3):545–9.
19. Krishnan-Sarin S, Reynolds B, Duhig AM, et al. Behavioral impulsivity predicts treatment outcome in a smoking cessation program for adolescent smokers. Drug Alcohol Depend 2007;88(1):79–82.
20. Chambers RA, Taylor JR, Potenza MN. Developmental neurocircuitry of motivation in adolescence: a critical period of addiction vulnerability. Am J Psychiatry 2003;160(6):1041–52.
21. Moeller FG, Barratt ES, Dougherty DM, et al. Psychiatric aspects of impulsivity. Am J Psychiatry 2001;158(11):1783–93.
22. Potenza MN. Should addictive disorders include non-substance-related conditions? Addiction 2006;101(s1):142–51.
23. Potenza MN, Taylor J. Found in translation: understanding impulsivity and related constructs through integrative preclinical and clinical research. Biol Psychiatry 2009;66(8):714–6.
24. Verdejo-García A, Lawrence AJ, Clark L. Impulsivity as a vulnerability marker for substance-use disorders: review of findings from high-risk research, problem gamblers and genetic association studies. Neurosci Biobehav Rev 2008;32(4):777–810.
25. Belin D, Mar AC, Dalley JW, et al. High impulsivity predicts the switch to compulsive cocaine-taking. Science 2008;320:1352–5.
26. Dalley JW, Fryer TD, Brichard L, et al. Nucleus accumbens D2/3 receptors predict trait impulsivity and cocaine reinforcement. Science 2007;315:1267–70.

27. Diergaarde L, Pattij T, Poortvliet I, et al. Impulsive choice and impulsive action predict vulnerability to distinct stages of nicotine seeking in rats. Biol Psychiatry 2008;63(3):301–8.
28. Nasralla NA, Yang TWH, Bernstein IL. Long-term risk preference and suboptimal decision making following adolescent alcohol use. Proc Natl Acad Sci U S A 2009;106(41):17600–4.
29. Lejuez CW, Read JP, Kahler CW, et al. Evaluation of a behavioral measure of risk taking: the balloon analogue risk task (BART). J Exp Psychol Appl 2002;8(2):75–84.
30. Aklin WM, Lejuez CW, Zvolensky MJ, et al. Evaluation of behavioral measures of risk taking propensity with inner city adolescents. Behav Res Ther 2005;43(2):215–28.
31. Dahl RE. Adolescent brain development: a period of vulnerabilities and opportunities. Ann N Y Acad Sci 2004;1021(1):1–22.
32. Steinberg L. Risk taking in adolescence: new perspectives from brain and behavioral science. Curr Dir Psychol Sci 2007;16(2):55–9.
33. Steinberg L. Risk taking in adolescence: what changes, and why? Ann N Y Acad Sci 2004;1021(1):51–8.
34. Bardo MT. High-risk behavior during adolescence: comments on part I. Ann N Y Acad Sci 2004;1021(1):59–60.
35. Casey BJ, Getz S, Galvan A. The adolescent brain. Dev Rev 2008;28(1):62–77.
36. Knutson B, Adams CM, Fong GW, et al. Anticipation of increasing monetary reward selectively recruits nucleus accumbens. J Neurosci 2001;21(159RC):1–5.
37. Kuhnen CM, Knutson B. The neural basis of financial risk taking. Neuron 2005; 47(5):763–70.
38. Galvan A, Hare TA, Parra CE, et al. Earlier development of the accumbens relative to orbitofrontal cortex might underlie risk-taking behavior in adolescents. J Neurosci 2006;26(25):6885–92.
39. Green L, Myerson J, Ostaszewski P. Discounting of delayed rewards across the life span: age differences in individual discounting functions. Behav Processes 1999;46(1):89–96.
40. Ernst M, Nelson EE, Jazbec S, et al. Amygdala and nucleus accumbens in responses to receipt and omission of gains in adults and adolescents. Neuroimage 2005;25(4):1279–91.
41. O'Doherty JP. Reward representations and reward-related learning in the human brain: insights from neuroimaging. Curr Opin Neurobiol 2004;14(6):769–76.
42. Gallagher M, McMahan RW, Schoenbaum G. Orbitofrontal cortex and representation of incentive value in associative learning. J Neurosci 1999;19(15):6610–4.
43. Romeo RD, McEwen BS. Stress and the adolescent brain. Ann N Y Acad Sci 2006;1094:202–14.
44. McEwen BS. Glucocorticoids, depression, and mood disorders: structural remodeling in the brain. Metabolism 2005;54(5):20–3.
45. Cerqueira JJ, Mailliet F, Almeida OFX, et al. The prefrontal cortex as a key target of the maladaptive response to stress. J Neurosci 2007;27(11):2781–7.
46. Giedd JN. Structural magnetic resonance imaging of the adolescent brain. Ann N Y Acad Sci 2004;1021(1):77–85.
47. Monti PM, Miranda R Jr, Nixon K, et al. Adolescence: booze, brains, and behavior. Alcohol Clin Exp Res 2005;29(2):207–20.
48. Smith RF. Animal models of periadolescent substance abuse. Neurotoxicol Teratol 2003;25(3):291–301.
49. Shapiro ML, Eichenbaum H. Hippocampus as a memory map: synaptic plasticity and memory encoding by hippocampal neurons. Hippocampus 1999;9(4): 365–84.

50. De Bellis MD, Clark DB, Beers SR, et al. Hippocampal volume in adolescent-onset alcohol use disorders. Am J Psychiatry 2000;157(5):737–44.
51. Nagel BJ, Schweinsburg AD, Phan V, et al. Reduced hippocampal volume among adolescents with alcohol use disorders without psychiatric comorbidity. Psychiatry Res 2005;139(3):181–90.
52. Medina KL, Schweinsburg AD, Cohen-Zion M, et al. Effects of alcohol and combined marijuana and alcohol use during adolescence on hippocampal volume and asymmetry. Neurotoxicol Teratol 2007;29(1):141–52.
53. Tapert SF, Theilmann RJ, Schweinsburg AD, et al. Reduced fractional anisotropy in the splenium of adolescents with alcohol use disorder. Proceedings for the International Society for Magnetic Resonance in Medicine. Toronto, 2003. p. 431. [abstract 2241].
54. De Bellis MD, Van Voorhees E, Hooper SR, et al. Diffusion tensor measures of the corpus callosum in adolescents with adolescent onset alcohol use disorders. Alcohol Clin Exp Res 2008;32(3):395–404.
55. Verdejo-Garcia A, Bechara A, Recknor EC, et al. Executive dysfunction in substance dependent individuals during drug use and abstinence: an examination of the behavioral, cognitive and emotional correlates of addiction. J Int Neuropsychol Soc 2006;12(3):405–15.
56. Bava S, Frank LR, McQuenny T, et al. Altered white matter microstructure in adolescent substance users. Psychiatry Res Neuroimaging 2009;173(3):228–37.
57. De Bellis MD, Narasimhan A, Thatcher DL, et al. Prefrontal cortex, thalamus, and cerebellar volumes in adolescents and young adults with adolescent-onset alcohol use disorders and comorbid mental disorders. Alcohol Clin Exp Res 2005;29(9):1590–600.
58. Medina KL, McQueeny T, Nagel BJ, et al. Prefrontal cortex volumes in adolescents with alcohol use disorders: unique gender effects. Alcohol Clin Exp Res 2008;32(3):386–94.
59. Tapert SF, Schweinsburg AD, Barlett VC, et al. Blood oxygen level dependent response and spatial working memory in adolescents with alcohol use disorders. Alcohol Clin Exp Res 2004;28(10):1577–86.
60. Caldwell LC, Schweinsburg AD, Nagel BJ, et al. Gender and adolescent alcohol use disorders on BOLD (blood oxygen level dependent) response to spatial working memory. Alcohol Alcohol 2005;40(3):194–200.
61. Tapert SF, Brown GG, Kindermann SS, et al. fMRI measurement of brain dysfunction in alcohol-dependent young women. Alcohol Clin Exp Res 2001;25(2):236–45.
62. Schweinsburg AD, Schweinsburg BC, Cheung EH, et al. fMRI response to spatial working memory in adolescents with comorbid marijuana and alcohol use disorders. Drug Alcohol Depend 2005;79(2):201–10.
63. Jacobsen LK, Mencl WE, Westerveld M, et al. Impact of cannabis use on brain function in adolescents. Ann N Y Acad Sci 2004;1021(1):384–90.
64. Jacobsen LK, Mencl WE, Pugh KR, et al. Preliminary evidence of hippocampal dysfunction in adolescent MDMA ("ecstasy") users: possible relationship to neurotoxic effects. Psychopharmacology (Berl) 2004;173(3–4):383–90.
65. Banich MT, Crowley TJ, Thompson LL, et al. Brain activation during the Stroop task in adolescents with severe substance and conduct problems: a pilot study. Drug Alcohol Depend 2007;90(2):175–82.
66. Clark CP, Brown GG, Eyler LT, et al. Decreased perfusion in young alcohol-dependent women as compared with age-matched controls. Am J Drug Alcohol Abuse 2007;33(1):13–9.

67. Tapert SF, Cheung EH, Brown GG, et al. Neural response to alcohol stimuli in adolescents with alcohol use disorder. Arch Gen Psychiatry 2003;60(7):727–35.
68. Britton JC, Phan KL, Taylor SF, et al. Neural correlates of social and nonsocial emotions: an fMRI study. Neuroimage 2006;31(1):397–409.
69. Bjork JM, Knutson B, Fong GW, et al. Incentive-elicited brain activation in adolescents: similarities and differences from young adults. J Neurosci 2004;24(8): 1793–802.
70. Hommer D, Bjork JM, Knutson B, et al. Motivation in children of alcoholics. Alcohol Clin Exp Res 2004;28:22A.
71. Wrase J, Schlagenhauf F, Kienast T, et al. Dysfunction of reward processing correlates with alcohol craving in detoxified alcoholics. Neuroimage 2007;35(2): 787–94.
72. Beck A, Schlagenhauf F, Wustenberg T, et al. Ventral striatal activation during reward anticipation correlates with impulsivity in alcoholics. Biol Psychiatry 2009;66(8):734–42.
73. Bechara A, Van Der Linden M. Decision-making and impulse control after frontal lobe injuries. Curr Opin Neurobiol 2005;18(6):734–9.
74. Bardo MT, Donohew RL, Harrington NG. Psychobiology of novelty seeking and drug seeking behavior. Behav Brain Res 1996;77(1–2):23–43.
75. Galvan A, Hare T, Voss H, et al. Risk-taking and the adolescent brain: who is at risk? Dev Sci 2007;10(2):8–14.
76. George MS, Anton RF, Bloomer C, et al. Activation of prefrontal cortex and anterior thalamus in alcoholic subjects on exposure to alcohol-specific cues. Arch Gen Psychiatry 2001;58(4):345–52.
77. Volkow N, Li T. The neuroscience of addiction. Nat Neurosci 2005;8(11):1429–30.
78. Clayton RR, Cattarello AM, Johnstone BM. The effectiveness of drug abuse resistance education (Project DARE): 5-Year follow-up results. Prev Med 1996; 25(3):307–18.
79. Cahill L. Why sex matters for neuroscience. Nat Rev Neurosci 2006;7(6):477–84.
80. Lynch WJ, Potenza MN, Cosgrove KP, et al. Sex differences in the vulnerability to stimulant abuse: a translational perspective. In: Brady KT, Back S, Greenfield SF, editors. Women and addiction. New York: Guilford; 2009. p. 407–18.
81. Nolen-Hoeksema S. Gender differences in risk factors and consequences for alcohol use and problems. Clin Psychol Rev 2004;24(8):981–1010.
82. Nolen-Hoeksema S, Girgus JS. The emergence of gender differences in depression during adolescence. Psychol Bull 1994;115(3):424–43.
83. Nock MK, Kazdin AE, Hiripi E, et al. Prevalence, subtypes, and correlates of DSM-IV conduct disorder in the National Comorbidity Survey Replication. Psychol Med 2006;36(5):699–710.
84. Mayes LC, Suchman N. Developmental pathways to substance abuse. In: Cicchetti D, Cohen D, editors. Developmental psychopathology. New York: John Wiley and Sons; 2006. p. 599–619.
85. Tsuang M, Lyons MJ, Meyer JM, et al. Co-occurrence of abuse of different drugs in men. Arch Gen Psychiatry 1998;55(11):967–72.

Development and Vulnerability Factors in Adolescent Alcohol Use

Karen G. Chartier, PhD[a], Michie N. Hesselbrock, PhD[b],
Victor M. Hesselbrock, PhD[b],*

KEYWORDS

- Adolescents • Alcohol use • Vulnerability factors
- Deviance proneness

Early adolescence is the key developmental period for the initiation of alcohol use that progresses on to regular use and problem drinking in midadolescence, later adolescence, and young adulthood. This article provides an overview of the characteristics of adolescent alcohol use, normative and subgroup variations in drinking, and the factors associated with increased risk for developing alcohol problems. The authors present the deviance prone model as a tool for examining the complex interactions between the risk factors reviewed.

Early adolescence (10–15 years) is associated with first alcohol use. Findings from 3 national surveys point to the seventh and eighth grades, when students are typically 13 to 14 years old, as the peak years for the initiation of alcohol use.[1] Late adolescence (16–20 years) is characterized by more risky alcohol use patterns, including binge drinking (ie, consuming more than 5 drinks on a single occasion). Normative rates of youth drinking increase with age, accelerating among older adolescents and leveling off in the 20s at around 21 to 22 years for heavy drinking and 25 to 26 years for current drinking.[2,3] **Fig. 1** shows past-year rates of drinking based on the 2007 National Survey on Drug Use and Health (NSDUH) for the US population. The highest incidence and prevalence of alcohol abuse and dependence is seen in those drinkers aged 18 to 23 years, followed by those aged 12 to 17 years.[4]

This work was supported by NIAAA Grant No. P60AA03510.
[a] University of Texas School of Public Health, 6011 Harry Hines Boulevard, V8.112, Dallas, TX 75390, USA
[b] Department of Psychiatry, University of Connecticut School of Medicine, 263 Farmington Avenue, MC-2103, Farmington, CT 06030, USA
* Corresponding author.
E-mail address: Hesselbrock@uchc.edu

Child Adolesc Psychiatric Clin N Am 19 (2010) 493–504
doi:10.1016/j.chc.2010.03.004
1056-4993/10/$ – see front matter

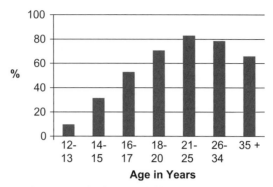

Fig. 1. US prevalence of past-year drinking in children aged 12 years and older. (*Data from* 2007 National Survey on Drug Use and Health (NSDUH), Substance Abuse and Mental Health Services Administration (SAMHSA), Office of Applied Studies.)

VARIATIONS IN ADOLESCENT DRINKING

Alcohol use behaviors vary by several sociodemographic characteristics, including ethnicity and gender, during adolescence.[5] **Table 1** provides estimates of 30-day alcohol use and binge drinking and the age of first use for the 3 largest US ethnic groups. According to the 2007 NSDUH, the prevalence of 30-day alcohol use and binge drinking was highest for whites, followed by Hispanics and then blacks. Relative to blacks, Hispanics and whites had somewhat earlier ages of drinking onset. Gender differences in the rate of 30-day alcohol use vary by ethnic group (ie, white males = white females, black females < black males, and Hispanic females > Hispanic males), but binge drinking was more prevalent in males than females for all ethnic groups. Females, particularly black females, also showed a later age of first alcohol use compared with males.

Regardless, recent research findings suggest that the gender gap in drinking behaviors has narrowed. Several studies have demonstrated secular trends in alcohol use behavior. More recently, Grucza and colleagues[6] showed an increase in the risk for drinking and alcohol dependence among women born after World War II. These

Table 1
US ethnic group and gender variations in alcohol use in youth aged 12 to 20 years

	2007				2005–2007	
	Percentage of 30-day Alcohol Use		Percentage of 30-day Binge Drinking		Mean Age of First Use	
	M	F	M	F	M	F
White[a]	32.8 (0.9)	31.3 (0.8)	24.8 (0.7)	19.4 (0.7)	13.95 (0.04)	14.10 (0.03)
Black[a]	17.3 (1.2)	20.2 (1.3)	9.2 (0.9)	7.1 (0.8)	14.22 (0.09)	14.35 (0.10)
Hispanic	27.5 (1.4)	23.4 (1.1)	19.2 (1.3)	12.3 (1.2)	13.84 (0.10)	14.08 (0.07)

Abbreviations: M, male; F, female.
[a] Non-Hispanic; estimates are percentage or Mean (standard error) as specified.
Data from Chen CM, Yi H, Williams GD, et al. Surveillance report #86, trends in underage drinking in the United Sates, 1991–2007. Bethesda (MD): National Institute on Alcohol Abuse and Alcoholism; 2009.

changes were observed in white and Hispanic females, but not in black females, and are attributed to a sharper decrease in the age of onset of drinking for women compared with men born between 1954 and 1983.[7] Consequently, early-onset alcohol use is associated with the early development of a variety of alcohol use problems and a more severe course of alcohol dependence.[8–10] Adolescent drinking behaviors appear to dependably predict later drinking and drinking problems in young adulthood.[11]

Different trajectories of alcohol use (ie, patterns of drinking overtime) have been identified among adolescents once drinking begins. Maggs and Schulenberg[12] summarized several adolescent drinking trajectories into young adulthood, including a stable abstainer or low-risk drinking course, a chronic heavy-use course, a late-onset heavy-use course, and a developmentally limited drinking course. Most adolescents drink at low-risk levels or age out of alcohol involvement as they transition toward family and career but other adolescents do not (ie, those in the chronic and late-onset heavy-use groups). A variety of explanatory factors for the development of alcohol problems have been proposed. A family history of alcoholism, temperament traits, cognitive functioning, conduct problems, and peer and family relationships are among the factors most frequently cited as being associated with an increased risk for adolescent alcohol use and problem drinking. These factors are reviewed in the following sections.

RISK FACTORS FOR PROBLEM DRINKING
Family History of Alcoholism

A variety of family pedigree, twin, and adoption studies have provided significant evidence of an increased risk for developing alcohol problems when a biologic parent is affected. The nature of the risk due to a family history of alcoholism has been grouped into genetic and environmental factors.[10,13] Although the proportion of the risk for developing alcohol dependence determined by either environmental or genetic factors has not been conclusively determined, it seems that genetic factors account for about 50% of the variance.[13] Twin, sibling pair, family (eg, Collaborative Study on the Genetics of Alcoholism [COGA]), and case-control studies are currently ongoing to identify candidate genes related to the susceptibility for developing alcoholism. Among others, *GABRA2, CHRM2,* and *ADH4* are associated with alcohol dependence in adults in the COGA study, findings that have been replicated by other researchers in other samples.[14,15]

High-risk environments may also interact with genetic vulnerability to increase an individual's risk of alcohol dependence. Stressful life events, childhood maltreatment, family violence, and poor social support combined with genetic vulnerability are associated with increased risk for alcoholism, depressive symptoms, and conduct problems.[16] Dick and colleagues[17,18] showed that genetic influences on adolescent substance use were enhanced in environments characterized by lower parental monitoring and substance-using friends. Genetic influences appear to have larger effects on the development of drinking frequency and alcohol dependence, whereas the onset of drinking is largely affected by environmental factors.[19,20]

Temperament Traits

Temperament has been identified as an important contributor to several theoretical formulations related to the development of alcohol use behaviors, including problem drinking.[21,22] Although prior research has shown that the vulnerability for the development of alcoholism lies, in part, in an individual's genetic makeup, several studies suggest that this genetic propensity may be partially expressed through the individual's temperament. Temperament is a set of behavioral and emotional reactions that varies among individuals, has moderate temporal and situational stability, and appears early in childhood.[23] In particular, behavioral undercontrol and negative affectivity, as temperament traits, have been linked to the development of alcohol-use problems.

Behavioral undercontrol is often conceived as including a wide range of traits, such as aggressiveness, delinquency, impulsivity, risk taking, sensation seeking, and disinhibition.[11] Further, the propensity to be disinhibited or easily bored may encourage the expression of externalizing behaviors, such as conduct problems, alcohol, and drug use.[24–26] For example, a negative association between age of first drink and disinhibitory behavior, including oppositionality, impulsiveness, and inattention assessed at 11 years to predict alcohol use at 14 years, was reported by McGue and colleagues.[27] Similarly, higher levels of disinhibition, risk taking, and boredom susceptibility also predict an earlier age of regular alcohol use, earlier marijuana use, and more frequent drinking.[28] Behavioral undercontrol may affect alcohol involvement and an earlier onset of adolescent substance use by increasing conduct problems and positive expectancies for alcohol consumption.[29,30]

Negative affectivity (ie, the tendency toward depression and neuroticism; internalizing behaviors) has been found to be overrepresented in samples of offsprings of alcoholics and individuals who later become alcoholic.[31] Some individuals may use drugs and alcohol to cope with and relieve the unpleasant symptoms of negative affect.[32,33] However, the evidence supporting the role of negative affectivity as a contributor to the development of alcohol and drug involvement is inconsistent.[11] Ohannessian and Hesselbrock[29,34] found that negative affectivity has no effect in predicting substance use in high-risk adolescents, whereas conduct problems and risk taking did play significant roles. Negative affectivity did not predict the age of onset of alcohol use but predicted conduct problems and the quantity and frequency of drinking once drinking behavior and problems were established among adolescents.[35] Further, different components of negative affectivity (ie, sadness, fear, guilt, and hostility) seem to differentially affect substance use in adolescents, with higher levels of hostility and lower levels of guilt associated with earlier marijuana use initiation in adolescents.[36]

Conduct Problems

Both cross-sectional[37,38] and longitudinal investigations have found that childhood conduct problems predict alcohol use and alcohol-related problems among adolescents and young adults.[39–42] Typically, both boys and girls with conduct problems have an early onset of alcohol and substance use problems and often manifest a more chronic and severe course of the disorder that continues well into middle age.[35,43–45] Further, when childhood and adolescent conduct problems lead to adult antisocial personality disorder (ASPD), the effects of ASPD on both the course and consequences of alcoholism are independent and additive to the effects of a family history of alcoholism.[43,46,47]

Childhood conduct disorder, like alcoholism, may not be a homogeneous disorder. A study of conduct problems among a community sample of girls found group differences in relation to symptom severity. Minimal or mild symptoms among girls typically show a developmental trajectory with possible dissipation of symptoms during adolescence and young adulthood. Girls having more severe symptoms in childhood continued to display disruptive behaviors well into adolescence and were at increased risk for developing *DSM-III-R* (*Diagnostic and Statistical Manual of Mental Disorders*

[Third Edition Revised]) conduct disorder.[48] Further, for adult men and women, the more severe the subtype of conduct or antisocial behavior the earlier the onset of alcohol or drug use and the more severe the substance dependence problems.[49,50] The relationship of childhood conduct problems to adolescent drinking behaviors may also vary by ethnic group. Increased childhood conduct problems predicted an earlier age of regular drinking onset for blacks but not for whites and Hispanics.[51] In general, studies of both clinical and nonclinical samples have found a positive association between the frequency of childhood conduct problems and an early onset of alcohol or drug use. Clearly, though, not all persons with childhood conduct problems go on to develop alcohol use problems.

Cognitive Functioning

Neuropsychologic deficiencies (eg, impulsivity, inability to use language to cognitively regulate behavior, and poor foresight) may influence the development of alcohol problems by compromising educational attainment and impairing psychosocial development among high-risk individuals. Differences in cognitive functioning as measured by electroencephalographic and event-related potential (EEG/ERP) methods have been reported among children and adolescents at risk for developing alcoholism before the onset of heavy drinking.[52,53] The age of first drink was associated with a reduced P300 ERP amplitude in 17-year-old twins.[27] Similarly, a reduced P300 amplitude and deficits in reading achievement predicted an early onset of drinking, which is separate from the contribution of familial density for alcoholism.[54] Differences in EEG and ERP brain wave patterns are typically found in the frontal brain region,[55] an area thought to be responsible for the cognitive skills of attention, planning, and foresight. Tests of frontal and temporal lobe functioning among high-risk young adult males were predictive of the age of first drink initiation and the frequency of drinking to intoxication.[56,57] However, some studies have failed to find an association between poor cognitive skills and alcohol use. For example, Sher and colleagues[30] showed that cognitive functioning as measured by verbal ability did not predict alcohol involvement in college students with a family history of alcoholism.

Alcohol Expectancies

The role of expectancies has been demonstrated in the production of a variety of behaviors, including the effect of certain positive and negative expectations on alcohol use.[58,59] Social learning theory suggests that expectancies about alcohol's effects on sexual enhancement, physical and social pleasure, increased social assertiveness, and relaxation[60] likely reflect a person's own experience with alcohol and result from exposure to beverage alcohol advertising and from observing the behavior of others when they are drinking. Repeated exposure to these events can begin even in childhood. For example, the positive expectancies of alcohol's effects among elementary school children have been found to increase across the first through fifth grades, most notably among 8- to 10-year-old children.[61] Shifts in alcohol expectancies occurring later in childhood typically reflect the changes in alcohol involvement observed across age groups. Positive alcohol expectancies increase during adolescence but decrease in early adulthood.[62] Similarly, positive alcohol expectancy seems to be a better predictor of drinking among individuals younger than 35 years, whereas negative alcohol expectancy better predicts drinking status for most individuals older than 35 years.[63]

Importantly, though, positive expectancies of alcohol's effects do predict the initiation of drinking, intention to drink, and drinking rates among both middle school[64] and college students.[65] Previous studies of college-aged offspring of an alcoholic parent have identified alcohol expectancies as key mediators for a family history of alcoholism and behavioral undercontrol in predicting alcohol involvement, relationships that hold equally for males and females.[30] Differences by race and grade, but not by gender, have been reported in the relationships between alcohol expectancies and alcohol use in children from 6th, 8th, and 11th grades.[66] Positive alcohol expectancies showed a stronger positive association in predicting alcohol use initiation in older adolescents compared with younger adolescents and for white and Hispanic adolescents in predicting alcohol initiation, drinking, and binge drinking. Chartier and colleagues[51] similarly reported a stronger association for white and Hispanic adolescents compared with black adolescents in the relationship of alcohol expectancies to the age of regular drinking onset.

Peer and Other Social Relations

Those to whom one can turn in times of trouble and from whom a person can confidently expect caring, valuing, and love can be defined as a social network. A strong social network has been reported to decrease the vulnerability to both mental and physical health problems, help moderate the need for medication, and help an individual recover more quickly after an illness.[67,68] Conversely, an increase in health problems has been reported in the context of high life stresses in the absence of social support.[67] The role of social support both from family[69–71] and from friends[70,72] has been examined in relation to the initiation of alcohol use, maintenance of drinking behavior, and onset of alcohol-related problem behaviors among both alcoholics and adolescents susceptible to developing alcoholism. The relationship of family and peer social support to alcohol and drug use in adolescents has been examined.[73] Adolescents reporting heavy marijuana and tobacco use perceived lower social support from friends and family compared with light users, whereas heavy alcohol users compared with light drinkers reported higher social support from friends. The connection between social relationships with peers and adolescent alcohol use is complex, because a certain level of alcohol involvement may indicate greater social success, whereas no alcohol use may be associated with less social success with peers.[11]

Three forms of peer influence have been suggested as contributing to the risk for adolescent alcohol use and problems: (1) the direct modeling or encouragement of alcohol use, (2) a self-sustaining affiliation with like-minded peers, and (3) the overestimation by adolescents of the prevalence of their peers' drinking.[74] Older siblings and parents may similarly influence adolescent alcohol and drug use through modeling, approval of drinking, and also by providing access to alcohol.[74,75] Further, family relationships, parenting styles, and other family-related factors may affect adolescent alcohol initiation, use, and the development of problems. At-risk adolescents living apart from their biologic father were shown to fare worse than those living with their father in terms of increased conduct problems and an earlier onset of alcohol and drug use.[76] Kramer and colleagues[77] similarly identified that the relationship of adolescents with their father is an important predictor of alcohol symptoms in young adults; a negative relationship with the father predicted increased alcohol symptoms in adulthood. Poor family management, inconsistent discipline, and inadequate supervision and monitoring among parents with an alcohol use disorder are also associated with increased problem behaviors in children.[78]

THE DEVIANCE PRONE MODEL

A single vulnerability factor may be insufficient to precipitate problematic alcohol involvement in an adolescent. More likely, multiple factors act synergistically to

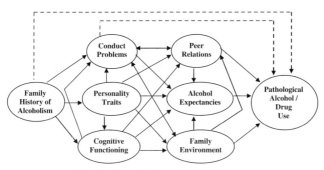

Fig. 2. Deviance prone model of vulnerability.

increase the probability of an adolescent developing alcohol problems. A variety of different theoretical models, using the risk factors cited earlier, have been proposed over time to explain the initiation and development of alcohol use and problems during adolescence. Typically, these models include a parental history of alcoholism, peer influences, externalizing behaviors, internalizing behaviors, and environmental and biologic factors as risk factors.[11,21,35,78,79] One of the more frequently cited models uses early childhood conduct problems or the propensity for deviant behavior as a major explanatory variable. The deviance prone model (**Fig. 2**) examines the complex interactions between a family history of alcoholism and mediating factors in predicting alcohol use problems. Sher[32] originally proposed the model as a heuristic device to examine the development of pathologic alcohol use. Many elements of the model have also been widely cited in the literature as predictors of both an early-onset and early regular use of alcohol and other drugs among adolescents.

Proneness is defined as the likelihood of occurrence of a normative transgression or problem behavior.[80] Early and regular adolescent drinking are problem behaviors that frequently co-occur with other problem behaviors, including tobacco and marijuana use, sexual behavior, and delinquency. Donovan and Jessor[81] suggest that unconventionality, a common factor, underlies these problem behaviors. Unconventionality is defined by placing a lower value on academic achievement, as a greater tolerance of deviance, as having a greater orientation toward friends than family, and as perceiving parental and friends' approval of problem behavior. The major features of the deviance prone model (ie, parental history of alcoholism, certain temperament traits, childhood conduct problems, cognitive difficulties, alcohol expectancies, and social relations) correspond with these and other characteristics of unconventionality and theoretically link the liability of familial alcoholism to the development of alcohol-related problems.

SUMMARY

This article demonstrates that alcohol use typically starts in early adolescence and increases with age into late adolescence and young adulthood. Ethnic and gender differences and different trajectories of alcohol use have been observed in large national epidemiologic samples. However, most adolescents drink at low-risk levels and mature out of risky drinking patterns during their mid-20s. Several putative susceptibility factors (ie, family or parental alcoholism, behavioral undercontrol, childhood conduct problems, neuropsychologic problems, alcohol expectancies, and peer and family relations) singly and in combination contribute to the initiation and frequency of alcohol use and to the development of alcohol use behavior, including pathologic alcohol involvement. Further, some studies have found that other putative risk factors such as negative affectivity did not consistently contribute to youth drinking but may be important in predicting continued heavy alcohol use or alcohol problem behavior in adulthood. Multiple risk factors likely interact among themselves, with the environment, and possibly with genetic factors to increase the probability for alcohol problems developing in adolescence. The deviance prone model provides an important tool for testing possible relationships and the sequencing of vulnerability factors for adolescent alcohol and drug use and allows for an examination of the complex interplay of risk factors that lead to the development of alcoholism and related alcohol problems.

REFERENCES

1. Faden VB. Trends in initiation of alcohol use in the United States 1975 to 2003. Alcohol Clin Exp Res 2006;30(6):1011–22.
2. Chen CM, Dufour MC, Yi H. Alcohol consumption among young adults ages 18–24 in the United States: results from the 2001–2002 NESARC survey. Alcohol Res Health 2004–2005;28(4):269–80.
3. Muthen BO, Muthen LK. The development of heavy drinking and alcohol-related problems from ages 18 to 37 in a U.S. national sample. J Stud Alcohol 2000; 61(2):290–300.
4. Harford TC, Grant BF, Yi HY, et al. Patterns of DSM-IV alcohol abuse and dependence criteria among adolescents and adults: results from the 2001 National Household Survey on Drug Abuse. Alcohol Clin Exp Res 2005;29(5):810–28.
5. Chen CM, Yi H, Williams GD, et al. Surveillance report #86, trends in underage drinking in the United States, 1991–2007. Bethesda (MD): National Institute on Alcohol Abuse and Alcoholism; 2009.
6. Grucza RA, Bucholz KK, Rice JP, et al. Secular trends in the lifetime prevalence of alcohol dependence in the United States: a re-evaluation. Alcohol Clin Exp Res 2008;32(5):763–70.
7. Grucza RA, Norberg K, Bucholz KK, et al. Correspondence between secular changes in alcohol dependence and age of drinking onset among women in the United States. Alcohol Clin Exp Res 2008;32(8):1493–501.
8. Grant BF, Dawson DA. Age at onset of alcohol use and its association with DSM-IV alcohol abuse and dependence: results from the National Longitudinal Alcohol Epidemiologic Survey. J Subst Abuse 1997;9:103–10.
9. Hingson RW, Heeren T, Winter MR. Age at drinking onset and alcohol dependence: age at onset, duration, and severity. Arch Pediatr Adolesc Med 2006; 160(7):739–46.
10. Prescott CA, Kendler KS. Age at first drink and risk for alcoholism: a noncausal association. Alcohol Clin Exp Res 1999;23(1):101–7.
11. Zucker RA. Anticipating problem alcohol use developmentally from childhood into middle adulthood: what have we learned? Addiction 2008;103(Suppl 1): 100–8.
12. Maggs J, Schulenberg J. Trajectories of alcohol use during the transition to adulthood. Alcohol Res Health 2004–2005;28(4):195–201.
13. Heath AC, Bucholz KK, Madden PA, et al. Genetic and environmental contributions to alcohol dependence risk in a national twin sample: consistency of findings in women and men. Psychol Med 1997;27(6):1381–96.
14. Edenberg HJ, Foroud T. The genetics of alcoholism: identifying specific genes through family studies. Addict Biol 2006;11(3–4):386–96.

15. Dick DM, Bierut LJ. The genetics of alcohol dependence. Curr Psychiatry Rep 2006;8(2):151–7.
16. Enoch MA. Genetic and environmental influences on the development of alcoholism: resilience vs. risk. Ann N Y Acad Sci 2006;1094:193–201.
17. Dick DM, Pagan JL, Holliday C, et al. Gender differences in friends' influences on adolescent drinking: a genetic epidemiological study. Alcohol Clin Exp Res 2007; 31(12):2012–9.
18. Dick DM, Pagan JL, Viken R, et al. Changing environmental influences on substance use across development. Twin Res Hum Genet 2007;10(2):315–26.
19. Dick DM, Bernard M, Aliev F, et al. The role of socioregional factors in moderating genetic influences on early adolescent behavior problems and alcohol use. Alcohol Clin Exp Res 2009;33(10):1739–48.
20. Barnow S, Schuckit MA, Lucht M, et al. The importance of a positive family history of alcoholism, parental rejection and emotional warmth, behavioral problems and peer substance use for alcohol problems in teenagers: a path analysis. J Stud Alcohol 2002;63(3):305–15.
21. Tarter RE, Vanyukov M. Alcoholism: a developmental disorder. J Consult Clin Psychol 1994;62(6):1096–107.
22. Blackson TC. Temperament: a salient correlate of risk factors for alcohol and drug abuse. Drug Alcohol Depend 1994;36(3):205–14.
23. Kagan J. Galen's prophecy: temperament in human nature. New York: Basic Books; 1994.
24. Sher KJ, Trull TJ. Personality and disinhibitory psychopathology: alcoholism and antisocial personality disorder. J Abnorm Psychol 1994;103(1):92–102.
25. Tarter RE, Laird SB, Kabene M, et al. Drug abuse severity in adolescents is associated with magnitude of deviation in temperament traits. Br J Addict 1990; 85(11):1501–4.
26. Windle M. A longitudinal study of antisocial behaviors in early adolescence as predictors of late adolescent substance use: gender and ethnic group differences. J Abnorm Psychol 1990;99(1):86–91.
27. McGue M, Iacono WG, Legrand LN, et al. Origins and consequences of age at first drink. I. Associations with substance-use disorders, disinhibitory behavior and psychopathology, and P3 amplitude. Alcohol Clin Exp Res 2001;25(8): 1156–65.
28. Ohannessian CM, Hesselbrock VM. Do personality characteristics and risk taking mediate the relationship between paternal substance dependence and adolescent substance use? Addict Behav 2007;32(9):1852–62.
29. Ohannessian CM, Hesselbrock VM. A comparison of three vulnerability models for the onset of substance use in a high-risk sample. J Stud Alcohol Drugs 2008;69(1):75–84.
30. Sher KJ, Walitzer KS, Wood PK, et al. Characteristics of children of alcoholics: putative risk factors, substance use and abuse, and psychopathology. J Abnorm Psychol 1991;100(4):427–48.
31. Barnes GE. Clinical and personality characteristics. In: Begleiter H, editor, The pathogenesis of alcoholism: psychosocial factors, vol. 6. New York: Plenum Press; 1983. p. 113–96.
32. Sher KJ. Children of alcoholics: a critical appraisal of theory and research. Chicago: University of Chicago Press; 1991.
33. Sher KJ, Levenson RW. Risk for alcoholism and individual differences in the stress-response-dampening effect of alcohol. J Abnorm Psychol 1982;91(5): 350–67.

34. Ohannessian CM, Hesselbrock VM. Paternal alcoholism and youth substance abuse: the indirect effects of negative affect, conduct problems, and risk taking. J Adolesc Health 2008;42(2):198–200.
35. Schuckit MA, Windle M, Smith TL, et al. Searching for the full picture: structural equation modeling in alcohol research. Alcohol Clin Exp Res 2006;30(2):194–202.
36. Ohannessian CM, Hesselbrock VM. A finer examination of the role that negative affect plays in the relationship between paternal alcoholism and the onset of alcohol and marijuana use. J Stud Alcohol Drugs 2009;70(3):400–8.
37. Hesselbrock MN. Childhood behavior problems and adult antisocial personality disorder in alcoholism. In: Meyer RE, editor. Psychopathology and addictive disorders. New York: Guilford Press; 1986. p. 78–94.
38. Ohannessian CM, Hesselbrock VM. An examination of the underlying influence of temperament and problem behaviors on drinking behaviors in a sample of adult offspring of alcoholics. Addict Behav 1994;19(3):257–68.
39. Kuperman S, Chan G, Kramer JR, et al. Relationship of age of first drink to child behavioral problems and family psychopathology. Alcohol Clin Exp Res 2005; 29(10):1869–76.
40. Rohde P, Lewinsohn PM, Seeley JR. Psychiatric comorbidity with problematic alcohol use in high school students. J Am Acad Child Adolesc Psychiatry 1996;35(1):101–9.
41. Brown SA, Gleghorn A, Schuckit MA, et al. Conduct disorder among adolescent alcohol and drug abusers. J Stud Alcohol 1996;57(3):314–24.
42. Johnson EO, Arria AM, Borges G, et al. The growth of conduct problem behaviors from middle childhood to early adolescence: sex differences and the suspected influence of early alcohol use. J Stud Alcohol 1995;56(6):661–71.
43. Cadoret RJ, Yates WR, Troughton E, et al. Adoption study demonstrating two genetic pathways to drug abuse. Arch Gen Psychiatry 1995;52(1):42–52.
44. Robins LN. Deviant children grown up: a sociological and psychiatric study of sociopathic personality. Baltimore (MD): Williams & Wilkins; 1966.
45. Vaillant GE. A long-term follow-up of male alcohol abuse. Arch Gen Psychiatry 1996;53(3):243–9.
46. Slutske WS, Heath AC, Dinwiddie SH, et al. Common genetic risk factors for conduct disorder and alcohol dependence. J Abnorm Psychol 1998;107(3): 363–74.
47. Hesselbrock VM, Hesselbrock MN. Alcoholism and antisocial personality disorder: are they different? Alcohol Alcohol Suppl 1994;2:479–84.
48. Cote S, Zoccolillio M, Tremblay RE, et al. Predicting girls' conduct disorder in adolescence from childhood trajectories of disruptive behaviors. J Am Acad Child Adolesc Psychiatry 2001;40(6):678–84.
49. Cottler LB, Price RK, Compton WM, et al. Subtypes of adult antisocial behavior among drug abusers. J Nerv Ment Dis 1995;183(3):154–61.
50. Bucholz KK, Hesselbrock VM, Heath AC, et al. A latent class analysis of antisocial personality disorder symptom data from a multi-centre family study of alcoholism. Addiction 2000;95(4):553–67.
51. Chartier KG, Hesselbrock MN, Hesselbrock VM. Ethnicity and adolescent pathways to alcohol use. J Stud Alcohol Drugs 2009;70(3):337–45.
52. Begleiter H, Porjesz B, Bihari B, et al. Event-related brain potentials in boys at risk for alcoholism. Science 1984;225(4669):1493–6.
53. Bauer LO, Hesselbrock VM. Subtypes of family history and conduct disorder: effects on P300 during the stroop test. Neuropsychopharmacology 1999;21(1): 51–62.

54. Hill SY, Shen S, Lowers L, et al. Factors predicting the onset of adolescent drinking in families at high risk for developing alcoholism. Biol Psychiatry 2000; 48(4):265–75.
55. Bauer LO, Hesselbrock VM. CSD/BEM localization of P300 sources in adolescents "at-risk": evidence of frontal cortex dysfunction in conduct disorder. Biol Psychiatry 2001;50(8):600–8.
56. Hesselbrock V, Bauer LO, Hesselbrock MN, et al. Neuropsychological factors in individuals at high risk for alcoholism. Recent Dev Alcohol 1991;9:21–40.
57. Deckel AW, Hesselbrock V, Bauer L. Relationship between alcohol-related expectancies and anterior brain functioning in young men at risk for developing alcoholism. Alcohol Clin Exp Res 1995;19(2):476–81.
58. Ajzen I. The theory of planned behavior. Organ Behav Hum Decis Process 1991; 50:179–211.
59. Brown SA, Goldman MS, Christiansen BA. Do alcohol expectancies mediate drinking patterns of adults? J Consult Clin Psychol 1985;53(4):512–9.
60. Brown SA, Christiansen BA, Goldman MS. The Alcohol Expectancy Questionnaire: an instrument for the assessment of adolescent and adult alcohol expectancies. J Stud Alcohol 1987;48(5):483–91.
61. Miller PM, Smith GT, Goldman MS. Emergence of alcohol expectancies in childhood: a possible critical period. J Stud Alcohol 1990;51(4):343–9.
62. Sher KJ, Gotham HJ. Pathological alcohol involvement: a developmental disorder of young adulthood. Dev Psychopathol 1999;11(4):933–56.
63. Leigh BC, Stacy AW. Alcohol expectancies and drinking in different age groups. Addiction 2004;99(2):215–27.
64. Christiansen BA, Smith GT, Roehling PV, et al. Using alcohol expectancies to predict adolescent drinking behavior after one year. J Consult Clin Psychol 1989;57(1):93–9.
65. Stacy AW, Widaman KF, Marlatt GA. Expectancy models of alcohol use. J Pers Soc Psychol 1990;58(5):918–28.
66. Meier MH, Slutske WS, Arndt S, et al. Positive alcohol expectancies partially mediate the relation between delinquent behavior and alcohol use: generalizability across age, sex, and race in a cohort of 85,000 Iowa schoolchildren. Psychol Addict Behav 2007;21(1):25–34.
67. Sarason B, Sarason I, Pierce G. Social support. New York: Wiley & Sons; 1990.
68. Holahan CJ, Moos RH. Risk, resistance, and psychological distress: a longitudinal analysis with adults and children. J Abnorm Psychol 1987;96(1):3–13.
69. Wolin SJ, Bennett LA, Noonan DL, et al. Disrupted family rituals; a factor in the intergenerational transmission of alcoholism. J Stud Alcohol 1980;41(3): 199–214.
70. Jacob T, Krahn GL, Leonard K. Parent-child interactions in families with alcoholic fathers. J Consult Clin Psychol 1991;59(1):176–81.
71. Windle M. The difficult temperament in adolescence: associations with substance use, family support, and problem behaviors. J Clin Psychol 1991;47(2):310–5.
72. Zucker RA, Gomberg ES. Etiology of alcoholism reconsidered. The case for a biopsychosocial process. Am Psychol 1986;41(7):783–93.
73. Averna S, Hesselbrock V. The relationship of perceived social support to substance use in offspring of alcoholics. Addict Behav 2001;26(3):363–74.
74. Brown SA, McGue M, Maggs J, et al. A developmental perspective on alcohol and youths 16 to 20 years of age. Pediatrics 2008;121(Suppl 4):S290–310.
75. Donovan JE. Adolescent alcohol initiation: a review of psychosocial risk factors. J Adolesc Health 2004;35(6):529 e527–18.

76. Averna S, Hesselbrock V. Parenting style moderates familial risk and adolescent outcomes. Alcohol Clin Exp Res 2001;25(5):45A.
77. Kramer JR, Chan G, Dick DM, et al. Multiple-domain predictors of problematic alcohol use in young adulthood. J Stud Alcohol Drugs 2008;69(5):649–59.
78. Sher KJ, Grekin ER, Williams NA. The development of alcohol use disorders. Annu Rev Clin Psychol 2005;1:493–523.
79. Brook JS, Whiteman M, Finch SJ, et al. Young adult drug use and delinquency: childhood antecedents and adolescent mediators. J Am Acad Child Adolesc Psychiatry 1996;35(12):1584–92.
80. Jessor R. Problem-behavior theory, psychosocial development, and adolescent problem drinking. Br J Addict 1987;82(4):331–42.
81. Donovan JE, Jessor R. Structure of problem behavior in adolescence and young adulthood. J Consult Clin Psychol 1985;53(6):890–904.

Evidence-Based Interventions for Preventing Substance Use Disorders in Adolescents

Kenneth W. Griffin, PhD, MPH*, Gilbert J. Botvin, PhD

KEYWORDS

- Prevention • Substance abuse • Adolescence • School
- Community • Family

Substance use and abuse continue to be important public health problems that contribute greatly to morbidity and mortality rates throughout the United States, Canada, and globally. For several decades, substantial research efforts have been undertaken to understand the epidemiology and etiology of substance use and abuse. The knowledge gained from this work has been important in identifying and developing effective prevention and treatment approaches. From person to person, there is great variability in patterns of substance use and abuse. Some individuals face lifelong struggles with addiction, whereas others go through life without experimenting with any substances; however, from a population perspective, the epidemiologic patterns are consistent and predictable. According to national datasets, the prevalence of alcohol, tobacco, and other drug use increases rapidly from early to late adolescence, peaks during the transition to young adulthood, and declines though the remainder of adulthood. Furthermore, there is accumulating evidence showing that the initiation of substance use early in life contributes to higher levels of use and abuse later in life. Early onset is also associated with a host of later negative health, social, and behavioral outcomes including physical and mental health problems, violent and aggressive behavior, and adjustment problems in the workplace and family.[1]

The well-established pattern of onset and progression of substance use and abuse during adolescence has led to the development of a variety of prevention initiatives for

Disclosure: Dr Botvin is President of National Health Promotion Associates (NHPA), which markets the Life Skills Training program. Dr Griffin is a consultant to NHPA.
Division of Prevention and Health Behavior, Department of Public Health, Weill Cornell Medical College, Cornell University, 402 East 67th Street, New York, NY 10065, USA
* Corresponding author.
E-mail address: kgriffin@med.cornell.edu

Child Adolesc Psychiatric Clin N Am 19 (2010) 505–526
doi:10.1016/j.chc.2010.03.005
1056-4993/10/$ – see front matter © 2010 Elsevier Inc. All rights reserved.

children and adolescents. Most adults with substance abuse problems begin to use substances during their adolescent years and therefore relatively few prevention efforts have focused on adults. Youth-focused prevention initiatives include educational and skills training programs for young people in school settings; programs that teach parents effective ways to monitor and communicate with their children and establish and enforce family rules regarding substance use; and community-based programs that combine these components with additional mass media or public policy components (eg, restricting access though enforcement of minimum purchasing age requirements). Preventing early-stage substance use or delaying the onset of use is a goal of many of these prevention initiatives. They typically focus on alcohol, tobacco, and marijuana use because these are the most widely used substances in our society. Because of their widespread use, these substances pose the greatest risk to public health. Middle or junior high school age students are most often targeted in prevention efforts because early adolescence is the time of life when substance use experimentation often begins to occur. A large body of research has examined the efficacy and effectiveness of prevention programs for adolescent substance abuse. Findings show that the most effective programs target salient risk and protective factors at the individual, family, and/or community levels, and are guided by relevant psychosocial theories regarding the etiology of substance use and abuse.[2,3]

EPIDEMIOLOGY AND PROGRESSION OF USE

National survey data demonstrate that the prevalence rates of alcohol, tobacco, and other forms of substance use among adolescents peaked during the period of the late 1970s and early 1980s. Prevalence rates generally declined during the late 1980s, only to begin to increase again during the 1990s. In recent years, prevalence rates for many substances have gradually declined among adolescents, although they remain a source of concern. Among high school seniors, the 2008 Monitoring the Future (MTF) study[4] found that the 30-day prevalence rate for cigarette smoking was 22% and the lifetime rate was 47%. The annual and lifetime prevalence rates for alcohol use among high school seniors were 67% and 73%, respectively. About 37% of high school seniors reported having used 1 or more illicit drugs over the past year and 48% reported having done so during their lifetime. The annual and lifetime prevalence rates among high school seniors were 32% and 42%, respectively, for marijuana use; 5% and 9%, respectively, for hallucinogen use; and 8% and 12%, respectively, for amphetamine use.

Although MTF trend data have shown gradual decreases in prevalence rates of smoking, alcohol use, and many forms of illicit drug use among adolescents, there have been increases in some forms of substance use and abuse as well. MTF findings reveal that nonmedical prescription drug abuse is a growing problem among adolescents. Prevalence rates for the nonmedical use of several prescription opiates have increased in recent years. Data on rates of abuse for hydrocodone (Vicodin), oxycodone (OxyContin), and oxycodone/acetaminophen (Percocet) began to be collected in 2002 in the MTF study. Among high school seniors, annual prevalence rates for hydrocodone abuse have gone from 4.1% in 2002 to 5.7% in 2008; rates of oxycodone abuse have gone from 1.6% in 2002 to 3.7% in 2008; and rates of oxycodone/acetaminophen abuse among high school seniors have gone from 1.9% in 2002 to 2.9% in 2008. The abuse of over-the-counter medications (including cough syrup to get high) is another growing problem among adolescents.[4] It is important that prevention efforts remain flexible enough to address the sometimes variable and changing nature of adolescent substance use and abuse as trends change over time.

In contemporary American society, it has become commonplace among young people to engage in some level of experimentation with substances. Substance use occurs almost exclusively in a social context during early adolescence and typically involves substances that are readily available. These include alcohol, tobacco, and inhalants. Some individuals become regular users and/or progress to marijuana, hallucinogens, and other illicit drugs in a fairly predictable pattern.[5] However, many individuals discontinue use after a brief period of experimentation, or fail to progress to the use of other substances. Unfortunately, some adolescents will develop patterns of substance abuse characterized by both psychological and physiologic dependence. Progressing to more serious levels of substance abuse and disorder can be best understood in terms of probabilities. At each step farther along the developmental progression from experimentation with alcohol and tobacco to the regular use of illicit drugs, an individual's risk of developing an alcohol or substance use disorder increases. Additionally, the initial social motivations for alcohol, tobacco, and other drug use eventually yield to motives primarily driven by pharmacologic and psychological factors.[6] Knowledge of the usual patterns and the progression of substance use has important implications for the focus and timing of preventive interventions. Prevention programs that effectively target risk factors for alcohol and tobacco use may not only prevent the use of these substances, but may also decrease or eliminate the risk of using other substances farther along the progression.

RISK AND PROTECTIVE FACTORS

In many respects, substance use and abuse can be considered developmental phenomena. First, there are the predictable epidemiologic patterns of adolescent substance use onset and progression. Second, research demonstrates that substance use is frequently linked to important developmental goals and transitions. The degree of involvement in substance use for any teenager is often a function of the negative pro-drug social influences that they are exposed to combined with their individual developmental vulnerabilities to these influences.

Social Influence Factors

One of the most consistent findings in research on the etiology of adolescent substance use is that social influences are central, powerful factors that promote experimentation or initiation of use. Along with exposure to positive attitudes and expectations regarding substance use, the modeling of substance use behavior by important others (eg, parents, older siblings, and peers) is a critical negative social influence.[7] Other powerful negative influences involve the positive portrayal of substance use and abuse by celebrities in movies, television, and music videos.[8] Advertisements that communicate positive messages about alcohol and tobacco use promote pro-substance use attitudes, expectancies, and perceived positive consequences of use that can translate into an increase of cigarette smoking and alcohol use behavior among young people.[9]

Developmental Factors

A developmental perspective on the etiology of substance use is instructive in our understanding of how to best prevent early experimentation with alcohol, tobacco, and other drugs. The second decade of life involves physical, biologic, social, and psychological changes that are profound and numerous. Adolescence is a key period for experimentation with a wide range of behaviors and lifestyle patterns. An adolescent's drive to experiment with new behaviors occurs for a number of reasons that are typically linked to psychosocial development. Trying out new and different behaviors is part of a natural process of separating from parents, gaining acceptance and popularity with peers, developing a sense of identity, autonomy, independence, and maturity, seeking fun and adventure, and/or rebelling against authority. Unfortunately, from an adolescent's point of view, engaging in alcohol, tobacco, and other drug use may be seen as a functional way of achieving independence, maturity, or popularity, along with other developmental goals. The most effective prevention approaches incorporate an understanding that substance use behaviors can fulfill a variety of developmental needs. Therefore, teaching children to "just say no" to substance use is necessary but not sufficient for behavior change.

Multiple Levels of Influence

Risk and protective factors contribute to the initiation, maintenance, and escalation of alcohol, tobacco, and illicit drug use, and these factors can be identified and addressed at the level of the individual, family, school, and community.

Individual factors

Individual level factors encompass cognitive, attitudinal, social, personality, pharmacologic, biologic, and developmental factors.[10] Cognitive risk factors for substance use include a deficiency of knowledge regarding the risks of use and abuse, along with the misperception that substance use is "normal" and that most people engage in use. As described in the self-medication hypothesis, affect regulation plays a central role in the etiology of substance use.[11] Psychological characteristics associated with substance use include poor self-esteem, low assertiveness, and poor behavioral self-control. Pharmacologic risk factors become increasingly important as an individual's substance use increases in frequency and quantity. Drugs of abuse such as cocaine, amphetamine, and morphine, as well as nicotine and alcohol, have different pharmacologic mechanisms of action. However, research shows that each of these substances affects the brain in a similar way. Drug use typically increases the activity of excitatory synapses on midbrain dopamine neurons.[12] Furthermore, there are likely to be important individual differences in terms of neurochemical reactivity to drugs, placing some individuals at higher risk.

Family factors

One central risk factor within families is the role that social learning processes play in terms of the modeling of behaviors and attitudes regarding substance use. A second important risk factor is the role that genetic heritability plays in the development of substance use disorders. Parenting practices need to be considered as well. Parenting can affect substance use both directly and indirectly by influencing established precursors of substance use such as aggressive behavior and other conduct problems. In particular, harsh disciplinary practices, poor parental monitoring, low levels of family bonding, and high levels of family conflict contribute to both internalizing and externalizing behaviors including substance use and abuse. Of course, family and parenting factors can also play a key beneficial or protective role in preventing adolescent substance use. Examples of protective parenting practices include firm and consistent limit-setting, careful monitoring, nurturing, and open communication patterns with children.[13]

School and community factors
Findings show that environmental factors and degree of bonding to conventional institutions are associated with adolescent substance use.[14] Students who are not engaged in school, fail to develop or maintain relationships with their teachers, and those who fail academically are more likely to engage in substance use. Similarly, when young people feel disengaged from their communities or feel unsafe in their neighborhoods, not only is this associated with greater substance use, but it also creates greater levels of community disorganization.[15] Youth who maintain active involvement in community institutions such as school and church are less likely to engage in substance use. Schools and communities can play a protective role by taking active steps to engage young people to avoid drug use and other problem behaviors.

PREVENTION TERMINOLOGY

Contemporary terminology for classifying interventions, initially proposed by the Institute of Medicine in 1994,[16] incorporates a continuum of care that includes prevention, treatment, and maintenance. In this framework, prevention refers only to interventions occurring before the onset of a disorder. Prevention is further categorized into 3 types: universal, selective, and indicated interventions. Universal prevention programs focus on the general population, with the aim of deterring or delaying the onset of a condition. Selective prevention programs target selected high-risk groups or subsets of the general population believed to be at high risk because of membership in a particular group (eg, pregnant women or children of drug users). Indicated prevention programs are created for those already showing early danger signs, such as the initial stages of engaging in a high-risk behavior or other related behaviors. Recruitment and participation in a selective intervention is based on membership in a high-risk subgroup. Recruitment and participation in an indicated intervention is based on an individual's warning signs or behaviors.

EVIDENCE-BASED PREVENTION PROGRAMS

In the following sections, contemporary evidence-based approaches to drug abuse prevention for children and adolescents at the school, family, and community levels are described. Several model preventive intervention programs are reviewed, including universal, selected, and indicated programs for schools and families, along with comprehensive community-based prevention programs. Descriptions of the model programs, including information on their primary goals, target audiences, implementation methods, program components, provider training, and evidence of effectiveness, were adapted in part from the Substance Abuse and Mental Health Services Administration (SAMHSA) Model Program *Fact Sheets*[17] and the SAMHSA National Registry of Evidence-Based Programs and Policies (NREPP) Web site.[18] Our review of the effectiveness of these model programs is focused on intervention effects on substance use behaviors as described on the National Registry of Evidence-based Programs and Practices (NREPP) Web site. We also state each intervention's readiness for dissemination score. The NREPP Web site rates each intervention on its readiness for dissemination based on the availability of implementation materials, training and support resources, and quality assurance procedures. Scores range from 0 to 4, where 4 is the highest rating given, representing highest readiness for dissemination.

SCHOOL-BASED PREVENTION

Schools are the focus of most attempts to develop and test evidence-based approaches to adolescent drug abuse prevention. School-based efforts are efficient in that they offer access to large numbers of students. Additionally, substance use is seen as inconsistent with the goals of educating our youth. However, many initial attempts at prevention were ineffective because they focused primarily on lecturing students about the dangers and long-term health consequences of substance use. Some programs used fear-arousal techniques designed to dramatize the dangers of drug use and scare individuals into not using drugs. These initial attempts were not theory-based and failed to incorporate information about the developmental factors and social influences and other etiologic factors that contribute to adolescent substance use. These approaches were based on a simple cognitive conceptual model: that people make decisions about substance use and abuse based on their knowledge of the adverse consequences involved. Over time, more effective contemporary approaches to school-based prevention were developed and tested. Programs became available that were derived from psychosocial theories on the etiology of adolescent drug use and focused primary attention on the risk and protective factors that promote the initiation and early stages of substance use.[2,3] Contemporary approaches to school-based prevention of substance use can be categorized into 3 types: (1) social resistance skills training; (2) normative education; and (3) competence enhancement skills training. Within a single preventive intervention, 1 or more of these approaches or components may be combined.

Social Resistance Skills

These interventions are designed with the goal of increasing adolescents' awareness of the various social influences that support substance use and teaching them specific skills for effectively resisting both peer and media pressures to smoke, drink, or use drugs.[19] Resistance skills training programs teach adolescents ways to recognize situations where they are likely to experience peer pressure to smoke, drink, or use drugs. Students are taught ways to avoid or otherwise effectively deal with these high-risk situations. Participants are taught that they can effectively respond to direct pressure to engage in substance use by knowing what to say (ie, the specific content of a refusal message) and how to deliver what they say in the most effective way possible. Resistance skills programs also typically include content to increase students' awareness of the techniques used by advertisers to promote the sale of tobacco products or alcoholic beverages. Students are taught techniques for formulating counterarguments to the appealing but misleading messages used by advertisers.

Normative Education

Normative education approaches include content and activities to correct inaccurate perceptions regarding the high prevalence of substance use. Many adolescents overestimate the prevalence of smoking, drinking, and the use of certain drugs, which can make substance use seem to be normative behavior. Educating youth about actual rates of use, which are almost always lower than the perceived rates of use, can reduce perceptions regarding the social acceptability of drug use. One way to present this information would be to collect and provide findings from classroom, school, or local community survey data that show actual prevalence rates of substance use in the immediate social environment. Otherwise, this can be taught using national survey data that typically show prevalence rates that are considerably lower than what teens believe. Additionally, normative education attempts to undermine popular but inaccurate beliefs that substance use is considered acceptable and not particularly dangerous. This can be done by highlighting evidence from national studies that shows strong antidrug social norms and generally high perceived risks of drug use in the population. Normative education materials are often included in social resistance programs.

Competence-Enhancement

Competence-enhancement programs recognize that social learning processes are important in the development of drug use in adolescents. Further, they recognize that youth with poor personal and social skills are more susceptible to influences that promote drug use. These youth may also be more motivated to use drugs as an alternative to more adaptive coping strategies.[19] Typically, competence enhancement approaches teach some combination of the following life skills: (1) general problem-solving and decision-making skills; (2) general cognitive skills for resisting interpersonal or media influences; (3) skills for increasing self-control and self-esteem; (4) adaptive coping strategies for relieving stress and anxiety through the use of cognitive coping skills or behavioral relaxation techniques; and (5) general social skills and general assertive skills. Competence enhancement programs are designed to teach the kind of generic skills that can be applied broadly in many areas of a young person's life, in contrast to the more task-focused drug resistance skills training approaches. The most effective competence-enhancement programs teach personal and social skills and emphasize the application of general skills to situations related to substance use as well as how they are used in other important situations. These same skills can be used for dealing effectively with the many challenges one confronts in everyday life.

MODEL SCHOOL-BASED PROGRAMS

In the following section, the authors review 3 model school-based substance abuse prevention programs for adolescents (**Table 1**). The 3 programs represent different tiers of prevention: *Life Skills Training* is a *universal* program designed for all students in a particular setting; *Project Toward No Drug Abuse* is a *selective* program designed for students attending alternative or continuation high schools; and *Brief Alcohol Screening and Intervention for College Students* is an *indicated* program designed for college students who are heavy drinkers.

Life Skills Training

The Life Skills Training (LST) program seeks to influence major social and psychological factors that promote substance use. Separate curricula have been developed for elementary school students (grades 4 to 6), middle or junior high students (grades 6 to 8, or grades 7 to 9), and high school students (grades 9 or 10). The Life Skills Training Middle School (LST-MS) program has been studied most extensively and is the focus of the following review. The LST-MS program is designed for 11- to 14-year-old students and is delivered in 15 class periods (typically 40 to 45 minutes long) in the first year of middle or junior high school. Booster interventions are taught in 10 class periods in the second year and 5 in the third year of middle or junior high school. Optional violence prevention units are available for each year of the program. LST-MS can be taught 1 or more times a week until the program is complete. The program content is delivered using cognitive-behavioral skills training techniques including instruction, demonstration, behavioral rehearsal (practice), feedback, social reinforcement, and extended practice in the form of behavioral homework assignments. The

Table 1
Sample school-based drug abuse prevention programs

	Universal (for Everyone in Population)	Selected (for Members of At-risk Groups)	Indicated (for At-risk Individuals)
Program	Life Skills Training (LST)	Project Toward No Drug Abuse (TND)	Brief Alcohol Screening and Intervention for College Students (BASICS)
Web Site	http://www.lifeskillstraining.com	http://tnd.usc.edu	http://depts.washington.edu/abrc/basics.htm
Target Population	Middle or junior high school students, additional programs available for elementary and high school students	Students attending alternative or continuation high schools; has also been tested in students attending traditional high schools	College students engaging in heavy alcohol use and/or at risk for negative consequences of alcohol use
Providers	Classroom teachers, peer leaders, or health professionals	Classroom teachers, health education staff	College counselor or personnel proficient in motivational interviewing techniques
Provider Training	One-and-a-half-day workshops train LST providers to implement the program with fidelity; activities and teaching strategies used in the program are used in the training sessions	One- to 2-day workshops provide TND teachers with an understanding of the theoretical basis, content, instructional techniques, and objectives of the program	One- to 2-day training workshop, depending on staff experience; practitioner training video is available
Goals	Prevent alcohol, tobacco, marijuana, other drug use, and violence by targeting multiple risk and protective factors and providing skills training in drug resistance skills, personal self-management, and social competence skills to build resilience and help youth navigate developmental tasks	Prevent tobacco, alcohol, other drug use, violence-related behaviors, and other problem behaviors by addressing motivation factors (ie, students' attitudes, beliefs, expectations, and desires regarding drug use); skills (social, self-control, and coping skills); and decision-making (ie, how to make decisions that lead to health-promoting behaviors)	Motivate students to reduce alcohol use to decrease the negative consequences of drinking; reveal discrepancies between the student's risky drinking behavior and his or her goals and values

Materials	Teachers manual and student guide for each year, relaxation audiotape, optional multimedia materials for smoking and biofeedback	Teacher manual, student workbooks, optional videotape, and a TND board game	Program manual, program workbook with sample tools, a training video, and personalized assessment and feedback sheets and handouts
Sessions	30 class sessions over 3 years	12 class sessions	Two 1-hour sessions
Teaching Methods	Facilitated discussion, structured small group activities, and role-playing scenarios are used to stimulate participation and promote the acquisition of skills	Program sessions are highly participatory and interactive. The sessions provide opportunities for interactions among students and between students and the teacher	Based on principles of motivational interviewing, program is delivered in an empathetic, nonjudgmental one-on-one session by trained counselor or staff
Findings	Three large-scale randomized effectiveness trials have shown reductions in tobacco, alcohol, marijuana, other illicit drug use, and violence/delinquency for a diverse range of adolescents, with duration of effects lasting up to 6 years, among LST participants compared with controls	Several randomized trials have been conducted showing reductions in tobacco, alcohol, and marijuana for up to 2 years; 1 study demonstrated effects on "hard drug" use 4 and 5 years after the intervention among TND participants compared with controls	Students receiving BASICS had significantly greater reductions in drinking frequency and quantity compared with control group students, with the greatest intervention impact observed in the first year after the intervention

LST program received a score of 4.0 (out of 4.0) on readiness for dissemination by NREPP.

Program components
The LST program consists of 3 major components that address critical domains found to promote substance use. Each component focuses on a different set of skills: (1) Drug Resistance Skills enable young people to recognize and challenge common misconceptions about substance use, as well as deal with peer and media pressure to engage in substance use; (2) Personal Self-Management Skills help students to examine their self-image and its effects on behavior, set goals and keep track of personal progress, identify everyday decisions and how they may be influenced by others, analyze problem situations, and consider the consequences of alternative solutions before making decisions; and (3) General Social Skills give students the necessary skills to overcome shyness, communicate effectively and avoid misunder-standings, use both verbal and nonverbal assertiveness skills to make or refuse requests, and recognize that they have choices other than aggression or passivity when faced with tough situations.

Program providers and training requirements
The LST program is implemented by a trained classroom teacher, counselor, or health professional. Program materials consist of a Teacher's Manual, Student Guide, and relaxation audiotape or CD. Provider training is recommended for all program providers in the form of a face-to-face training workshop, CD-ROM, or online training. The standard face-to-face training workshops consist of a day and a half training session conducted by certified LST trainers who teach the background, theory, and rationale for the program; familiarize participants with the program; teach participants the skills needed to implement LST; provide an opportunity to practice teaching selected portions of the program; and provide opportunities to discuss practical implementation issues.

Evidence of effectiveness
In support of the quality of research on LST, the NREPP Web site lists 7 peer-reviewed outcome papers from 4 demographically diverse cohorts of students, along with 10 replication studies. All the outcomes studies were randomized controlled trials comparing LST to control group participants. One long-term study followed a cohort of predominantly White suburban students from seventh grade to the end of high school. Students who received LST were compared with controls 6 years after the intervention, and findings revealed a significant decrease in cigarette smoking; alcohol use (drunkenness); and concurrent tobacco, alcohol, and marijuana use in the LST group. The strongest intervention effects were observed among students exposed to at least 60% of the intervention; these students had significantly lower rates than controls for use of tobacco, alcohol, marijuana, and multiple drugs. A separate randomized controlled trial of a predominantly urban minority sample found less smoking, alcohol use, inhalant use, and multiple drug use at the posttest and 1-year follow-up among students who received LST relative to controls as well as a 50% reduction in binge drinking at both the 1- and 2-year follow-up assessments. A subsample of adolescents considered to be at high risk for substance use initiation were found to engage in less smoking, drinking, inhalant use, and multiple drug use compared with similarly matched controls. A third randomized controlled trial of a rural predominantly White sample found a significantly slower rate of increase in substance use initiation from at the posttest, 1-year follow-up, and 5.5 years past baseline compared with controls. The LST group was found to engage in less

methamphetamine use in the 11th and 12th grade follow-up assessments, relative to controls. When growth over time was examined in a high-risk subsample, the LST group had slower increases in the rates of marijuana use and multiple drug use compared with controls. In addition, LST was found to produce effects on violence and delinquency, normative beliefs about substance use, and substance use refusal skills.

Project Toward No Drug Abuse

Project Toward No Drug Abuse (TND) is a high school–based program designed to help high-risk students (14 to 19 years old) resist substance use and abuse. TND consists of twelve 40- to 50-minute lessons that focus on motivational activities, social skills training, and decision-making components. The program content is delivered through group discussions, games, role-playing exercise, videos, and student worksheets. Project TND was initially developed for high-risk students attending alternative or continuation high schools. It has been adapted and tested among students attending traditional high schools as well. Project TND's lessons are presented over a 4- to 6-week period. Project TND received a score of 3.1 (out of 4.0) on readiness for dissemination by NREPP.

Program components
Project TND was developed to fill a gap in substance abuse prevention programming for senior high school youth. Project TND addresses 3 primary risk factors for tobacco, alcohol, and other drug use; violence-related behaviors; and other problem behaviors among youth. These include motivation factors such as attitudes, beliefs, and expectations regarding substance use; social, self-control, and coping skills; and decision-making skills with an emphasis on how to make decisions that lead to health-promoting behaviors. Project TND is based on an underlying theoretical framework proposing that young people at risk for substance abuse will not use substances if they (1) are aware of misconceptions, myths, and misleading information about drug use that lead to use; (2) have adequate coping, self-control, and other skills that help them lower their risk for use; (3) know about how substance use may have negative consequences in their own lives as well as in the lives of others; (4) are aware of cessation strategies for quitting smoking and other forms of substance use; and (5) have good decision-making skills and are able to make a commitment to not use substances. Program materials for Project TND include an implementation manual for providers covering instructions for each of the 12 lessons, a video on how substance abuse can impede life goals, a student workbook, an optional kit containing evaluation materials, the book *The Social Psychology of Drug Abuse*,[20] and Project TND outcome articles.

Program providers and training requirements
A 1- to 2-day training workshop conducted by a certified trainer is recommended for teachers before implementing Project TND. The training workshops are designed to build the skills that teachers need to deliver the lessons with fidelity, and inform them of the theoretical basis, program content, instructional techniques, and objectives of the program.

Evidence of effectiveness
In support of the quality of research on Project TND, the NREPP Web site lists 5 peer-reviewed outcome papers with study populations consisting of primarily Hispanic/Latino and White youth, along with 4 replication studies. Across 3 randomized trials, students in Project TND schools exhibited a 25% reduction in rates of hard drug

use relative to students in control schools at the 1-year follow-up; in addition, those who used alcohol before the intervention exhibited a reduction in alcohol use prevalence of between 7% and 12% relative to controls. In a study testing a revised 12-session TND curriculum, students in Project TND schools (relative to students in control schools) exhibited a reduction in cigarette use of 27% at the 1-year follow-up and 50% at the 2-year follow-up, a reduction in marijuana use of 22% at the 1-year follow-up, and at the 2-year follow-up students in TND schools were about one-fifth as likely to use hard drugs. In this study, males who were nonusers at pretest were about one-tenth as likely use marijuana relative to similar students in control schools. At the 4- and 5-year follow-up assessments, students in Project TND schools were less likely to report using hard drugs, compared with students in control schools. In addition, Project TND was found to produce effects on risk of victimization and frequency of weapons-carrying.

Brief Alcohol Screening and Intervention for College Students

The Brief Alcohol Screening and Intervention for College Students (BASICS) program is an indicated prevention program for college students who drink alcohol heavily and have had or are at risk for alcohol-related problems including poor class attendance, missed assignments, accidents, sexual assault, or violent behavior. It is not designed for students who are alcohol dependent. The goal of BASICS is to motivate students to reduce their alcohol use to decrease the negative consequences of drinking. BASICS is delivered in two 1-hour interviews. Students complete a brief online assessment survey between the first session and second session. BASICS received a score of 3.9 (out of 4.0) on readiness for dissemination by NREPP.

Program components

BASICS is based on principles of motivational interviewing, a directive, client-centered counseling style that is focused on eliciting behavior change by helping clients to explore and resolve ambivalence. BASICS is delivered in an empathetic, nonconfrontational, and nonjudgmental manner and is aimed at providing personal feedback to the student that reveals discrepancies between a student's risky drinking behavior and his or her life goals and values. The first of 2 interviews gathers information about the student's drinking patterns and history, beliefs about alcohol, and provides instructions for self-monitoring drinking between the 2 interview sessions. Between interviews, students complete an online assessment survey that is used to develop a customized feedback profile that is reviewed in the second interview. The assessment survey compares an individual's alcohol use with alcohol use norms, and assesses negative consequences and risk factors for heavy drinking along with perceived risks and benefits of drinking. The assessment results are discussed in the second interview, which takes place approximately 1 or 2 weeks later. The counselor provides personalized feedback and works with the student to review options in terms of how the student can make changes to decrease or abstain from alcohol use.

Program providers and training requirements

Providers are counselors and other college personnel proficient in motivation interviewing techniques. Provider training can be completed in 1 to 2 days, and is conducted by the program developers either onsite or offsite. Training reviews the relevant information about alcohol use among college students along with principles of motivational interviewing. A training workbook provides the information and charts needed for conducting the interviews.

Evidence of effectiveness

In support of the quality of research on the BASICS program, the NREPP Web site lists 4 peer-reviewed outcome papers (representing 3 cohorts of students) with study populations consisting of primarily White youth, along with 4 replication studies. The first study evaluated the impact of BASICS on students engaging in high-risk drinking over a 4-year follow-up period. Findings indicated that students receiving BASICS had significantly greater reductions in drinking frequency and quantity compared with control group students, with the greatest intervention impact observed in the first year after the intervention. A second study evaluated the short-term effects of BASICS on college students engaging in binge drinking. Controlling for gender, BASICS reduced the number of times alcohol was consumed and the frequency of binge drinking episodes from baseline to a 6-week follow-up assessment. At the 6-month follow-up, students receiving BASICS had greater reductions in drinking quantity and peak quantity compared with students in the control group. At the 2-year follow-up assessment, students in the intervention group reported drinking an average of 3.6 drinks per drinking occasion, compared with 4.0 drinks per occasion for controls, a small effect size that was statistically significant. A third study evaluated the effectiveness of the BASICS program among fraternity members. In this study, students in the control group received a required 1-hour didactic presentation on alcohol use. Findings indicated that students receiving BASICS had significantly greater reductions in average drinks per week and typical peak blood alcohol content levels at the 1-year follow-up. In addition, BASICS was found to produce effects on negative consequences of alcohol use.

FAMILY-BASED PREVENTION

There are a variety of effective family-based prevention approaches for adolescent substance abuse. Some focus exclusively on providing parents with the skills needed to keep their children away from drugs. These programs, provided to parents without children present, teach specific parenting skills such as ways to nurture, bond, and communicate with children; how to help children develop prosocial skills and social resistance skills; training on rule-setting and techniques for monitoring activities; and ways to help children reduce aggressive or antisocial behaviors. A second type of family-based prevention focuses on teaching family skills with parents and children together. These programs aim to improve family functioning, communication skills, and provide training to help families discuss and develop family policies on substance abuse, along with teaching parents how to effectively enforce these rules.[13] Interventions that focus on both parenting skills and family bonding appear to be the most effective in reducing or preventing substance use. However, an important limitation of family-based prevention lies in the difficulty of getting parents to participate, particularly the parents of teens most at risk for drug abuse.

MODEL FAMILY-BASED PREVENTION PROGRAMS

In the following section, the authors review 3 model family-based substance abuse prevention programs for adolescents (**Table 2**). Again, programs are selected at each prevention tier: *Family Matters* is a universal program designed for all families that include young adolescents; *Creating Lasting Family Connections* is a selective program designed for youth and families in high-risk environments; and *Brief Strategic Family Therapy* is an indicated program designed for families in which children and adolescents exhibit early substance use, rebelliousness, and/or delinquency.

Table 2
Sample family-based drug abuse prevention programs

	Universal (for Everyone in Population)	Selected (for Members of At-risk Groups)	Indicated (for At-Risk Individuals)
Program	Family Matters (FM)	Creating Lasting Family Connections (CLFC)	Brief Strategic Family Therapy (BSFT)
Web Site	http://familymatters.sph.unc.edu/index.htm	http://copes.org/index.php	http://www.brief-strategic-family-therapy.com
Target Population	Children aged 12–14 years and their parents	Adolescents aged 9–17 years and their families from high-risk environments	Children and adolescents (aged 6–17 years) who engage in substance use and/or delinquent behaviors; families with behavior management issues
Providers	Implemented at home by parents; 4 follow-up telephone technical assistance calls by health educators	Implemented by 2 or more trained facilitators	Counselor should have master's level training in social work or marriage/family therapy; individuals with bachelor's level training with experience working with families can implement the intervention
Provider Training	Health educators who conduct follow-up telephone calls receive 2 days of training before making telephone calls.	Five to 10 days of facilitator training focus on teaching the skills needed to implement the program and fully engage participants; a community mobilization component focuses on recruitment and retention planning	Training, supervision, and certification is required for agencies implementing the program; advanced training consists of four 3-day workshops (12 days total) over several months
Goals	Address issues related to family/adult substance use; the availability of substances; and social attitudes about substance use in the media and among peers. Help families improve parental monitoring, family support, rule-setting, and communication.	Enhance family bonding and communication skills among parents and youth and other skills for personal growth; facilitate the use of appropriate community resources and services in resolving family problems and addressing youth problem behavior	Provides families with the tools to overcome individual and family risk factors through focused interventions to improve maladaptive family interaction and skills building strategies to strengthen families

Materials	Four instructional booklets are mailed to parents, 1 every 2 weeks	Facilitator manual, participant notebooks, program posters	Videotape equipment is needed during supervision phase of provider training
Sessions	Booklets contain readings/activities to get participants to identity and address family characteristics, behaviors, and attitudes that influence adolescent substance use	Weekly 2.5-hour parent and youth training sessions for a 20-week period, or sessions can be offered in 5-week increments throughout the year	Counselor and family typically meet for 12 to 17 weekly sessions that are 60 to 90 minutes each
Teaching Methods	Self-administered at home by parents; some activities are for adult family members only; others are for adults and adolescents together	It is recommended that 2 or more facilitators run each of the parent and youth sessions to facilitate a team approach that enhances learning	Family therapy
Findings	A randomized controlled trial compared participating families with controls and found that the intervention reduced the prevalence of smoking and drinking among teens, after adjusting for demographic variables and pretest rates of use. These effects were maintained at 3 and 12-month follow-up assessments, although effect sizes were small.	Compared with youth in the comparison group, CLFC children reported less frequent alcohol use in the previous 3-month period; as family pathology decreased, CLFC reduced the frequency of alcohol and other drug use at the 12-month assessment; CLFC parents used more community services when a personal or family problem arose	A series of randomized trials showed that participation in BSFT produced reductions in youth marijuana use and overall substance use, compared with control group participants; a study of adolescent girls showed significantly greater reductions in substance use at posttest and at the 1-year follow-up compared with similar girls in the control group

Family Matters

Family Matters is a universal prevention program designed to prevent tobacco and alcohol use in children 12 to 14 years old. The program is implemented at home by parents, who receive 4 instructional booklets that are successively mailed to the home along with follow-up telephone calls from trained health educators after each mailing. During the telephone calls, health educators answer questions and encourage parents to complete each booklet and the included parent-child activities. The first booklet is mailed 24 days after an introductory letter is sent to parents; health educators telephone the parent 13 days after each booklet is mailed; and the next booklet in the series of 4 is mailed after each phone call is completed. One complete program cycle is scheduled to take 79 days. Family Matters received a score of 3.3 (out of 4.0) on readiness for dissemination by NREPP.

Program components

The Family Matters booklets contain readings and activities designed to get families to identify and address family characteristics, behaviors, and attitudes that can influence adolescent substance use. These include levels of adult supervision and support, family rule-setting and communication, family time spent together, parental monitoring, family/adult substance use, the availability of substances, and social attitudes about substance use in the media and among peers. The 4 Family Matters booklets are (1) *Why Families Matter,* which describes the program and encourages participation; (2) *Helping Families Matter to Teens,* which discusses how family factors such as communication patterns and parenting styles influence adolescent alcohol and tobacco use; (3) *Alcohol and Tobacco Rules Are Family Matters,* which addresses issues such as the availability of tobacco and alcohol in the home and developing family rules about child substance use; and (4) *Non-Family Influences That Matter,* which deals with nonfamily influences on adolescent substance use, such as friends who use and the media. Some of the Family Matters materials and activities are for adult family members only, whereas others are for adult and adolescent family members together.

Program providers and training requirements

The health educators who conduct follow-up telephone calls after each mailing can be paid staff or volunteers. It is recommended that they participate in a 2-day training session before making telephone calls. They do not interact with the adolescent as part of program delivery.

Evidence of effectiveness

In support of the quality of research on Family Matters, the NREPP Web site lists 2 peer-reviewed outcome papers with study populations consisting of primarily White youth (no replication studies were listed). In a randomized controlled trial comparing families participating in Family Matters with those not participating, findings indicated that the intervention reduced the prevalence of smoking and drinking among both users and nonusers, after adjusting for demographic variables and pretest rates of use. Further, these effects were maintained at 3- and 12-month follow-up assessments, although the effect sizes were small. The intervention reduced smoking onset among adolescents; at the 12-month follow-up, 16.4% fewer participating adolescents had initiated smoking compared with a control group of adolescents who did not receive the program.

Creating Lasting Family Connections

Creating Lasting Family Connections (CLFC) is a selective intervention that is designed to prevent substance abuse and violence among adolescents and families in high-risk environments. CLFC is designed to enhance family bonding and communication skills among parents and youth, while promoting healthy beliefs and attitudes that are inconsistent with drug use and violence. CLFC has been implemented in schools, churches, community centers, and other settings. Facilitators provide weekly parent and youth training sessions for a 20-week period, or the sessions can be offered in 5-week increments throughout the year. Facilitators are trained to be knowledgeable about local community service providers and make referrals when appropriate and necessary. CLFC received a score of 3.7 (out of 4.0) on readiness for dissemination by NREPP.

Program components

A coordinator planning to implement CLFC trains a small staff of volunteers to recruit and retain participating families from high-risk environments, and then identifies, recruits, and selects the relevant community collaborators for the program. The program facilitator administers 6 interactive modules, 3 to parents and 3 to youth. Each module contains 5 to 6 sessions lasting up to 2.5 hours each. The sessions focus on substance use issues, personal and family responsibilities, and communication and refusal skills. In addition to the parent and youth training sessions, the CLFC program aims to foster greater use of community services in resolving family problems and addressing youth problem behavior.

Program providers and training requirements

It is recommended that 2 or more facilitators run each of the parent and youth sessions to facilitate a team approach that enhances learning. If CLFC is provided over a 20-week period, these 4 facilitators can work with up to 30 families (1 day per week, 4 hours a day). Preparation for implementing the program can take up to 3 months, including 5 to 10 days of facilitator training that focuses on methods to fully engage participants, followed by the recruitment of families, and the planning and organization regarding community mobilization activities.

Evidence of effectiveness

In support of the quality of research on CLFC, the NREPP Web site lists 2 peer-reviewed outcome papers reporting results of 1 cohort of youth and parents (no replication studies were listed). Findings indicated that when resiliency factors targeted by the program improved, the program produced effects on substance use frequency at the 3- and 12-month assessments. Compared with youth in the comparison group, those receiving the CLFC intervention reported less frequent alcohol use in the previous 3-month period. As family pathology decreased, CLFC reduced the frequency of alcohol and other drug use at the 12-month assessment. In addition, CLFC was found to produce effects on other outcomes, including use of community services and parent knowledge and beliefs about alcohol and other drug use.

Brief Strategic Family Therapy

Brief Strategic Family Therapy (BSFT) is an indicated family-based prevention program that aims to decrease individual and family risk factors through skills building and by improving and strengthening family relationships. BSFT targets children and adolescents (6 to 17 years of age) who engage in rebellious, truant, or delinquent behaviors, as well as those who are engaging in substance use and/or associating with peers exhibiting these behaviors. The program is also beneficial for families experiencing problematic relationships, parental discord, or behavior management issues. BSFT is designed for a variety of settings, and has been implemented in community-based health and social services agencies and clinics. The program is designed to be delivered over an 8- to 12-week period, and the sessions are 60 to 90 minutes each. The BSFT counselor meets with family members at their home or in the program office. BSFT received a score of 3.3 (out of 4.0) on readiness for dissemination by NREPP.

Program components
The BFST counselor implements the intervention in 4 distinct steps. The first step is to develop a therapeutic alliance by accepting and demonstrating respect for each individual family member and the family as a whole. The second step is to assess family strengths and supportive relationships as well as problematic relationships within the family that affect youth behavior or parenting abilities. The third step is to develop an approach to change that takes advantage of family strengths and that addresses problematic relationships. The fourth and final step is to implement change strategies that may include reframing to change the meaning of interactions, shifting interpersonal boundaries as needed, building conflict resolution skills, and providing parental coaching. The overall goal of these change strategies is to increase and reinforce competent family interactions and behaviors.

Program providers and training requirements
One full-time BFST counselor can provide the program to 15 to 20 families for in-office sessions and 10 to 12 families for in-home sessions. To successfully implement BSFT in-office, an agency should be open at times that are convenient for participating families and provides transportation and child-care services if needed. In BSFT, the counselor is trained to be problem-focused and practical, with a goal of moving the family from problematic to competent interactions. An ideal BFST counselor has master's level training in social work or marriage and family therapy; however, individuals with bachelor's level training with experience working with families can implement the intervention. Certification is required for agencies implementing the BFST program. Advanced training consists of four 3-day workshops (12 days total) over a period of several months.

Evidence of effectiveness
In support of the quality of research on BSFT, the NREPP Web site lists 7 peer-reviewed outcome papers and 1 replication study. Three of the outcome studies reported on adolescent drug use outcomes. Adolescents who participated in BSFT showed significantly greater reductions in marijuana use compared with adolescents in the comparison group in 1 study, and less overall substance use in another study. In a third study, adolescent girls who participated in BSFT showed significantly greater reductions in substance use at posttest and at the 1-year follow-up than adolescent girls in the comparison group. In addition, BSFT was found to produce effects on other outcomes, including engagement in therapy, conduct problems and aggression, and family functioning.

COMMUNITY-BASED PREVENTION

Evidence-based drug abuse prevention programs delivered to entire communities typically have multiple components. These often include a school-based component and family or parenting components, along with mass media campaigns, public policy initiatives, and other types of community organization and activities. These interventions require a significant amount of resources and coordination, given the broad scope of the activities involved. The program components are often managed by a coalition of stakeholders including parents, educators, and community leaders. Research has shown that community-based programs that deliver a coordinated, comprehensive message about prevention can be effective in preventing adolescent substance use.

MODEL COMMUNITY-BASED PREVENTION PROGRAM
Community Trials Intervention to Reduce High-risk Drinking

Community Trials Intervention to Reduce High-Risk Drinking (RHRD) is a universal intervention that aims to alter community-wide alcohol use patterns such as drinking and driving, underage drinking, binge drinking, and related problems. This multicomponent program uses several environmental intervention strategies to increase community awareness, prevent access to alcohol for underage drinkers, and enforce laws regarding alcohol use and sales. RHRD received a score of 2.8 (out of 4.0) on readiness for dissemination by NREPP.

Program components
The RHRD program uses 5 prevention components. The first is reducing alcohol access, which is accomplished by helping communities use zoning and municipal regulations to control the density of bars, liquor stores, and so forth. The second component is responsible beverage service, which involves training alcohol beverage servers and assisting retailers develop policies and procedures to reduce drunkenness and driving after drinking. The third component aims to reduce drinking and driving through increased law enforcement and sobriety checkpoints. The fourth component reduces underage alcohol access by training alcohol retailers to avoid selling to minors and those who provide alcohol to minors, and through increased enforcement of laws regarding alcohol sales to minors. The fifth component provides communities with the tools to form the coalitions needed to implement and support the interventions that will address all RHRD prevention components. To properly implement RHRD, project staff must assess community priorities and decide which interventions to use and how to adapt them. Typically, this involves working closely with local community organizations, opinion leaders, law enforcement, zoning and planning commissions, policy makers, and the public to collect this information.

Program providers and training requirements
Recommended project staff for RHRD include a director who is responsible for developing the initiative, seeking funding, building coalitions, and hiring project staff; an assistant director who manages office operations and staff and implements the program; along with 1 or more data managers, administrative assistants, and volunteers. Training and consultation target the specific needs and problems of the individual community. Training manuals for RHRD are available along with brochures that offer strategies and tactics for reducing alcohol use within the community. The RHRB project Web site is located at http://www.pire.org/communitytrials/index.htm.

Evidence of effectiveness
In support of the quality of research on RHRD, the NREPP Web site lists 2 peer-reviewed outcome papers and 1 replication study. One of the outcome studies reported on alcohol use outcomes. In the study, alcohol consumption was assessed via telephone surveys to randomly selected individuals from households in the intervention and comparison communities. Findings indicated that individuals living in the intervention community sites had significant reductions in drinking quantities, rates

of driving when having had too much to drink, and rates of driving over the legal limit, when compared with individuals living in comparison sites. In addition, RHRD was found to produce effects on other outcomes, including alcohol-related traffic accidents and alcohol-related assaults.

SUMMARY

Prevalence rates of alcohol, tobacco, and other drug use increase rapidly during the years from early to late adolescence, and typically peak during young adulthood. Prevention programs for adolescents have been developed and implemented in school, family, and community settings. The most effective programs are guided by relevant psychosocial theory regarding the etiology of substance abuse and target key risk and protective factors that have been shown to be associated with substance abuse behavior. Among adolescents, substance use involvement is typically a function of the negative pro-drug social influences in their social environment combined with individual psychosocial vulnerabilities to these influences.

School-based prevention programs that have been tested and proven effective focus on building drug-resistance skills, general self-regulation and social skills, and/or changing normative expectations regarding inaccurate beliefs about the high prevalence of substance use. The most effective programs are highly interactive in nature, skills-focused, and implemented over multiple years. Literature reviews and meta-analytic studies have shown that programs with these characteristics can reduce smoking, alcohol, and other forms of substance use in young people, compared with youth who do not participate in such programs. Several rigorous outcome studies of school-based prevention programs have demonstrated clear evidence of short- and long-term effects on substance use behavior. Family-based prevention programs typically emphasize parenting skills training and/or improving family functioning, communication, and family rules regarding substance abuse. Those family interventions that combine parenting skills and family bonding components appear to be the most effective. Community-based drug abuse prevention programs include some combination of school, family, mass media, public policy, and community organization components. Community programs that present a coordinated, comprehensive message across multiple delivery components are most effective in terms of changing behavior.

Although there are a growing number of evidence-based prevention programs for adolescent substance use and abuse, it is important that prevention efforts remain flexible and responsive to changing trends in use. For example, the abuse of prescription and over-the-counter medications among adolescents is a growing problem that requires a coordinated and comprehensive response. This is especially true because these medications are often readily accessible to teenagers, either from medicine cabinets at home, from friends or relatives, or for purchase at the local pharmacy or through the Internet. Multiple stakeholders can address the issue of ready access. Parents can limit access by safeguarding medications in a secure location, keeping an inventory of medications in the home, and disposing of unused or old medications. Physicians can limit access by documenting and monitoring prescription histories and refill requests for all patients and ensuring that prescription pads are secured. Pharmacists can limit access by identifying and addressing the issue of forged prescriptions. Of course, in addition to reducing access, each of these stakeholders can play a key role in raising awareness of the dangers of abusing medications.

As we move forward, it is important to address several factors that reduce the public health impact of effective prevention programming. It is still the case that most schools use non–evidence-based prevention programs, family-based prevention programs often do not reach the families in greatest need, and starting community prevention programs requires substantial resources. It is clear that more research is needed to facilitate the wide dissemination of effective prevention programs into our schools, families, and communities.

REFERENCES

1. Newcomb MD, Locke T. Health, social, and psychological consequences of drug use and abuse. In: Sloboda Z, editor. Epidemiology of drug abuse. New York: Springer; 2005. p. 45–59.
2. Hawkins JD, Catalano RF, Miller JY. Risk and protective factors for alcohol and other drug problems in adolescence and early adulthood: implications for substance abuse prevention. Psychol Bull 1992;112:64–105.
3. Petraitis J, Flay BR, Miller TQ. Reviewing theories of adolescent substance use: organizing pieces in the puzzle. Psychol Bull 1995;117:67–86.
4. Johnston LD, O'Malley PM, Bachman JG, et al In: Monitoring the future national survey results on drug use, 1975–2008, vol. I. Bethesda (MD): National Institute on Drug Abuse; 2009. Secondary school students.
5. Kandel D. Stages and pathways of drug involvement: examining the gateway hypothesis. New York: Cambridge University Press; 2002.
6. Hartel CR, Glantz MD. Drug abuse: origins and interventions. Washington, DC: American Psychological Association; 1997.
7. Mayberry ML, Espelage DL, Koenig B. Multilevel modeling of direct effects and interactions of peers, parents, school, and community influences on adolescent substance use. J Youth Adolesc 2009;38:1038–49.
8. Villani S. Impact of media on children and adolescents: a 10-year review of the research. J Am Acad Child Adolesc Psychiatry 2001;40:392–401.
9. Tye J, Warner K, Glantz S. Tobacco advertising and consumption: evidence of a causal relationship. J Public Health Policy 1987;8:492–507.
10. Swadi H. Individual risk factors for adolescent substance use. Drug Alcohol Depend 1999;55:209–24
11. Khantzian EJ. The self-medication hypothesis of substance use disorders: a reconsideration and recent applications. Harv Rev Psychiatry 1997;4: 231–44.
12. Saal D, Dong Y, Bonci A, et al. Drugs of abuse and stress trigger a common synaptic adaptation in dopamine neurons. Neuron 2003;37:577–82.
13. Lochman JE, van den Steenhoven A. Family-based approaches to substance abuse prevention. J Prim Prev 2002;23:49–114.
14. Fletcher A, Bonell C, Hargreaves J. School effects on young people's drug use: a systematic review of intervention and observational studies. J Adolesc Health 2008;42:209–20.
15. Hays SP, Hays CE, Mulhall PF. Community risk and protective factors and adolescent substance use. J Prim Prev 2003;24:125–42.
16. Institute of Medicine. Reducing risks for mental disorders: frontiers for preventive intervention research. Washington, DC: National Academy Press; 1994.
17. Schinke S, Brounstein P, Gardner S. Science-based prevention programs and principles, 2002. DHHS Pub. No. (SMA) 03-3764. Rockville (MD): Center for Substance Abuse Prevention; 2002. Substance Abuse and Mental Health Services Administration.

18. National Registry of Evidence-based Programs and Practices (NREPP web site). Substance Abuse and Mental Health Services Administration (SAMHSA). Available at: http://www.nrepp.samhsa.gov. Accessed November 15, 2009.
19. Botvin GJ. Preventing drug abuse in schools: social and competence enhancement approaches targeting individual-level etiological factors. Addict Behav 2000;25:887–97.
20. Sussman S, Ames SL. The social psychology of drug abuse. Philadelphia: Open University Press; 2001.

Evidence for Optimism: Behavior Therapies and Motivational Interviewing in Adolescent Substance Abuse Treatment

Mark J. Macgowan, PhD, LCSW[a,*], Bretton Engle, PhD, LCSW[b]

KEYWORDS

- Motivational interviewing • Behavior therapy
- Cognitive behavioral therapy • Substance abuse • Adolescents

Behavior therapies and motivational interviewing approaches have been widely used in clinical and nonclinical, and primary and secondary medical settings for the treatment of alcohol and other drug (AOD) problems among adolescents. Behavior therapy (BT), or more appropriately behavior therapies, is used here to include a wide range of cognate therapies, such as cognitive therapy, cognitive-behavior therapy, and social learning-based treatments, all of which have been widely used in the treatment of AOD problems. More recently, motivational interviewing (MI) has been developed and applied with adolescents and is similarly diverse, with a number of MI adaptations. This article reviews BTs and MIs, including therapies that combine BT and MI, or uses one or the other in conjunction with another psychosocial therapy. The focus of this article is on treatment studies involving clinical samples in which AODs are used. Thus, studies on prevention are excluded. Also not included are contingency management approaches, which are covered in the article by Stanger and Budney elsewhere in this issue.

Support was received from the National Institute of Alcoholism and Alcohol Abuse (1 R21AA15679-01).

[a] Community-Based Intervention Research Group, College of Public Health and Social Work, Florida International University, GL 485, 11200 SW 8th Street, Miami, FL 33199, USA
[b] School of Social Work, Barry University, 11300 NE Second Avenue, Miami Shores, FL 33161, USA
* Corresponding author.
E-mail address: Macgowan@fiu.edu

Child Adolesc Psychiatric Clin N Am 19 (2010) 527–545
doi:10.1016/j.chc.2010.03.006
1056-4993/10/$ – see front matter © 2010 Elsevier Inc. All rights reserved.

The first section describes the methods used to find the studies, which is followed by separate critical reviews of BTs, MI, and combined approaches. We then offer an integrative discussion of relevant research and treatment issues emerging from the review with recommendations. The primary aim of this article was to determine the state of the science of BT and MI therapies in the treatment of adolescent AOD use and make recommendations for clinical practice and research.

METHOD

This article reports findings from published, peer-reviewed journals in the English language. Studies must have included adolescents (mean age 19 years or younger) with AOD use but not tobacco, explicitly used BT, MI, or adaptations either separately or together, and must have been controlled and compared 2 conditions within the same study (but not necessarily randomized). We conducted an extensive literature search in academic databases (Academic OneFile, and more specific databases, Psychinfo and PubMed). We included any published study that met the criteria up to mid-2009. In addition to these sources, we consulted recent reviews of controlled studies for potentially missing articles.[1–9]

We report descriptive findings about each study and evaluate the efficacy of the approaches. The studies were evaluated according to the standards developed by the American Psychological Association's (APA) Division 12 Task Force[10,11] that defined "well-established" and "probably efficacious" treatments. According to these criteria, well-established treatments

1. Have at least 2 good between-group design experiments demonstrating efficacy in at least 1 of the following ways:
    Superior (statistically significantly so) to placebo or to another treatment or equivalent to an already established treatment in experiments with adequate statistical power (about 30 per group)
2. Must be conducted with treatment manuals
3. Must specify the characteristics of the client samples
4. Have effects that have been demonstrated by at least 2 different investigators or investigating teams.

The criteria for probably efficacious treatments should include the following:

1. Two experiments showing the treatment is superior (statistically significant so) to a waiting-list control group or
2. One or more experiments meeting the well-established treatment criteria 1a or 1b, 2, and 3, but not 4.

In addition, Chambless and colleagues[12] described methodological criteria that each study should have when determining efficacy. The criteria include the following:

1. Use of outcome assessment measures with demonstrated reliability and validity
2. Use of multiple methods of assessment (favored but not required)
3. Include follow-up results that demonstrate the enduring effects of different interventions, especially for disorders that have variable courses
4. Include all clients initially assigned to treatment in final analysis (especially when attrition is high)
5. Report on treatment adherence (favored but not required)
6. Report findings of between-group differences rather than draw conclusions based on pretest to posttest differences within each condition.

Because the APA Task Force was focused mostly on treatments for adults, Division 12 appointed a second task force with an emphasis on treatments for children and adolescents. In addition to preserving the first 2 categories, the task force developed a third category called "promising interventions."[13] To meet those criteria,

1. There must be positive support from 1 well-controlled study and at least 1 other less-well-controlled study;

OR

2. There must be positive support from a small number of single-case design experiments;

OR

3. There must be positive support from 2 or more well-controlled studies by the same investigator.

This study will identify treatments that meet the criteria for "well-established," "probably efficacious," and "promising." In addition, the findings from this review will be compared with 2 recent systematic reviews of adolescent AOD treatments.[1,7] This is advisable when there are conflicting results not only across studies but also within studies where there may be significant differences on some but not all measures.[12]

RESULTS
Behavioral Therapies

BTs include, among others, behavior therapy, cognitive therapy, social learning, and cognitive-behavior therapy. These therapies tend to modify behaviors, cognitions, or environmental reinforcers related to adolescent AOD use. These therapies often borrow and blend from each other, so classifying behavior therapies into particular camps is often difficult. BTs for AOD use are often offered as a package of treatments combining different techniques from behavior theories. In the treatment of AOD problems among adolescents, the BTs reviewed in this article incorporate a variety of techniques including self monitoring, cravings management, mood regulation such as relaxation training, skills-building such as problem-solving and assertiveness training, relapse prevention, modeling, behavior rehearsal, feedback, and homework. This article includes studies that used BTs or their major components or techniques as a major part of treatment.

Studies of BTs first began in any significant numbers with adults. With a few exceptions (eg, relaxation training), reviews have reported that BTs have been generally effective for adults with alcohol problems.[14] The evidence for drug abuse treatment has lagged, but the evidence for adults is that BTs are effective.[15,16] With adolescents, reviews of the early outcome literature yielded some promising BT treatments.[17,18] However, the studies included in these reviews were largely uncontrolled and there was insufficient evidence to support the differential effectiveness of any particular treatment. Only in the past 10 to 15 years have rigorous controlled studies of BTs involving adolescents been published.

The first controlled BT study was by Azrin and colleagues.[19] In that study, 26 youths with illegal drug use were randomly assigned to either a behavioral-based individual intervention (BT-I, n = 15) or to a supportive group counseling comparison condition (n = 11), both of which were 15 sessions. The BT-I treatment consisted of rehearsal, self-monitoring, with specific techniques that included stimulus and urge control, and contracting that included family involvement. There were both statistically and clinically significant differences between conditions in reductions in drug use. The behavioral treatment condition had a greater reduction in illegal drug use (across measures) compared with the supportive counseling program (large effects). Youth in BT had significantly better improvements in other areas such as school attendance, parent relationship satisfaction, conduct ratings, and depression ratings.

Building on his earlier study, Azrin and colleagues[20] undertook a second study, but this time compared family behavior therapy (n = 29) with an individual cognitive problem-solving therapy (ICPS, n = 27). The problem-solving treatment used in the study differed from previous efforts in that this effort was more purely cognitive. The use of problem-solving steps was reinforced and there was no emphasis on behavioral features such as rehearsal, homework, or behavioral recording charts. Both interventions included 15 sessions. This study included a sample of dually diagnosed youth with conduct disorder and substance dependence. Both groups had significant decreases in their average number of days using drugs per month from pretest to 6 months during treatment, and the results were maintained by the 6-month follow-up. Both groups also experienced significant improvements in conduct through follow-ups. Within ICPS, there were significant reductions in AOD and other problems through 6-month follow-up. Although youth in both conditions demonstrated similar decreases in their drug use over time; there was no differential benefit of one treatment over the other.

Conrod and colleagues[21] examined the efficacy of a cognitive behavioral group therapy (CBT-G) intervention targeting youths with personality factors that placed them at high risk for drinking and drinking problems. The researchers characterized the intervention as selective, targeting not a clinical sample with AOD use disorders, but youth with reported alcohol use in the past 4 months, and a personality profile placing them at risk of subsequent alcohol problems and comorbid psychopathology. The personality profiles included anxiety sensitivity, hopelessness, and sensation seeking. Youth were randomly assigned to a 2-session CBT-G intervention (n = 166) or to a no-treatment control condition (n = 131). The CBT-G consisted of psychoeducation, behavioral coping skills training, and cognitive coping skills training. By 4-month follow-up, youth in the CBT condition had significantly lower levels of alcohol consumption, number of problem drinking symptoms, and binge drinking, when compared with youth in the control condition. The brief CBT-G intervention had significant but small effects in reducing alcohol use and problems among selected high risk drinking youth.

Kaminer and colleagues[22] undertook a series of studies that included youth with comorbid disorders. The first study[22] compared CBT-G (n = 13) and interactional group treatment (IGT, n = 10) for up to 3-month follow-up. The primary purpose of the study was to test whether youth could be matched to particular treatments based on diagnostic condition. The study's aim was to determine whether youth with externalizing disorders would have better outcomes when treated with CBT-G than with IGT, and youths with internalizing disorders would do better in IGT. The CBT approach viewed AOD abuse as a maladaptive way of coping with problems or meeting certain needs. AOD use was related to a sequence of learned behaviors that can be changed through the application of behavior modification. Thus, treatment focused on the factors that precipitated and maintained episodes of AOD use, and involved didactic presentations, modeling, role-playing, and homework exercises. Thirty-two dually diagnosed adolescents released from an outpatient aftercare treatment facility were randomly assigned to CBT-G or IGT. Both groups consisted of 12 weekly, 90-minute sessions. At 3-month follow-up no matching effects were found, but an unexpected finding was noted: adolescents in the CBT-G condition demonstrated a significant reduction in severity of substance use compared with those assigned to IGT. CBT-G demonstrated greater reduction in substance use compared with IGT. In a 15-month follow-up study, Kaminer and Burleson[23] reported that youths maintained significant treatment gains on measures of AOD use and psychiatric status, but there were no significant differences between therapy types.

In a third and larger study, Kaminer and colleagues[24] examined the effects of a briefer version of the CBT group (n = 51) versus a psychoeducational group therapy (PET, n = 37), which included 3- and 9-month follow-ups. The sample consisted of 88 predominately dually diagnosed youth referred to outpatient AOD treatment who were randomly assigned to 8 weeks of CBT or PET groups. Self-reported AOD use measures showed significant improvement through 3- and 9-month follow-up across conditions. A greater reduction in other drug use occurred among older youth and male youth in the CBT-G condition at 3-month follow-up, compared with the PET condition, but this was not maintained at 9-month follow-up.

Liddle and colleagues[25] included a CBT intervention as an active comparison group for the development and testing of Multidimensional Family Therapy (MDFT) in 3 studies. In the first clinical trial,[25] 152 multiethnic adolescents were assigned to MDFT (n = 47), Adolescent Group Therapy (AGT, n = 53), or Multifamily Educational Intervention (MEI, n = 52). AGT was based on CBT and emphasized social skills training, such as communication, self-control, self-acceptance, and problem solving. Statistically significant reductions were achieved in all 3 conditions, although the biggest reductions and across more domains (eg, family functioning, school performance) were in the MDFT condition. However, the findings also provided support for the AGT intervention. At the 12-month follow-up, drug use in the AGT condition gradually declined from pretest and was as low as for those who were in the MDFT condition, demonstrating a "sleeper effect." In addition, the AGT at 12-month follow-up had significantly lower rates of drug use than the MEI condition.

A second study compared MDFT (n = 39) with peer group treatment (PGT, n = 41), which was based on social learning and behavior therapy.[26] This study was focused on including younger (mean age 13.7 years) diverse youth and reported findings through discharge from treatment. Both conditions demonstrated significant improvements in youth alcohol and marijuana use over the course of treatment until discharge from treatment. MDFT had more rapid decreases in cannabis use over treatment than AGT, and for adolescents who reported using alcohol during treatment, those in the MDFT condition demonstrated significantly better changes in alcohol use than youth in AGT.

In a follow-up study, Liddle and colleagues[27] reported 12-month outcomes for MDFT and PGT (now called adolescent group therapy, AGT). Both treatments showed significant reductions in the number of youths reporting any AOD problems during the 12-month follow-up and the proportion of youth abstaining from AOD use significantly increased over time. There were also clinically significant reductions in AOD problems over time, but the frequency of their use by the end of treatment was not clinically significant, in contrast with MDFT, which had more clinically meaningful reductions in AOD frequency. MDFT had more rapid decreases in reported problems over time than AGT, and youths in the MDFT condition reported fewer days of AOD use and increased abstinence from AOD. MDFT also had greater improvements in reducing delinquency, internalized distress, and risk in the areas of family, peer, and school functioning.

Najavits and colleagues[28] examined the efficacy of Seeking Safety (SS), a coping skills program adapted for youth, which targeted both posttraumatic stress disorder

(PTSD) and AOD disorders among female adolescents. All participants had AOD and PTSD diagnoses, with most experiencing trauma in the form of sexual or physical abuse. In the small study, youth were randomly assigned to either SS combined with usual treatment (SS+TAU, n = 18), or to usual treatment (TAU, n = 15). According to the researchers, the SS manual included 25 topics representing cognitive, behavioral, and interpersonal domains, and each topic included a "safe coping skill" relevant for both AOD and PTSD, such as Asking for Help. The researchers used full intent-to-treat analyses, including all data available at each time point (pretest, posttest, 3-month follow-up). The results were that youth in the SS+TAU condition had significantly better outcomes on 7 of 10 subscales of the AOD measure than those in TAU. In addition, youth in the treatment condition had significantly fewer substance use disorders (SUDs) than TAU by follow-up. The SS+TAU condition experienced significantly better outcomes on trauma-related symptoms (sexual, physical abuse), cognitions related to SUD and PTSD (but not PTSD), and all differences favored treatment over TAU.

In a randomized clinical trial, Smith and colleagues[29] evaluated the efficacy of strengths-oriented family therapy (SOFT, n = 58) and The Seven Challenges program (7C, n = 40). The 7C program was a combination of group (10 sessions) and individual (5 sessions) CBT treatment that incorporated cognitive-emotional, decision-making processes, which included decision-making exercises, skills training, and interactive journaling with clinicians, with motivational interviewing concepts. Both groups experienced significant reductions in AOD use at 3- and 6-month follow-ups. Specifically, youth in both groups were significantly more likely to abstain or be in full remission at follow-ups compared with baseline. Within the 7C condition, the odds of AOD use at the 3- and 6-month follow-ups were reduced by 93% and 95% respectively, and the odds of AOD problems were reduced by 52% and 69%, respectively. Neither treatment was superior to the other in reducing the odds of continued use or continued AOD symptoms.

Stice and colleagues[30] tested the efficacy of a brief CBT-G intervention in reducing depression symptoms and AOD use. In a randomized controlled trial (RCT), the CBT-G intervention (n = 89) was compared with 3 other conditions, a group supportive-expressive intervention (GS-EI, n = 88), bibliotherapy (n = 80), and an assessment-only control condition (n = 84). The study's primary area of interest was depression and AOD use. CBT-G focused on increasing participant involvement in pleasant activities and replacing negative cognitions with positive cognitions, and involved homework to reinforce the skills taught in the sessions, and behavioral techniques to reinforce the use of new skills. Motivational enhancement exercises were also included to maximize willingness to use the new skills. Youth in the CBT-G condition had significantly greater reductions in depressive symptoms than those in GS-EI, bibliotherapy, and assessment-only conditions at posttest. The CBT-G intervention yielded significantly greater reductions in depressive symptoms than in assessment-only at 6-month follow-up and the changes were clinically significant. Youth in the CBT-G condition demonstrated significantly greater reductions in AOD use at posttest for all conditions but GS-EI, and by 6-month follow-up than youth in all 3 other conditions.

Waldron and colleagues[31] randomly assigned 114 multiethnic adolescents to 4 treatment conditions: functional family therapy (FFT, n = 30), individualized cognitive-behavior therapy (CBT-I) with motivational enhancement therapy (CBT-I/MET, n = 31), combined FFT with CBT-I/MET (joint, n = 29), and a psychoeducation group intervention that included drug and alcohol education and skills training (n = 30). The CBT-I intervention included a 2-session MET followed by 10 skills modules, which included communication training, problem-solving, refusal skills, negative mood management, and relapse prevention. The group intervention included behavioral elements such as exploration of expectancies and consequences of AOD use and assertiveness and refusal skills training. The intervention has been classified as CBT in the researcher's subsequent studies,[7] and is thus classified as CBT-G in this article. Thus, 3 of the interventions included elements of BTs, but only the group condition was exclusively CBT. Two outcomes were used in the study, percentage days of marijuana use and changes from heavy to minimal marijuana use. Youth in FFT and joint condition had significantly fewer days of marijuana use from pretreatment to the 4-month follow-up. However, only youths in the joint and CBT-G conditions maintained significant reduction in percentage of days of marijuana use through to the 7-month follow-up. Thus, there seemed to be a delay effect in the CBT-G condition in that gains were not observed at 4- but rather 7-month follow-up. Youths in the CBT-I/MET did not have significant reductions in marijuana use at either 4- or 7-month follow-up. With respect to changes from heavy to minimal marijuana use, significantly more youths achieved minimal use in the FFT, joint, and CBT-I/MET conditions at the 4-month follow-up. At 7 months, significant changes from heavy to minimal use were seen in the FFT, joint, and CBT-G conditions, but not in the CBT-I/MET condition. When comparing treatments, the FFT condition had a significantly lower rate of marijuana use than did the CBT-I/MET and CBT-G treatments at 4 months, but there were no differences between conditions by the 7-month posttest.

Summary of Behavior Therapies

Thirteen articles tested 12 different BT interventions in group or individual modalities, either as the primary or comparison condition. Most were delivered in outpatient settings but 2 were school-based.[21,30] Treatment lengths ranged from 2 to 25 sessions, with a median of 12 sessions. Most (8 of 12) were group interventions.

With respect to problem severity, most of the treatments tended to target youth with at least moderate AOD use. Several targeted youth with comorbidity that included PTSD,[28] elevated depression,[30] and both internalizing and externalizing disorders including conduct disorder.[20,22–24] With respect to effectiveness, most had significant changes from pretest through follow-ups. The BT condition had superior outcomes than at least 1 comparison condition on an AOD variable in half of the interventions.[19,21,22,25,28,30] One study noted a superior outcome versus the comparison condition among older youths and males at short-term follow-up.[24] The studies involving youth with comorbidity demonstrated that in most cases, CBT-based interventions reduced AOD use over time, and in some cases, over comparison conditions. When examining the criteria from Chambless and colleagues,[10–12] only 2 studies, both group-based, had sufficient sample sizes and a treatment that performed better than the comparison condition on many if not all indicators of AOD use.[21,30] The other 4 studies that demonstrated significant differences compared with comparison conditions[19,22,25,28] suffered from small sample sizes or had only one measure or outcome point that was significantly different from the comparison condition. Thus, although the body of research did not meet the criteria for "well established" the BT interventions met the criteria for "probably efficacious," given that they were better than comparison groups on some or all AOD measures.

Motivational Interviewing

Motivational interviewing (MI) includes a number of different approaches that use motivational processes. MI was originally developed by William Miller[32] for adult alcohol drinkers. It has theoretical roots in social learning and CBT[33] but is humanistic at its core. MI is defined as a "collaborative, person-centered form of guiding to elicit and strengthen motivation for change."[34(p137)] This "form of guiding" is characterized by the therapist's emphasis on collaborating with the client, supporting client autonomy, and evoking the client's own views of behavior change.[35] In addition, MI consists of techniques that are often described with the acronym, OARS: open questions, affirmations, reflections, summaries. These techniques are used to increase motivation and strengthen commitment to behavior change. Because it values client autonomy, MI does not require than an individual "admit" to an AOD problem before considering behavior change. Thus, it is thought that adolescents may respond more favorably to MI approaches than to "confrontation of denial" approaches.

MI principles have been incorporated into a number of different versions. Adapted motivational interviewing (AMI) has been used to describe interventions based partially but not solely on MI. Motivational enhancement therapy (MET) is based on MI but typically incorporates client feedback regarding the targeted behavior. Although MI tends to be a brief intervention, brief motivational interventions (BMI) are explicitly so. Finally, most brief interventions (BI) are also MI-based.

With adults, MI and its adaptations have good strong empirical support for treating AOD disorders,[36,37] although other reviews have noted that the effects for reducing other drugs is mixed and that stronger effects are seen for interventions that combine MI with other approaches.[15] The literature on MI with adolescents is much more recent. The first published report of MI in the literature with adolescents with nontobacco AOD use was by Monti and colleagues in 1999.[38] Since then, there have been a number of controlled studies.

Twelve different controlled studies that draw upon MI principles and techniques are presented in the following sections according to treatment setting. The first set of 5 studies were in schools, followed by 4 in community settings that serve either heavy AOD users or homeless youth, and 3 in primary health care settings (ie, health care clinic, emergency departments).

School-based studies

The first 2 studies were in high schools in the United States. The other 3 were in "further education colleges" in the United Kingdom, which enroll older adolescents. In the first study, Walker and colleagues[39] examined the feasibility and efficacy of a school-based MET with an ethnically diverse sample of adolescents. Youth were randomly assigned either to MET (n = 47) or to delayed treatment control (n = 50). MET did not significantly reduce marijuana use compared with a 3-month delayed control condition, but both conditions significantly reduced use from baseline. A nonstatistical difference in number of participants exhibiting a meaningful change (ie, having reduced baseline marijuana use by at least 50% or no longer reporting symptoms of abuse and/or dependence at 3-month follow-up) was also noted for the MET condition. This study provided some support for the usefulness and appropriateness of the school setting to intervene in heavy adolescent AOD use and suggested that assessment alone may reduce use, but provided no conclusive evidence for the efficacy of MET.

Winters and Leitten[40] tested 2 BIs, a brief intervention adolescent only (BI-A, n = 26) and a brief intervention with adolescents and a parental component (BI-AP, n = 26). A delayed treatment group served as a control condition (n = 27). Both BI conditions were associated with reduced drug use and related consequences, and these improvements exceeded the changes in the assessment-only control group. BI-AP exhibited greater and more consistent intervention effects compared with the BI-A condition. This study provided additional support for intervening in adolescent AOD use in the school setting. It also found clear empirical support for the efficacy of BI with mild to moderate AOD using adolescents particularly when a parental component was added.

In the first of 3 RCTs in schools in the United Kingdom, McCambridge and Strang[41] tested the effects of a single 1-hour MI (n = 105) against an "education as usual" condition (n = 95). At the 3-month follow-up, those in the MI condition had significant reductions of AOD use compared with the control group (Cohen's d effect sizes = 0.34 and 0.75 for alcohol and cannabis, respectively). A follow-up study noted that after 12 months these differential effects diminished to nonsignificant levels.[42] However, both groups achieved a small but statistically significant reduction in marijuana use frequency at 12 months.

A second study by McCambridge and colleagues[43] trained youth workers with the intervention model used in the first study.[41,42] In this quasi-experimental study, the MI group (n = 59) exhibited a statistically significant reduction in alcohol use compared with an assessment only condition (n = 103), but there was no evidence of impact on cannabis use.

A third study[44] focused on reducing marijuana use and for a comparison condition, the researchers developed a standardized protocol called drug information and advice-giving (DIA). The MI intervention (n = 94) did not reduce marijuana use outcomes more than the DIA intervention (n = 104). In this study, MI fidelity was assessed using the Motivational Interviewing Treatment Integrity instrument. Scores fell below proficiency and competency thresholds.[45] There were also practitioner-interaction effects such that clients seen by certain practitioners in the MI condition were significantly more likely to decrease their marijuana use. Thus, this study suffered from methodological limitations.

The 5 MI studies in schools produced mixed results. Three studies reported beneficial effects, but in 1 study, the initial positive effects[41] diminished at the 12-month follow-up.[42]

Community settings for homeless and other "hard to reach" youth

Two randomized studies targeted youth with hard AOD use in the United Kingdom and in Thailand. The first[46] evaluated an AMI intervention targeted for youth with moderate to heavy substance use. AMI included a self-assessment questionnaire, a single-session intervention, and standard printed information about the health risks of stimulant drugs and hazardous alcohol consumption. Both the intervention group (n = 166) and the control group consisting of health risk information only (n = 176) reported significant reductions in their stimulant use. However, there were no significant between-subjects effects for abstinence or changes in frequency and amount used.

The second study[47] examined the effects of BI (n = 24) compared with a psychoeducation control (n = 24) with methamphetamine abusing or dependent youth in Thailand. Results were mixed with some indication of superior effects of the BI group, including a statistically significant difference in the number of days per week of use compared at the 8-week follow-up assessment. Differences between conditions on other outcomes, such as amount used per occasion, were not significant but reductions from baseline were. This study supported the effectiveness of BI in reducing methamphetamine use relative to an assessment control. Moreover, this difference was found despite a significant reduction achieved by both conditions from baseline to the follow-up assessment.

Peterson and colleagues conducted 2 clinical trials with homeless adolescents. The first randomized trial[48] studied the effects of a single session ME (n = 92) compared with 2 control conditions: assessment only (AO, n = 99) and assessment at 1-month follow-up only (AFO, n = 94). ME was informed by the transtheoretical model of behavior change, the theory of reasoned action, and norm confrontation models.[49] An AFO was offered in addition to AO condition to address potential assessment reactivity or Hawthorne effects. ME participants reduced use of hard substances significantly more than the AO control condition at the 1-month (but not 3-month) follow-up, and no differences were found for marijuana or alcohol. Post hoc analyses within the ME group suggested that those who were rated as more engaged and more likely to benefit showed greater drug use reduction than did those rated as less engaged.

Baer and colleagues[50] made several modifications to their previous protocol to increase engagement. For example, instead of a single session, the BMI included up to 4 sessions (n = 66), which was compared with treatment as usual (n = 61). Youth experienced significant reductions in AOD use over time. However, there were no significant differences between conditions in AOD use.

These studies involving homeless and other "hard to reach" youth highlight the challenges associated with intervening with this high-risk population. It is likely that BMIs alone are not enough to cause lasting change in AOD use with these youth with many unmet needs. Thus, a more comprehensive intervention that also targets more needs may be needed.

Primary medical care settings

Three studies involving MI have been done in primary medical care settings. The first randomized study[51] tested a BMI intervention (Project CHAT, n = 38), against a standard care (SC, n = 26) control condition with a mostly Hispanic adolescent sample. Participants in the MI condition versus the SC condition exhibited statistically significant reductions in marijuana use as well as intentions to use marijuana, and prevalence estimates of marijuana use, with large reported effect sizes. Although trends for reductions in alcohol use were found, these effects were not statistically significant.

Two studies by the same research group were done in emergency departments in hospitals. The first randomized study[38] tested a BMI (n = 52) against standard care (SC, n = 42) with adolescents who had been drinking before the event that precipitated emergency medical attention. Both conditions resulted in reduced alcohol use, but BMI significantly outperformed SC in reducing drinking and driving and alcohol-related injuries, alcohol-related problems, and moving violations than SC at 6-month follow-up.

The second study[52] examined the effects of BMI (n = 78) compared with SC (n = 74) on alcohol-related consequences and use. Both conditions resulted in reduced quantity of drinking during the 12-month follow-up; however, alcohol-related negative consequences, which were already relatively low, stayed low at follow-up. Adolescents who screened positive for problematic alcohol use at baseline and who received MI, reported significantly reduced average number of drinking days per month and frequency of high-volume drinking, compared with SC.

These studies highlighted the utility of health care settings for adolescent AOD use intervention. Intervening in AOD and other risk behaviors in these settings has unique potential to affect adolescents, capitalizing on a potentially significant life event or "teachable moment."

Summary of Motivation Interviewing Treatments

Twelve different MI interventions were reviewed. All were individualized interventions and the quality of the studies was generally strong. Most (n = 5) of the studies were in school settings, followed by 3 in primary medical care settings, and 4 for homeless and other "hard to reach" youth. Most of the MI interventions were single session (n = 8), followed by 2 sessions (n = 3), and 1 of 4 sessions. Most of the studies involved youth with moderate to heavy use, and no studies targeted dually diagnosed individuals, although some studies clearly involved a majority with an AOD disorder.[47,48]

Given the brevity of the interventions and the relatively serious AOD problems, it is significant that there were effects. All of the studies reported reductions in at least one AOD through follow-up. MI had superior outcomes than comparison conditions on all indicators through follow-ups in 2 studies.[38,40] Five studies [43,47,48,51,52] reported significantly better outcomes than comparison conditions on some but not all outcome measures at follow-ups. When examining the criteria from Chambless and colleagues,[10–12] 2 studies demonstrated significant differences with a comparison condition, had adequate sample sizes, and had a treatment that performed better on many if not all indicators of AOD than the comparison condition.[38,41] However one of the studies subsequently completed a 12-month follow-up,[42] and failed to find sustained effects. Two additional studies[40,47] reported significant differences between the treatment and comparison conditions, but were insufficiently powered.[1] Thus, the body of research did not meet the criteria for "well-established" or "probably efficacious" treatments, but the MI interventions met the criteria as a "promising" intervention.[13] Thus, MI is a promising treatment choice, particularly in circumstances in which youth with significant AOD problems are not likely to seek treatment on their own, and brief treatment is offered opportunistically, such as in a primary medical care setting when other services are sought, or in school during class time.

Behavior Therapies Combined with Other Approaches

Some studies have combined BTs and/or MIs with other psychosocial treatments. Sometimes the purpose of such combinations is to have treatment elements target different problem or risk areas. Twelve interventions have been combined.

One of the studies reviewed earlier in this article included 2 combined treatments. Waldron and colleagues[31] included 2 combined conditions, one that paired CBT-I with MET (CBT-I/MET, n = 31) and a second that paired CBT-I/MET with functional family treatment (joint, n = 29). Recall that youths in the CBT-I/MET did not have significant reductions in percentage of days of marijuana use at either 4- or 7-month follow-ups, but did experience changes from heavy to minimal marijuana use at the 4-month follow-up. Youths in the joint condition had significant reductions in both indicators of marijuana use at 4- and 7-month follow-ups, but there were no significant differences between conditions.

Bailey and colleagues implemented a pilot study in Australia[53] involving youth at risk for alcohol problems. Youth were randomly assigned to either 4 sessions of a group that combined MI with CBT (MI/CBT-G, n = 17) or to a no-treatment condition (n = 17). Youth in the MI/CBT-G condition significantly increased their readiness to reduce or quit drinking by the second follow-up. Youths reduced the frequency of their drinking at posttreatment and at 1-month follow-up, whereas the control group reported increases at 2-month follow-up. As a result, youth in the MI/CBT-G condition experienced significant reductions in their frequency of drinking at posttreatment through the 2-month follow-up relative to the control group (largely because of the control group increasing its frequency of drinking at 2-month follow-up). Both groups had significantly reduced number of drinks consumed per drinking occasion. There was a significant difference between groups in pretest to 2-month follow-up in frequency of binge drinking and in hazardous drinking (largely because of the control group increasing their drinking in both areas compared with the treatment group).

Battjes and colleagues[54] examined the effectiveness of a CBT-G intervention that incorporated elements of both social learning theory, which explained how adult and peer role models began and continued AOD use, and operant conditioning theory, which explained how AOD use progressed and was maintained. CBT-G was the foundation on which 2 conditions were created, namely, 19 sessions of CBT-G with 1 session of MI (n = 95), and CBT-G with a 1-session counseling overview (CO, n = 99). In this quasi-experimental study, low to moderate AOD-using youth were assigned to either condition. Main outcomes were AOD use and criminal behaviors at 6- and 12-month follow-ups. Youths in both conditions experienced significant reductions in their marijuana use at 6-month follow-up, with reductions largely sustained at 12-month follow-up. However, there were no changes in alcohol use or criminal involvement. Type of treatment preparation (MI or CO) was not associated with marijuana use outcomes. In this study, the addition of MI to CBT-G did not have an additive effect.

The Cannabis Youth Treatment Study was a major effort to compare the efficacy of a number of short (3 months) interventions for adolescents with cannabis use.[55,56] Five short-term manualized treatments were tested in 2 separate RCTs.[57] In the first, 3 treatments were compared; 2 sessions of individual motivational enhancement therapy plus 3 sessions of group cognitive behavioral therapy (MET/CBT5, n = 102); 2 sessions of MET plus 10 sessions of group CBT (MET/CBT12, n = 96); and MET/CBT12 plus the family support network (FSN, n = 102). In the second trial, 3 treatments were compared: MET/CBT-5 (n = 100), 12 weeks of adolescent community reinforcement approach (ACRA, n = 100), and multidimensional family therapy (MDFT, n = 100). Across both trials, all treatments demonstrated significant pre-post reductions in AOD use and there were no significant differences among groups. Across conditions, half relapsed at least once through 12-month follow-up and two thirds were using AOD or had related problems, pointing to the need for continued ongoing treatment. The economic analysis indicated that the MET/CBT5 condition across both trials was the most cost-effective (better than all in the first trial, second to ACRA in the second trial). Thus, of the 2 MET/CBT interventions, MET/CBT5 was superior.

Guided Self-Change (GSC) was developed as a brief outpatient CBT-MI that incorporated self-management to help participants formulate and implement their own treatment plans.[58–60] GSC was developed for problem drinkers, not dependent on alcohol but still demonstrating alcohol problems. Breslin and colleagues[61] evaluated the First Contact program (FC), a GSC intervention that combined an assessment-feedback session plus 4 group sessions in a quasi-experimental design. The study examined both the effectiveness of FC (n = 22) and also whether further community treatment after the intervention increased the effectiveness of FC (FC+, n = 28). The study reported that youth in FC, with or without extra treatment, experienced significant reductions in substance use and number of consequences, and significantly increased confidence in high-risk situations, up to 6 months after program entry.

Latimer and colleagues[62] evaluated an intervention consisting of family and group CBT, called integrated family and cognitive therapy (IFCBT, n = 21), which was compared with psychoeducation (n = 22) in a randomized trial. IFCBT was informed by ecological theory, social learning, and family systems theory and consisted of 4 modules: 3 CBT modules offered in a group format delivered over 32 sessions, and 1 module offered in a family format delivered over 16 sessions. Both the group and family sessions were delivered concurrently. The comparison condition was called drug harm psychoeducation group (DHPE), and emphasized the physiologic consequences of drug use. IFCBT had substantial reductions in alcohol and marijuana use from pretest through 6-month follow-ups. IFCBT was significantly better than DHPE in reducing alcohol and marijuana use, and in improving problem-solving and school learning skills, during the 6-month follow-up, with medium to strong effect sizes. Thus, the IFCBT appeared to be successful in targeting putative cognitive mechanisms related to AOD use.

Liddle and colleagues[63] compared MDFT (n = 112) with CBT-I plus family (n = 112). CBT-I incorporated elements of dialectical behavior therapy, along with social learning, classical and operant principles, and cognitive elements. Clinicians within the CBT-I condition used a modular approach in selecting treatment strategies. Examples of modules included providing information, contingency contracting, self-monitoring, problem-solving training, communication skills training, identifying cognitive distortions, and homework. The CBT-I also included a family-involved component in that parents attended the first 2 sessions. This study is notable because it included a large sample of African Americans (72%). Both treatments demonstrated statistically significant reductions in AOD problem severity and frequency of cannabis use at 12-month follow-up. There were no significant differences between conditions with respect to frequency of cannabis use or with alcohol use through 12-month follow-up. However, those in the MDFT condition reported significantly less AOD problem severity, other drug use, and a significantly higher proportion of youth reported minimal AOD use or abstinence at 6- and 12-month follow-ups. Thus, this study demonstrated that CBT-I was effective in reducing AOD use and problems, and on some AOD variables was as effective as MDFT, but that MDFT had superior effects across more AOD outcomes.

Martin and Copeland[64] compared a 2-session motivational and CBT intervention called the adolescent cannabis check-up (ACCU, n = 20) to a 3-month delayed-treatment control condition (DTC, n = 20). After an initial detailed assessment session, a feedback and skills intervention session was provided. An optional component of the second session included practical strategies for quitting and reducing use including a discussion of triggers, managing craving, goal setting, and relapse prevention. ACCU had significant and substantial reductions in cannabis use from baseline to 3-month follow-up, and when compared with DTC (medium to strong effect sizes).

A study in the Netherlands[65] compared the efficacy of a combined CBT-G and MI intervention (n = 53), compared with an information-only control (n = 54). The treatment consisted of 7 sessions that combined 6 sessions of group-based CBT followed by 1 session of an adapted form of MI based on the Brief Alcohol Screening and Intervention for College Students (BASICS) program.[66] The intervention was effective in changing several of the targeted cognitive determinants, such as a significant increase in the perception of risk factors for developing alcohol problems and a significant decrease in positive alcohol expectancies in the experimental versus control group. However, despite these changes in cognitive determinants of drinking, the treatment group failed to show a significant difference in decrease of drinking at posttest compared with the control group through follow-ups. Thus, the putative mechanisms for explaining alcohol use failed to suggest that targeting cognitive domain is sufficient.

Summary of Combined Treatments

Twelve combined interventions were reviewed. CBT was combined with MI in all but 3 cases, which combined family treatment with CBT.[31,62,63] Many of the combined approaches were done in groups. Not counting the replication of MET/CBT-5, half of the interventions involved some form of group treatment. The duration of treatments ranged from as low as 2 sessions (ACCU)[64] to 24 sessions (joint),[31] with a median of 10 sessions. In terms of outcomes, most of the studies had significant changes in AOD use from pretest through follow-ups, but only 3 had most or all outcomes significantly better than the other condition,[53,62,64] and only 1 with some differences in favor of a joint condition.[31] In terms of overall efficacy of the approaches using the criteria from Chambless and colleagues,[10–12] none of the studies could be considered "well-established" or "probably efficacious," largely because there was no replication of the same intervention by a different investigating team and/or because the intervention was not superior to the comparison or control condition. However, they met the criteria as "promising" interventions,[13] but marginally so, given the very low sample sizes in each condition. In all studies involving group treatment, there were positive changes in AOD use and not one report of iatrogenic effects.

DISCUSSION

This article reviewed 36 different interventions across 34 peer-reviewed publications; 12 each of BTs, MIs, and BT plus psychosocial approaches. Across interventions, most demonstrated significant changes from pretest to follow-ups. For the BTs, 12 different BT interventions were tested in group or individual modalities. Most of the BTs demonstrated significant changes from pretest through follow-ups. Although half of the BT interventions[19,21,22,25,28,30] had superior outcomes on at least 1 comparison condition on an AOD variable, only 2 had sufficient sample sizes and a treatment that performed better than the comparison conditions on many if not all indicators of AOD use.[21,30] Thus, the BT interventions met the criteria for "probably efficacious." This finding can be compared with the conclusions of 2 other recent reviews that examined the BT evidence. One that included a rigorous quality-of-study analysis[1] concluded that BTs have evidence of treatment superiority in at least 2 methodologically strong studies. Waldron and Turner[7] evaluated whether treatments included in their meta-analysis were significantly better than a minimally treated condition, which was derived from pooled findings from the studies included in their meta-analysis. Using such methodology, they reported that CBT-G was considered a "well-established" treatment and that CBT-I was considered "promising." Thus, the findings from this and the other 2 reviews support the efficacy of BTs in the treatment of adolescent AOD use. When considering both within and across treatment changes over time, most of the CBT interventions were helpful in significantly, and in many cases substantially, reducing AOD use over time, which makes individual and group-based BTs clear clinical choices.

For the 12 different MI interventions, all had significant reductions in at least one AOD indicator through follow-up. Except for 4 studies that demonstrated no significant differences between conditions on AOD outcomes,[39,42,44,46] most of the studies had superior outcomes than comparison conditions on some or all indicators through follow-ups. The body of MI research met the criteria as a "promising" intervention. Becker and Curry's review[1] noted that MIs had superior evidentiary support in 2 or more methodologically strong studies. Thus, MI approaches may be viewed as a good treatment option. Many of the MI studies indicated that both nontreatment-seeking but AOD-involved adolescents, and youth with SUDs can be recruited into treatment. As a stepped approach, this could be valuable. In addition, there is good evidence for the efficacy of MI treatments in health care settings.

There were 12 combined BT plus other psychosocial interventions. Most of these demonstrated significant changes in AOD use from pretest through follow-ups, but only 3 had most or all outcomes significantly better than the other condition, although the samples sizes were only about 20 in each condition.[53,62,64] Two of these were combined MI and CBT interventions, but given their very low sample sizes (mean of 18.5), combined approaches may be classified only marginally as a "promising" intervention.

Table 1 offers a summary of the level of evidence for the treatments reviewed, along with the support from the 2 recent systematic reviews. BTs are recommended and MI interventions are also a viable treatment choice. There is less evidence for combined psychosocial approaches. The most effective therapy for serious and comorbid disorders are BTs. For youth with mild AOD use, or for a treatment that is suitable for locations that are not primary AOD treatment settings, such as schools or medical settings, MI is perhaps the first choice. However, the 2 brief, group-based CBTs are also good options.[21,30] Most of the BT interventions and a few of the combined interventions were group-based. The evidence clearly supports the efficacy of group-based interventions in reducing alcohol and in some cases, related problems.

The findings should be interpreted in light of methodological issues that attenuated the findings, and which should inform future research. Overall, the studies used designs that were methodologically rigorous and used control (routine or standard treatment) and comparison conditions. In the case of BTs, clear methodological improvements have been made when compared with the studies before the 1990s. However, improvements in methodology are sorely needed, such as increasing the sample sizes in the conditions. Many of the BT and MI studies that demonstrated superior effects over the comparison condition did not have adequate sample sizes, many below 20. Adequately powered studies are important to detect differences and to meet the criteria of "well-established." In particular, studies continue to have

---

Table 1
Efficacy of behavior therapies, motivational interviewing, and combined psychosocial approaches

Treatment	Level of Evidence[a]	Settings	Problem Severity	Reports from Recent Systematic Reviews[b]
Behavior therapies[c]	Probably efficacious	Outpatient	Mild to heavy use; SUDs; DD	BTs: "Evidence of treatment superiority"[1]; BT-G: "Well-established"[7]; BT-I: "Promising"[7]
Motivational interviewing	Promising	Schools; Community clinics; Hospitals	Mild to heavy use, SUDs	"Evidence of treatment superiority"[1]
Behavior therapies + psychosocial	Promising[d]	Mostly outpatient	Mild to heavy use; SUDs	NA

Abbreviations: BTs, behavior therapies; BT-G, group-based behavior therapy; BT-I, behavior therapy with individuals; DD, dual-diagnosis; NA, not available; SUD, substance use disorder.
   [a] Levels of evidence: well-established, probably efficacious[10]; Promising.[13]
   [b] Systematic reviews since 2004.
   [c] Excludes contingency management approaches.
   [d] Marginally classified as "promising" because of low sample sizes.

insufficient sample sizes in the group condition. There is a critical need to sufficiently power group-based studies, to account not only for group-level phenomenon, such as cohesion or compositional variables, but also to manage the problem of nonindependence of observations, which can lead to spurious "significant" results.[67,68] Other methodological needs include strengthening the randomization process (eg, computerized generation, assignment concealment from investigators), more clear and complete reporting of study objectives and primary outcomes, wider use of intent-to-treat analyses, and outcome assessment by independent evaluators.[1]

REFERENCES

1. Becker SJ, Curry JF. Outpatient interventions for adolescent substance abuse: a quality of evidence review. J Consult Clin Psychol 2008;76(4):531–43.
2. Deas D, Thomas SE. An overview of controlled studies of adolescent substance abuse treatment. Am J Addict 2001;10(2):178–89.
3. Engle BC, Macgowan MJ. A critical review of adolescent substance abuse group treatments. J Evid Based Soc Work 2009;6(3):217–43.
4. Perepletchikova F, Krystal JH, Kaufman J. Practitioner review: adolescent alcohol use disorders: assessment and treatment issues. J Child Psychol Psychiatry 2008;49(11):1131–54.
5. Vaughn MG, Howard MO. Adolescent substance abuse treatment: a synthesis of controlled evaluations. Research On Social Work Practice 2004;14(5): 325–35.
6. Waldron HB, Kaminer Y. On the learning curve: the emerging evidence supporting cognitive-behavioral therapies for adolescent substance abuse. Addiction 2004;99(Suppl 2):93–105.
7. Waldron HB, Turner CW. Evidence-based psychosocial treatments for adolescent substance abuse: a review and meta-analysis. J Clin Child Adolesc Psychol 2008;37(1):236–59.
8. Williams RJ, Chang SY. A comprehensive and comparative review of adolescent substance abuse treatment outcome. Clinical Psychology: Science & Practice 2000;7(2):138–66.
9. Winters KC, Botzet AM, Fahnhorst T, et al. Adolescent substance abuse treatment: a review of evidence-based research. In: Leukefeld CG, Gullotta TP, Staton-Tindall M, editors. Adolescent substance abuse: evidence-based approaches to prevention and treatment. New York (NY): Springer; 2009. p. 73–96.
10. Chambless DL, Baker MJ, Baucom DH, et al. Update on empirically validated therapies. II. Clin Psychol 1998;51(1):3–16.
11. Chambless DL, Sanderson WC, Shoham V, et al. An update on empirically validated therapies. Clin Psychol 1996;49(2):5–18.
12. Chambless DL, Hollon SD. Defining empirically supported therapies. J Consult Clin Psychol 1998;66(1):7–18.
13. Spirito A. Introduction to the special issue on empirically supported treatments in pediatric psychology. J Pediatr Psychol 1999;24(2):87–90.
14. Miller WR, Wilbourne PL, Hettema JE. What works? A summary of alcohol treatment outcome research. In: Hester RK, Miller WB, editors. Handbook of alcoholism treatment approaches: effective alternatives. 3rd edition. Boston: Allyn & Bacon; 2003. p. 13–63.
15. Carroll KM, Onken LS. Behavioral therapies for drug abuse. Am J Psychiatry 2005;162(8):1452–60.

16. Finney JW, Wilbourne PL, Moos RH. Psychosocial treatments for substance use disorders. In: Nathan PE, Gorman JM, editors. A guide to treatments that work. New York: Oxford University Press; 2007. p. 179–202.

17. Catalano RF, Hawkins JD, Wells EA, et al. Evaluation of the effectiveness of adolescent drug abuse treatment, assessment of risks for relapse, and promising approaches for relapse prevention. Int J Addict 1990;25(9A–10A): 1085–140.

18. Davidge AM, Forman SG. Psychological treatment of adolescent substance abusers: a review. Child Youth Serv Rev 1988;10(1):43–55.

19. Azrin NH, Donohue B, Besalel V, et al. Youth drug abuse treatment: a controlled outcome study. J Child Adolesc Subst Abuse 1994;3:1–16.

20. Azrin NH, Donohue B, Teichner GA, et al. A controlled evaluation and description of individual-cognitive problem solving and family-behavior therapies in dually-diagnosed conduct-disordered and substance-dependent youth. J Child Adolesc Subst Abuse 2001;11(1):1–43.

21. Conrod PJ, Stewart SH, Comeau N, et al. Efficacy of cognitive-behavioral interventions targeting personality risk factors for youth alcohol misuse. J Clin Child Adolesc Psychol 2006;35(4):550–63.

22. Kaminer Y, Burleson JA, Blitz C, et al. Psychotherapies for adolescent substance abusers: a pilot study. J Nerv Ment Dis 1998;186(11):684–90.

23. Kaminer Y, Burleson JA. Psychotherapies for adolescent substance abusers: 15-month follow-up of a pilot study. Am J Addict 1999;8(2):114–9.

24. Kaminer Y, Burleson JA, Goldberger R. Cognitive-behavioral coping skills and psychoeducation therapies for adolescent substance abuse. J Nerv Ment Dis 2002;190(11):737–45.

25. Liddle HA, Dakof GA, Parker K, et al. Multidimensional family therapy for adolescent drug abuse: results of a randomized clinical trial. Am J Drug Alcohol Abuse 2001;27(4):651–88.

26. Liddle HA, Rowe CL, Dakof GA, et al. Early intervention for adolescent substance abuse: pretreatment to posttreatment outcomes of a randomized clinical trial comparing multidimensional family therapy and peer group treatment. J Psychoactive Drugs 2004;36(1):49–63.

27. Liddle HA, Rowe CL, Dakof GA, et al. Multidimensional family therapy for young adolescent substance abuse: twelve-month outcomes of a randomized controlled trial. J Consult Clin Psychol 2009;77(1):12–25.

28. Najavits LM, Gallop RJ, Weiss RD. Seeking safety therapy for adolescent girls with PTSD and substance use disorder: a randomized controlled trial. J Behav Health Serv Res 2006;33(4):453–63.

29. Smith DC, Hall JA, Williams JK, et al. Comparative efficacy of family and group treatment for adolescent substance abuse. Am J Addict 2006;15(Supp l1):131–6.

30. Stice E, Rohde P, Seeley JR, et al. Brief cognitive-behavioral depression prevention program for high-risk adolescents outperforms two alternative interventions: a randomized efficacy trial. J Consult Clin Psychol 2008;76(4):595–606.

31. Waldron HB, Slesnick N, Brody JL, et al. Treatment outcomes for adolescent substance abuse at 4- and 7-month assessments. J Consult Clin Psychol 2001; 69(5):802–13.

32. Miller WR. Motivational interviewing with problem drinkers. Behavioural Psychotherapy 1983;11(2):147–72.

33. Tevyaw TO, Monti PM. Motivational enhancement and other brief interventions for adolescent substance abuse: foundations, applications and evaluations. Addiction 2004;99(Suppl 2):63–75.

34. Miller WR, Rollnick S. Ten things that motivational interviewing is not. Behav Cogn Psychother 2009;37(2):129–40.
35. Rollnick S, Miller WR, Butler C. Motivational interviewing in health care: helping patients change behavior. New York: Guilford Press; 2008.
36. Burke BL, Arkowitz H, Menchola M. The efficacy of motivational interviewing: a meta-analysis of controlled clinical trials. J Consult Clin Psychol 2003;71(5): 843–61.
37. Vasilaki EI, Hosier SG, Cox WM. The efficacy of motivational interviewing as a brief intervention for excessive drinking: a meta-analytic review. Alcohol Alcohol 2006; 41(3):328–35.
38. Monti PM, Colby SM, Barnett NP, et al. Brief intervention for harm reduction with alcohol-positive older adolescents in a hospital emergency department. J Consult Clin Psychol 1999;67(6):989–94.
39. Walker DD, Roffman RA, Stephens RS, et al. Motivational enhancement therapy for adolescent marijuana users: a preliminary randomized controlled trial. J Consult Clin Psychol 2006;74(3):628–32.
40. Winters KC, Leitten W. Brief intervention for drug-abusing adolescents in a school setting. Psychol Addict Behav 2007;21(2):249–54.
41. McCambridge J, Strang J. The efficacy of single-session motivational interviewing in reducing drug consumption and perceptions of drug-related risk and harm among young people: results from a multi-site cluster randomized trial. Addiction 2004;99(1):39–52.
42. McCambridge J, Strang J. Deterioration over time in effect of motivational interviewing in reducing drug consumption and related risk among young people. Addiction 2005;100(4):470–8.
43. Gray E, McCambridge J, Strang J. The effectiveness of motivational interviewing delivered by youth workers in reducing drinking, cigarette and cannabis smoking among young people: quasi-experimental pilot study. Alcohol Alcohol 2005;40: 535–9.
44. McCambridge J, Slym RL, Strang J. Randomized controlled trial of motivational interviewing compared with drug information and advice for early intervention among young cannabis users. Addiction 2008;103(11):1809–18.
45. Moyers TB, Martin T, Manuel JK, et al. Assessing competence in the use of motivational interviewing. J Subst Abuse Treat 2005;28:19–26.
46. Marsden J, Stillwell G, Barlow H, et al. An evaluation of a brief motivational intervention among young ecstasy and cocaine users: no effect on substance and alcohol use outcomes. Addiction 2006;101(7):1014–26.
47. Srisurapanont M, Sombatmai S, Boripuntakul T. Brief intervention for students with methamphetamine use disorders: a randomized controlled trial. Am J Addict 2007;16(2):111–6.
48. Peterson PL, Baer JS, Wells EA, et al. Short-term effects of a brief motivational intervention to reduce alcohol and drug risk among homeless adolescents. Psychol Addict Behav 2006;20(3):254–64.
49. Baer JS, Peterson PL, Wells EA. Rationale and design of a brief substance use intervention for homeless adolescents. Addict Res Theory 2004;12(4):317–34.
50. Baer JS, Garrett SB, Beadnell B, et al. Brief motivational intervention with homeless adolescents: evaluating effects on substance use and service utilization. Psychol Addict Behav 2007;21(4):582–6.
51. D'Amico EJ, Miles JNV, Stern SA, et al. Brief motivational interviewing for teens at risk of substance use consequences: a randomized pilot study in a primary care clinic. J Subst Abuse Treat 2008;35(1):53–61.

52. Spirito A, Monti PM, Barnett NP, et al. A randomized clinical trial of a brief motivational intervention for alcohol-positive adolescents treated in an emergency department. J Pediatr 2004;145(3):396–402.

53. Bailey K, Baker A, Webster R, et al. Pilot randomized controlled trial of a brief alcohol intervention group for adolescents. Drug Alcohol Rev 2004;23(2):157–66.

54. Battjes RJ, Gordon MS, O'Grady KE, et al. Evaluation of a group-based substance abuse treatment program for adolescents. J Subst Abuse Treat 2004;27(2):123–34.

55. Dennis ML, Titus JC, Diamond G, et al. The Cannabis Youth Treatment (CYT) experiment: rationale, study design and analysis plans. Addiction 2002;97(s1): 16–34.

56. Diamond G, Godley SH, Liddle HA, et al. Five outpatient treatment models for adolescent marijuana use: a description of the Cannabis Youth Treatment Interventions. Addiction 2002;97(s1):70–83.

57. Dennis ML, Godley SH, Diamond G, et al. The Cannabis Youth Treatment (CYT) Study: main findings from two randomized trials. J Subst Abuse Treat 2004;27(3): 197–213.

58. Sobell MB, Sobell LC. Guided self-change model of treatment for substance use disorders. J Cogn Psychother 2005;19(3):199–210.

59. Sobell MB, Sobell LC. Problem drinkers: guided self-change treatment. New York: Guilford Press; 1993.

60. Sobell MB, Sobell LC. Guiding self-change treatment. In: Miller WR, Heather N, editors. Treating addictive behaviors: processes of change. 2nd edition. New York: Plenum; 1998. p. 189–202.

61. Breslin C, Li S, Sdao-Jarvie K, et al. Brief treatment for young substance abusers: a pilot study in an addiction treatment setting. Psychol Addict Behav 2002;16(1): 10–6.

62. Latimer WW, Winters KC, D'Zurilla T, et al. Integrated family and cognitive-behavioral therapy for adolescent substance abusers: a stage I efficacy study. Drug Alcohol Depend 2003;71(3):303–17.

63. Liddle HA, Dakof GA, Turner RM, et al. Treating adolescent drug abuse: a randomized trial comparing multidimensional family therapy and cognitive behavior therapy. Addiction 2008;103(10):1660–70.

64. Martin G, Copeland J. The adolescent cannabis check up: randomized trial of a brief intervention for young cannabis users. J Subst Abuse Treat 2008;34(4): 407–14.

65. Thush C, Wiers RW, Theunissen N, et al. A randomized clinical trial of a targeted intervention to moderate alcohol use and alcohol-related problems in at-risk adolescents. Pharmacol Biochem Behav 2007;86(2):368–76.

66. Dimeff LA. Brief Alcohol Screening and Intervention for College Students (BASICS): a harm reduction approach. New York: Guilford Press; 1999.

67. Johnson JE, Burlingame GM, Olsen JA, et al. Group climate, cohesion, alliance, and empathy in group psychotherapy: Multilevel Structural Equation Models. J Couns Psychol 2005;52(3):310–21.

68. Macgowan MJ. A guide to evidence-based group work. New York: Oxford University Press; 2008.

Contingency Management Approaches for Adolescent Substance Use Disorders

Catherine Stanger, PhD*, Alan J. Budney, PhD

KEYWORDS

- Contingency management • Adolescent substance abuse
- Marijuana • Parenting

An emerging literature indicates that adolescents in treatment for substance abuse have better outcomes than those not in treatment, and suggests that multiple types of behavioral interventions hold promise.[1] Treatments with empirical support from well-designed, randomized clinical trials include group and individual cognitive behavioral therapy (CBT), CBT combined with motivational enhancement therapy (MET), community reinforcement approach counseling (CRA), functional family therapy, multidimensional family therapy (MDFT), multisystemic therapy (MST), brief strategic family therapy, family support network (FSN), and family behavior therapy. The MET and CBT interventions that have been tested are similar in scope and duration to those used with adults. The family-focused interventions take advantage of social networks (parents, schools, and other social agencies) that are unique to adolescents. These interventions generally include efforts to address and alter maladaptive family patterns that contribute to substance use (eg, parent drug use, parent-child relationships, parent supervision), make use of resources in the school and criminal justice system, and address problems that might be associated with the child's peer network. Although they have yet to be clearly supported by the empirical literature,[2,3] some assert that these behaviorally based, family approaches produce a more potent effect than those that do not include a family component.

This work was supported by NIDA Grant DA15186, NIAAA Grant AA016917, and the Arkansas Biosciences Institute, the major research component of the Arkansas Master Tobacco Settlement.

Center for Addiction Research, Department of Psychiatry, University of Arkansas for Medical Sciences, 4301 West Markham Street #843, Little Rock, AR 72205, USA

* Corresponding author.

E-mail address: cstanger@uams.edu

Child Adolesc Psychiatric Clin N Am 19 (2010) 547–562

doi:10.1016/j.chc.2010.03.007

childpsych.theclinics.com

Even with the most potent interventions tested to date, reductions in substance use observed have been modest, and robust effects on abstinence rates have been difficult to prove. For example, the largest published clinical trial included adolescents aged 12 to 18 years who endorsed at least 1 criterion for cannabis abuse or dependence and had used cannabis in the previous 90 days.[2] Adolescents received 1 of 5 treatment treatments across 4 clinical sites: MET/CBT5 (2 individual and 3 group sessions), MET/CBT12 (2 individual and 10 group sessions), MET/CBT12 plus FSN, adolescent CRA, and MDFT. Significant decreases in drug use and symptoms of dependence were observed following each of the treatments. However, robust between-treatment differences in outcomes were not observed. Although reductions in drug use were promising compared with that observed in prior treatment studies, approximately two-thirds of the young people continued to experience significant substance-related symptoms. That is, many never achieve abstinence or substantial reductions in cannabis use, and many of those who are initially successful relapse. These findings, combined with the similarly modest effects reported in studies examining the family-focused and individual/group therapies mentioned earlier, indicate a strong need for continued exploration and development of more potent adolescent treatment models and interventions.[4] Moreover, few studies have attempted to isolate active components of multifaceted treatments and little is known about mechanisms of action for the positive effects observed across studies.[1]

One alternative candidate for enhancing outcomes with a strong probability of success is contingency management (CM) based interventions. CM interventions are based on extensive basic science and clinical research evidence showing that drug use and abuse are sensitive to systematically applied environmental consequences (ie, reinforcement and punishment contingencies).[5] CM approaches have become one of the most thoroughly researched and effective behavioral procedures to increase drug abstinence and other treatment targets across adult substance-dependence disorders[6–8]; however, such interventions have received only minimal attention in the adolescent treatment literature. Clinical studies across multiple, adult substance-dependent populations have shown the efficacy of various types of CM interventions for increasing (1) abstinence from alcohol, cannabis, cocaine, methamphetamine, and opiates; (2) counseling attendance and retention in treatment; (3) compliance with medications like naltrexone; and (4) completion of therapeutic activities.

CM CONCEPTUALIZATION AND BASIC PRINCIPLES

CM applications are derived from an operant framework, in which substance use is considered operant behavior that is maintained, in part, by the pharmacologic actions of the substance in conjunction with social and other nonpharmacologic reinforcement derived from a substance-using lifestyle. An important feature of this conceptual model is that it facilitates a direct connection between clinical practice and the scientific disciplines of behavior analysis and behavioral pharmacology. Those disciplines include an extensive research literature showing principles and procedures that can be applied to modify behavior of all kinds, including substance use and misuse. A major strength of conceptualizing substance abuse as an operant behavior is that, as such, it is amenable to change via the same processes and principles as other types of human behavior irrespective of its cause. The treatment goal is to systematically weaken the influence of reinforcement derived from substance use and its related lifestyle, and to increase the frequency and magnitude of reinforcement derived from healthier alternative activities, especially those that are incompatible with continued substance use.

The CM approach capitalizes on knowledge that drug seeking and drug use can be directly modified by manipulating the relevant environmental contingencies. Typically, CM interventions are used to engender therapeutic change within a comprehensive treatment program in a substance-abuse treatment clinic. CM programs arrange the therapeutic environment such that (1) target therapeutic behaviors such as drug abstinence, counseling attendance, and medication compliance are carefully monitored, and (2) reinforcing or punishing events (eg, tangible rewards or incentives, suspension of employment or school, loss of privileges) occur when the target behavior is or is not achieved.

Within the adult substance-abuse treatment literature, CM interventions have primarily involved the use of positive reinforcement; however, negative reinforcement, positive punishment, and negative punishment contingencies can also motivate increases and decreases in therapeutic target goals. This article provides clarification of these 4 basic processes that can be used to design effective CM interventions. Positive reinforcement involves delivery of a desired consequence (eg, tangible goods or services, social praise, increased privileges) contingent on meeting a therapeutic goal (eg, negative urinalysis test results, attendance at a counseling session). Negative reinforcement involves removing an aversive or confining circumstance (eg, criminal justice supervision, early curfew, grounding) contingent on meeting a therapeutic goal. Positive punishment involves delivery of a punishing consequence (eg, suspension for school, loss of phone or computer use, grounding) contingent on evidence of undesirable behavior (eg, positive urinalysis test result). Negative punishment involves removal of a positive circumstance or condition (eg, reduction in the value of rewards that could be earned, removal or reduction of privileges) contingent on evidence of the occurrence of an undesirable behavior.

Reinforcement and punishment contingencies can be effective tools in substance-abuse treatment programs. Typically use of positive reinforcement is preferred to punishment. Caution is indicated when considering use of punishment contingencies without careful planning, as these may inadvertently increase undesirable behaviors such as treatment dropout or negatively affect therapeutic relationships. Almost all CM applications developed for adults have used positive reinforcement principles.[5]

CM IMPLEMENTATION

Behavioral analytical theory and the empirical literature on behavior change suggest that the efficacy of CM interventions is influenced by 5 variables: the schedule used to deliver consequences, the magnitude of the consequence, the choice of the target behavior, the selection of the type of consequence, and the monitoring of the target behavior (**Fig. 1**).[9] The schedule of reinforcement or punishment refers to the temporal relation between the target behavior and the delivery of the consequence. Generally, efficacy is likely to improve as the temporal delay between the occurrence of the target behavior and delivery of the consequence decreases. For example, all else being equal, providing positive reinforcement for drug abstinence 5 minutes after a client submits a negative urine specimen would likely engender greater rates of abstinence than waiting a week before reinforcement is delivered. Similarly, more frequent schedules of reinforcement are usually preferable to less frequent schedules in establishing an initial target behavior like drug abstinence or regular attendance at counseling sessions. Frequent schedules allow multiple opportunities to reinforce and thereby strengthen the target behavior. Once a target behavior is established, less frequent schedules are typically considered for maintenance of behavior change. Two schedules that have shown efficacy across multiple substance-abuse treatment studies are

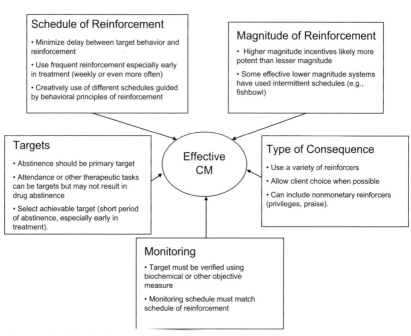

Schedule of Reinforcement

• Minimize delay between target behavior and reinforcement

• Use frequent reinforcement especially early in treatment (weekly or even more often)

• Creatively use of different schedules guided by behavioral principles of reinforcement

Magnitude of Reinforcement

• Higher magnitude incentives likely more potent than lesser magnitude

• Some effective lower magnitude systems have used intermittent schedules (e.g., fishbowl)

Targets

• Abstinence should be primary target

• Attendance or other therapeutic tasks can be targets but may not result in drug abstinence

• Select achievable target (short period of abstinence, especially early in treatment).

Effective CM

Type of Consequence

• Use a variety of reinforcers

• Allow client choice when possible

• Can include nonmonetary reinforcers (privileges, praise).

Monitoring

• Target must be verified using biochemical or other objective measure

• Monitoring schedule must match schedule of reinforcement

Fig. 1. Key principles in CM implementation.

a fixed schedule with escalating rewards and a reset contingency (typically referred to as abstinence-based vouchers or incentives[5]) and an intermittent schedule of rewards using the fishbowl method.[10] Both schedules are described in more detail later in the context of our adolescent CM program.

The magnitude of reinforcement or punishment is also an important factor that can affect the efficacy of CM interventions. For example, if the goal is drug abstinence, a $10 incentive for each negative drug test is likely to be more effective in increasing abstinence than one worth $2.00. Given the resilience of substance use, strong reinforcers may be necessary to compete with the reinforcement derived from well-established use patterns. Multiple studies have shown that greater magnitude schedules of reinforcement have resulted in better abstinence outcomes than lower magnitude.[11] Creative use of low-magnitude reinforcers and variable or intermittent schedules can successfully modify target behaviors among drug abusers.[12] However, as one would expect, the larger the incentives the higher the probability of motivating behavior change in a greater proportion of cases. In addition, larger magnitude incentives have been shown to be more cost-effective than lower magnitude incentives.[13,14]

The type of reinforcers or punishers used in a CM program can be critical to its success. Individuals vary greatly in the types of goods and services that serve as reinforcers. For example, a specific reinforcer (eg, pizza or movie theater passes) that serves as an effective incentive for one client may not be reinforcing for another. Use of a range of incentives or allowing clients to choose their incentive can increase the probability that the incentive serves as a reinforcer and facilitates the desired target behavior. Incentives used in adult CM programs have ranged from cash, choice of gift cards, on-site retail items, increased chance of receiving prizes, desirable clinic privileges, employment or housing opportunities, and refunds of treatment service fees.[8] Each of these has its strengths and drawbacks, and must be tailored to the needs and limitations of the clinic.

The most commonly selected target behavior used in adult CM programs has been drug abstinence. CM programs, however, have also targeted medication compliance, counseling attendance, and completion of lifestyle change activities. When choosing targets, one should be aware that successful change in one behavior may not result in change in another. For example, treatment attendance may improve by providing incentives for coming to sessions, but drug use might not be affected.[15] The extant adult CM literature suggests that the first choice of a target behavior should be drug use. When selecting other targets, these should be specific, individualized behavioral goals that have a high probability for successful completion.

Effective monitoring of the targeted behavior is essential to a CM program, because consequences (reinforcement or punishment) must be applied systematically. With substance abusers, this typically involves some form of biochemical verification of drug abstinence, usually via urinalysis testing. Such testing requires careful planning so that the schedule of testing (frequency) allows optimal detection of substance use and abstinence. The testing program used in our studies, which illustrates the multiple issues involved in and importance of choosing a monitoring schedule that optimizes efficacy, is described later. The importance of having a method for objectively and reliably verifying whether a target behavior occurred also pertains to other target behaviors. Reliance on self-reports of drug use or completion of other therapeutic tasks is not adequate for effective delivery of a CM program.

CM FOR ADOLESCENT SUBSTANCE ABUSE

Several factors indicate that CM interventions would likely enhance outcomes for adolescent substance abusers. First, the empirically based principles of behavior and behavior change from which CM strategies are derived are applicable to all humans and nonhuman species. Given the clear and robust data supporting CM for adult substance-use treatment outcomes, there is strong reason to expect that similar, CM-based intervention alternatives would be effective for adolescents. Second, adolescents rarely seek treatment on their own but instead enter treatment because their parents, school, or the judicial system require it. Most adolescents show low motivation to quit or remain abstinent and do not typically see their use as a significant problem in need of treatment.[16] CM interventions can offer clear incentives (eg, tangible positive reinforcers) for quitting that are designed to enhance or engender initial or long-term motivation to abstain. Third, these referral agents that direct adolescents into treatment (families, schools, legal authorities) are also potential sources for the implementation of CM strategies that could enhance initial motivation for abstinence and for maintaining treatment gains by continuing to provide CM following a treatment episode. Such interventions could be effective additions or alternatives to clinic-based treatments.

ADOLESCENT CM RESEARCH

Although not clearly labeled as such, CM strategies seem to be at least a small component of the empirically based family interventions mentioned earlier. Several studies describe use of CM-like procedures as part of the multicomponent intervention being examined (eg, instructing parents to provide rewards and consequences for abstinence or substance use, or other problem behavior targets or instructing therapists to reinforce abstinence).[3,17–19] The descriptions of these procedures typically do not provide enough detail to determine the type, schedule, magnitude, or monitoring procedures of the CM-type components being administered, and none of these early studies attempted to isolate and test the CM components. Azrin and colleagues[20] did provide such details about their CM program that included structured parental reinforcement of drug-incompatible activities (which could be monitored by parents at home), but did not specifically target drug abstinence per se.

There are a few recent examples of the use of CM to target adolescent tobacco use. Krishnan-Sarin and colleagues[21] found that young people participating in a school-based tobacco-cessation program who received an abstinence-based incentive intervention and CBT had greater rates of tobacco abstinence than young people who received CBT alone. A total of 53% of CM young people were abstinent for the entire 4-week intervention period, compared with 0% of the CBT-only group. The CM procedures were reported in a highly replicable fashion and they included twice-daily breath carbon monoxide (CO) assessment in week 1, fading to every other day in week 4, an escalating incentive schedule with a reset, payments to both groups for attending sessions, noncontingent payments to the CBT-only group for providing samples, earnings of up to $313.75 cash in the CM group for 4 weeks of abstinence, and objective and clearly specified definitions of abstinence. In a second trial, Cavallo and colleagues[22] compared the same CBT+CM protocol with 3 brief (10–15 minute) CBT sessions per week + the same CM protocol (frequent brief behavioral intervention [FBBI]). These investigators reported a 4-week abstinence rate of 57.1% in the weekly CBT+CM condition, not significantly different from the rate of 38.5% in the 3 times per week FBBI+CM condition. A 2-month follow-up found that 12.5% of the young people who received weekly CBT+CM and 28.6% of the young people who received FBBI+CM were abstinent, also not significantly different. Adding CM to CBT clearly boosts abstinence rates dramatically in the short-term; however, the high relapse rates suggest the need for longer duration interventions.

Another CM program for adolescent smoking, a Web-based 30-day intervention, was tested using a reversal design with 4 young people.[23] All 4 participants achieved abstinence, and 3 of the 4 participants met abstinence criteria when incentives were thinned and during a return to baseline phase. The CM procedures were reported in a highly replicable fashion and they included breath CO assessment 3 times per day, an escalating incentive schedule with a reset, earnings of up to $386.75 cash paid weekly for meeting criteria in all conditions, and objective and clearly specified definitions of abstinence. Across the 30 days, 97.2% of samples were obtained, showing high compliance with the Web-based submission of 3 video clips per day showing the use and results of breath CO tests. Although larger and longer-term studies need to be conducted, this promising method seems feasible and could extend the reach of CM.

There are also a few examples of the use of CM to target adolescent drug use. Henggeler and colleagues[24] tested whether an abstinence-based incentive intervention would enhance outcomes in adolescents participating in drug court. The CM procedure did not enhance outcomes when added to drug court and a comprehensive family-based therapy (MST). A possible reason for the lack of a positive CM effect was that all young people (including the comparison group) received incentives and consequences based on urine drug testing results through a 12-month drug court program. Also, the CM procedures, as detailed in the implementation manual,[25] involved use of some procedures that reflect significant differences from the typical CM procedures used in effective adult studies. Specifically, 4 weeks of abstinence had to be achieved before earning vouchers, earned points were taken away in the form of fines, drug use resulted in a loss of the opportunity to earn vouchers for at least 2 weeks, and the magnitude of clinic-based incentives was low ($150 maximum in a 12-month period).

Godley and colleagues[26] described a CM intervention for adolescent substance users during continuing care provided after residential treatment. The intervention involved weekly sessions for 12 weeks and used a fishbowl reinforcement program to increase participation in personal goal-related activities and abstinence, with young people completing 64% of the activities they specified. To date, they have reported only on the completion of activities by young people in the CM conditions as an index of the feasibility of identifying, verifying, and increasing prosocial, goal-oriented activities among substance-using young people.

DEVELOPMENT OF A COMPREHENSIVE CM-BASED TREATMENT

In an effort to enhance outcomes for adolescent substance abuse (primarily focusing on marijuana), we sought to create a developmentally appropriate outpatient CM-based intervention.[27,28] This model integrates 4 empirically based interventions. First, an abstinence-based reinforcement intervention (voucher program) is used to enhance motivation to engage in treatment and engender marijuana and other drug abstinence. Monetary-based incentives are provided by the clinic for abstinence documented by urine and breath testing. This procedure is similar to the oft-replicated abstinence-reinforcement programs effective in adult treatment studies.[29,30]

Second, a parent-directed CM program is used to further motivate initiation and maintenance of drug abstinence and to better manage other related behavior problems. Parents are likely to consider their adolescent's marijuana use as problematic, and are usually motivated to take action. However, they may not have the skills to effectively change their adolescent's behavior. With careful training and resources, parents (or guardians) are a natural choice for delivering a CM program that could also enhance or engender motivation to abstain. Our parent CM program includes 2 components. Parents implement a substance-monitoring contract (SMC) that specifies positive and negative consequences to be delivered by the parents in response to documented abstinence or use. The family management curriculum (FMC) from the adolescent transitions program (ATP) teaches parents basic principles and skills to decrease problem behaviors and increase prosocial behaviors, and has shown efficacy for treating conduct disorder.[31] Because conduct problems often predate and co-occur with adolescent substance abuse,[32,33] we reasoned that targeting conduct problems, in addition to drug abstinence, might further enhance outcomes in treatment of adolescent substance abuse. Parent compliance with family management treatment positively affects treatment outcome,[34] hence the third component of this model uses CM to motivate parent participation. Here, parents earn chances to win prizes via an innovative positive reinforcement program[35] for actively participating in each treatment component.

Fourth, adolescents receive individual therapy (MET/CBT) to enhance motivation and provide coping skills training focused on achieving and maintaining abstinence.[36,37] Weekly 90-minute sessions are held for 14 weeks, with approximately 45 minutes for the individual teen session, and 45 minutes for the parent training session. At the end of the 14 weeks, all families are offered an additional 12 weeks of once-weekly substance testing to facilitate parental monitoring and are referred, when appropriate, to other community resources. In summary, the combination of the individual therapy, voucher program, FMC, and incentives for parent participation is designed to increase (1) adolescents' motivation to achieve and maintain abstinence, (2) parents' abilities to use effective parenting to decrease substance use and other behavior problems, and (3) adolescents' coping skills to help them achieve and adapt to a substance-free lifestyle.

Adolescent CM Implementation Details

To facilitate evaluation, generalization, and dissemination of CM approaches to adolescent substance abuse, it is important to provide procedural details about the key implementation variables that influence the efficacy of any CM intervention: schedule, magnitude, type of consequence, target behavior, and monitoring. Our abstinence-based incentive program was designed so that (1) substance use and its absence are readily detected; (2) abstinence is reinforced; (3) substance use results in a loss of reinforcement; and (4) positive reinforcement gleaned from drug abstinence is used to increase nondrug reinforcement. We use the following schedule for our clinic-based CM intervention for marijuana and other substance abstinence. We offer teens the opportunity to earn rewards twice weekly for 14 weeks based on documented substance abstinence. This schedule allows for frequent opportunities for earning reinforcement, and makes it probable that any marijuana used at any time during a given week would be detected (see later detailed discussion of monitoring issues). Regarding magnitude, during weeks 1 to 2, participants receive $5 vouchers for each specimen provided independent of test results because of the issues summarized later with the prolonged presence of marijuana metabolites in urine. These vouchers reinforce the provision of the urine specimen (attendance and compliance with the program) and serve as priming reinforcers to show what can be gained via the voucher program. During weeks 3 to 14 adolescents earn vouchers only if they provide a substance-negative specimen and parents report abstinence (see later discussion of target). The voucher value starts at $1.50, escalates by $1.50 with each consecutive negative specimen, and a $10 bonus is earned for each 2 consecutive negative results. Vouchers are reset back to their initial value if results were positive, from which they escalate again after 3 consecutive negative results. This schedule and magnitude of reinforcement are specifically designed to encourage achievement of longer periods of continuous abstinence.[30] The total magnitude earnings for an adolescent who provides 4 valid urine specimens during the first 2 weeks of treatment and is abstinent throughout weeks 3 to 14 is $590. Voucher programs with this same schedule and magnitude have been used successfully with adult marijuana users.[29,38]

Monetary-based vouchers are the type of incentive used. Adolescents earned vouchers (coupons reflecting the amount earned that day and the total voucher balance available on that day), each time abstinence is documented as described later. Vouchers earned are redeemed for goods or services therapists deem in concert with the treatment goal of increasing prosocial, nondrug-related activities. Examples of voucher purchases include gift cards or certificates for clothing stores, large chain stores, restaurants, and movie theaters; no cash is provided to adolescents.

The target of this CM program is abstinence from marijuana, alcohol, and other drugs. Note that in adults, targeting multiple drugs simultaneously is generally a more difficult goal to achieve than targeting the primary abused substance only.[39] Nonetheless, with adolescents we target all substances for the following reasons. First, although marijuana is the primary drug of abuse for most teens enrolled in treatment, they frequently use alcohol, occasionally use other drugs such as opiates, cocaine, or amphetamines, and commonly report prescription drug misuse. In addition to the obvious potential for harm of these other substances, we believed that parents would not be receptive to a treatment that provides reinforcement for marijuana abstinence in situations in which we, or they, detect their teen using other substances typically considered even more harmful than marijuana. Our experience to date using this procedure suggests that placing voucher contingencies on all drugs of abuse with adolescents who primarily abuse marijuana is not problematic. Little other drug use is usually observed, attrition is low, and most adolescents earn incentives for drug abstinence during the intervention.

To monitor the target behavior (substance abstinence) we use the following procedures. Because the primary target substance is marijuana, and to develop an appropriate monitoring schedule to detect marijuana abstinence, we considered the following information in developing our schedule and monitoring procedure. Urinalysis testing provides the usual and typically best method for obtaining the documented evidence needed to effectively administer a CM program targeting drug abstinence. With marijuana, such testing poses some unique issues. First, regular, heavy marijuana users are likely to test positive for marijuana use for 1 to 3 weeks after cessation at detection levels of 50 ng/mL of 11-nor-9-carboxy-9-tetrahydrocannabinol (THCCOOH), the primary marijuana metabolite, which is an accepted cutoff level for documenting recent abstinence. Thus, in our voucher program, we provide a 2-week notice before initiating the voucher program that informs clients that it will take 2 weeks of abstinence from marijuana for them to achieve a negative urinalysis result. Thus, reinforcement for abstinence must be delayed, which is the reason for reinforcing participation only during weeks 1 to 2. Some clinical agencies and researchers have begun to use quantitative or semiquantitative testing for THCCOOH levels as a means to differentiate abstinence from residual THCCOOH in the urine. These methods could potentially reduce the need for delaying reinforcement. However, the accuracy of these procedures for differentiating recent abstinence from reduced use or past use depends heavily on frequent testing in the early weeks of abstinence (daily or almost daily testing is required to interpret the findings reliably), which would be costlier than the qualitative tests that rely on standardized cutoffs, and would pose additional burden for participants.

A second related concern less frequently encountered is the possibility that a participant can provide a urine specimen that is negative for cannabis use on one day and then positive for cannabis the next day during the early weeks of abstinence. This result can occur because marijuana metabolites are stored in the fatty cells and the rate of their release can vary depending on activities like exercise. We have observed this only a handful of times, but it is worth noting.

A third concern is that urinary THCCOOH levels are affected by the dilution factor of the specific urine specimen provided. Many clients either intentionally or inadvertently drink large quantities of liquid that dilute a urine specimen such that a false-negative test result might be obtained. If possible, a method to screen for dilute specimens should be used as part of the urine toxicology program. Measurement of creatinine level is one method to approximate the dilution factor. Invalid specimens (creatinine level less than 30 mg/dL) results in a request to provide a replacement specimen within 4 to 24 hours. Failure to submit a scheduled specimen or replacement specimen is treated as a positive result, unless the parent provides an appropriate reason for not being able to attend the clinic. Notwithstanding these issues, the methods to detect recent marijuana use described here have been used effectively and without substantial problems in multiple clinical trials. A comprehensive understanding of the urine toxicology process, however, is necessary to facilitate implementation of an effective program.

To accurately monitor substance abstinence, we conduct urine tests twice per week. This schedule has been used with marijuana-using adults, but differs from the original voucher program for cocaine. Our decision to modify the schedule was 2-fold. First, we felt it was more practical for participants to make 2 rather than 3 visits to the clinic per week. Second, we were concerned that a single instance of cannabis use would carry over to multiple urine tests with the more frequent schedule. The twice-a-week schedule is sufficient to detect almost any cannabis use without exacerbating the potential for carryover positive tests. In summary, we believed that the practical advantages and reduction in the carryover problem gained with the twice-per-week schedule outweighed the potential benefits that might come from using a voucher delivery schedule that reinforced abstinence more frequently.

An alcohol breath test is performed at each visit, and parents are provided with and trained to use disposable breathalyzers to test for alcohol use at home. All parents are given 5 disposable breathalyzers that detect breath alcohol levels at 0.02/bal and above each week to use at home to detect alcohol use. Parents in the CM condition were instructed to ask their children to take the breath test when parents suspected alcohol use, using the following procedure. Parents asked the teen if he or she used alcohol that day. If the answer was yes, parents did not administer a breath test, and followed steps outlined later for a positive test. If the teen said no, they did not use alcohol, the parent asked him or her to take the breath test. If the breath test was positive or the test was refused, parents implemented the agreed consequence (procedure described later) and reported the positive test to the clinic.

Urine specimens are obtained under same-gender, staff observation to minimize risk of provision of invalid or tampered specimens. Specimens are immediately tested on site for marijuana, cocaine, opioids, benzodiazepines, amphetamines, and methamphetamines using the enzyme-multiplied immunoassay technique (EMIT). Rapid or quick tests that can be easily obtained and used without extensive training are good alternatives to use of EMIT or other types of analyzers. If either the adolescent or parents report substance use, or a positive urine specimen or breath test is obtained, the adolescent is considered positive for the purpose of CM implementation.

CM Interventions Implemented by Parents

In addition to the CM procedures implemented by clinic staff, we provide explicit instruction to parents in how to use CM procedures at home. First, with guidance from the therapist, parents develop an SMC that focuses on substance use or abstinence. The contract specifies positive and negative consequences to be delivered by the parents in response to documented abstinence or use (based on results of the substance monitoring procedures mentioned earlier) (**Fig. 2**). The consequences are determined via a collaborative process between therapist, parent, and adolescent, and reevaluated each week during weekly counseling sessions. This contract uses the same target (abstinence), schedule (twice per week), and monitoring method (urine drug testing, breath alcohol testing, and self/parent reports) as our clinic-based CM. Parents individualize the type of consequence (monetary, voucher type system, privileges) and the magnitude of the consequences, and these factors change throughout treatment in response to treatment success or failure.

Parents also receive a comprehensive behavioral parent-training program delivered during weekly sessions. The FMC of the ATP is used to teach parents basic principles and skills designed to decrease problem behaviors and increase prosocial behaviors.[40] This program, designed to target young people's conduct problems, seemed likely to yield broad benefits because conduct problems are comorbid with and strong predictors of poor outcomes among treated adolescent substance abusers.[41,42] This curriculum is consistent with the CM model, as parents are taught to select and define problem (target) behaviors and track (monitor) those behaviors over time. Parents clearly specify in advance the type of consequences they will use to increase positive

Substance Monitoring Contract

If _____'s urine drug screen is negative (no drugs detected or reported) and there were no positive or refused alcohol breath tests since the last drug screen, I will:

1.   Praise their progress!
2.   Ask how I can help them keep up the good work.
3.   Celebrate their progress by:

        _____

        _____

        _____

If _____'s urine drug screen is positive (drugs detected or reported) and/or there were positive or refused alcohol breath tests since the last drug screen, and/or urine screen is refused, I will:

1.   Remain calm!
2.   Not give a lecture
3.   Ask how I can help them
4.   Express confidence that they can do better next time
5.   Use the following consequence:

        _____

_____   Date

Parent Signature   Date

_____   Date

Teen Signature   Date

_____   Date

Therapist Signature   Date

Fig. 2. Substance monitoring contract.

behaviors, similar to those used in the substance monitoring contract, the schedule on which consequences will be provided (eg, daily), and the magnitude of the consequence. Similar procedures are followed to identify consequences for negative behaviors.

We also use the fishbowl method[35] to enhance parent participation and compliance. Each week, parents are asked to complete 6 tasks: attend therapy, attend midweek urine testing appointments, implement the SMC (twice per week), complete homework, and administer breathalyzers. Parents earn 1 draw from the fishbowl for each task. Each draw results in obtaining a winning (75% chance) or nonwinning slip (25% chance). Winning slips range in value from small ($1–$2, 68% chance), to medium ($20, 7% chance), to large prizes ($100, 1% chance). Prizes are delivered immediately and include gift certificates to restaurants, ice-cream shops, movie theaters, and grocery stores.

Initial Adolescent CM Trial Results

We completed an initial 2-group randomized trial comparing CBT+CM (abstinence-based reinforcement and parent-based CM) with CBT+parent drug education (PDE; an attention control condition).[28] Of the 69 young people enrolled (14–18 years of age), 31 met DSM-IV criteria for marijuana abuse, 30 for marijuana dependence, and 8 adolescents did not meet criteria for abuse or dependence, but reported regular marijuana use. As hypothesized, CM enhanced continuous abstinence outcomes, engendering more weeks of continuous marijuana abstinence during treatment (7.6 weeks vs CBT+PDE 5.1 weeks; $P = .04$, $d = 0.48$, medium effect). Those in the CM group were also more likely to achieve 8 weeks or more of continuous abstinence (53% vs 30%, $P = .06$) and 10 weeks or more of continuous abstinence (50% vs 19%, $P = .006$).

Despite differences in abstinence during treatment, we did not observe a significant between-group difference in abstinence after treatment. There was an increase in marijuana use from discharge to the 9-month follow-up, which, although not returning to intake levels, is of significant concern. Across psychopathology and parenting measures, the CM condition tended to show better outcomes, with significant main effects of treatment condition on negative discipline and externalizing. However, the treatment × time effects were not significant on any scale, indicating that adolescents in both conditions improved on measures of internalizing and externalizing psychopathology, and parents in both conditions showed parenting improvements. There was some evidence of better parental monitoring in the CM condition. Although both groups were given free breathalyzers by their clinicians and instructed in their use, CM mothers administered significantly more breathalyzers during treatment than CBT+PDE mothers (mean = 12.9 for CBT+CM vs 2.97 for CBT+PDE, $t(67) = 3.66$, $P<.001$). We hypothesize that CBT+CM mothers administered more breathalyzers because they were instructed in contingency contracting, providing them with a clear plan to use the testing results.

The lack of significant treatment condition differences during posttreatment were unexpected and may have resulted from low power to detect differences, a more potent effect of the comparison treatment than expected (rates of abstinence seem good in both conditions compared with prior treatment studies), or simply a less potent intervention effect than expected. Particularly relevant to this discussion of CM, the comparison intervention included incentives for participation in counseling and twice-weekly urine testing, systematically provided test results to parents, and provided weekly counseling and case management to parents. Although this condition was meant to serve as an attention control for the CM intervention, we expect that it was active and enhanced outcomes that would have been achieved with MET/CBT alone and might be considered an alternative model warranting future study. In particular, parents in the comparison condition may have responded to the urine drug testing results in a similar manner to parents in the CM condition (ie, withdrawal of privileges or other punishment delivered contingently following positive drug tests, rewards delivered contingently following negative drug tests). The likely tendency for at least some parents to respond in this way may have served to make outcomes more similar across conditions. Moreover, the CM incentive program for attendance and participation may have positively affected retention, thereby facilitating the effect of the individual counseling and the parent program.

REAL-WORLD APPLICATION AND CHALLENGES

Despite only a handful of studies reporting the potential of CM for adolescent substance abuse, recent reports indicate that clinicians and provider systems have begun to find innovative ways to implement CM into community treatment settings. Lott and Jennicus[43] describe how they developed a low-cost CM program to enhance attendance, participation, and abstinence in their community-based, intensive outpatient day-treatment program. Reasoning that adolescents may be more sensitive to small, low-cost behavioral incentives than adults, they administered a fishbowl reinforcement program that cost less than $0.50 per day. Although acknowledging that this was not an experimentally rigorous study, the investigators point out that in addition to the positive effect of CM on outcomes, the clinical billings generated by increased retention easily exceeded the costs of implementing the CM program.

Henggeler and colleagues[44] have taken CM dissemination a step further. They trained 432 community therapists who attended a 1-day workshop to implement a CM program for adolescent substance abuse. Systematic follow-up interviewing showed that 58% of the therapists who treated a substance-abusing adolescent used CM with at least 1 young person. They reported little observable or reported resistance to CM adoption, in contrast with the common belief that practitioners are resistant to using these methods.

Before discussing potential barriers to dissemination, we offer a few caveats to consider when developing a CM intervention for general implementation. Like other forms of behavioral treatment, it is important to ensure delivery of an effective intervention. To do so with CM requires adequate knowledge of behavioral principles and the clinical aspects of substance-use testing and treatment to design a program with a high likelihood of success. That is, adequate attention needs to be paid to the schedule and magnitude of the reinforcement plan and to the selection of a target that is clinically appropriate and that can be objectively and accurately monitored. Implementation of a weak or poorly designed plan may result in failure and will provide an inadequate test of CM in general. The design and complexity of the plan also influence the ease with which it can be disseminated. Ideally, one must carefully balance these factors along with consideration of cost constraints when developing a CM program. The paucity of research on CM interventions with adolescents and on the parametrics of CM interventions in general poses challenges for selection of a CM model to apply in diverse settings. Providers must carefully extrapolate from existing studies and rely on a combination of clinical experience and expertise in behavioral principles when developing and implementing a CM program that will be effective in a specific treatment setting. A Blending Initiative from the National Institute on Drug Abuse and the Substance Abuse and Mental Health Services Administration, *Promoting Awareness of Motivational Incentives*, reflects one of a growing number of publicly available resources to guide the development of CM programs.[45]

The most probable and oft-discussed barrier to implementation of CM interventions is cost. Because most effective CM interventions involve tangible incentives with set costs, CM programing tends to be viewed differently from costs associated with more traditional types of clinical interventions (psychosocial therapies or medications). A common response to presentations showing the efficacy of CM is that the treatment system cannot afford incentives or the urine toxicology testing. As mentioned earlier, there may be many options for development of low-cost CM programs that can add to the efficacy of existing programs. However, if CM interventions can significantly enhance outcomes and are the treatment of choice for achieving optimal abstinence rates, it would seem incumbent on providers to revaluate the logistics of their clinical operations and budgets and work with the treatment reimbursement systems to develop plans to offer such potent options to their clients.

SUMMARY AND FUTURE DIRECTIONS

The addition of CM-based interventions to the menu of effective treatment alternatives for substance abuse has generated discussion and excitement in the research and treatment provider communities. Although the research base for applications in adolescent settings is only beginning to appear, the overwhelming positive evidence base for adult substance-abuse treatment gives much reason for high expectations.

Future research and clinical innovation must continue to stress the need to find even more potent CM models that delineate necessary and optimal parameters and components for effective implementation. A variety of options are needed for the multitude of clinical settings that must intervene with adolescents. Better understanding of the essential components and effective methods for training community providers in the behavioral principles that underlie CM must guide efforts to disseminate effective CM alternatives.

We now know that CM strategies can be effective for retaining clients in treatment, increasing treatment attendance, and promoting abstinence across multiple types of substance abuse and dependence with various clinical populations. We know that reinforcement schedule parameters such as frequency and magnitude affect the potency of CM interventions, and we know that clinicians are willing to learn and implement CM. What is now needed to maximize the effectiveness of CM interventions in the greater community is research to better isolate its active components, accumulation of data on its cost-effectiveness, and guidelines for how to best use resources to maximize cost-benefit ratios. We further suggest that dissemination efforts must include provider training in the basic principles guiding CM, especially if the provider needs to assist parents in developing and implementing a CM program. With adolescents, areas of future focus should include effective use of parental influence, potential application by systems mandating treatment (schools and judicial), and use of technology such as the Internet and cell phones to increase access to and reduce costs of effective interventions such as CM. Despite some promising examples of adolescent CM interventions, there remain large gaps in our knowledge about how to assist most adolescent substance abusers in achieving and maintaining abstinence. Paying close attention to the principles that underlie CM may facilitate the development of more effective interventions.

REFERENCES

1. Waldron HB, Turner CW. Evidence-based psychosocial treatments for adolescent substance abuse. J Clin Child Adolesc Psychol 2008;37(1):238–61.
2. Dennis M, Godley SH, Diamond G, et al. The cannabis youth treatment (CYT) study: main findings from two randomized trials. J Subst Abuse Treat 2004;27: 197–213.
3. Waldron HB, Slesnick N, Brody JL, et al. Treatment outcomes for adolescent substance abuse at 4- and 7-month assessments. J Consult Clin Psychol 2001; 69:802–13.
4. Compton WM, Pringle B. Services research on adolescent drug treatment. Commentary on "the cannabis youth treatment (CYT) study: main findings from two randomized trials". J Subst Abuse Treat 2004;27:195–6.
5. Higgins ST, Heil SH, Lussier JP. Clinical implications of reinforcement as a determinant of substance use disorders. Annu Rev Psychol 2004;55:431–61.
6. Petry NM, Simic F. Recent advances in the dissemination of contingency management techniques: clinical and research perspectives. J Subst Abuse Treat 2002;23:81–6.
7. Stitzer M. Contingency management and the addictions. Addiction 2006;101(11): 1536–7.
8. Higgins ST, Silverman K, Heil SH. Contingency management in substance abuse treatment. New York: The Guilford Press; 2008.
9. Sulzer-Azaroff B, Meyer GR. Behavior analysis for lasting change. Fort Worth (TX): Holt Rinehart and Winston; 1991.

10. Petry NM, Peirce JM, Stitzer ML, et al. Effect of prize-based incentives on outcomes in stimulant abusers in outpatient psychosocial treatment programs: a national drug abuse treatment clinical trials network study. Arch Gen Psychiatry 2005;62:1148–56.
11. Lussier JP, Heil SH, Mongeon JA, et al. A meta-analysis of voucher-based reinforcement therapy for substance use disorders. Addiction 2006;101(2):192–203.
12. Petry NM, Martin B. Low-cost contingency management for treating cocaine- and opioid-abusing methadone patients. J Consult Clin Psychol 2002;70(2):398–405.
13. Sindelar J, Elbel B, Petry NM. What do we get for our money? Cost-effectiveness of adding contingency management. Addiction 2007;102(2):309–16.
14. Olmstead TA, Sindelar JL, Easton CJ, et al. The cost-effectiveness of four treatments for marijuana dependence. Addiction 2007;102(9):1443–53.
15. Iguchi MY, Lamb RJ, Belding MA, et al. Contingent reinforcement of group participation versus abstinence in a methadone maintenance program. Exp Clin Psychopharmacol 1996;4:315–21.
16. Breda C, Heflinger CA. Predicting incentives to change among adolescents with substance abuse disorder. Am J Drug Alcohol Abuse 2004;30(2):251–67.
17. Liddle HA, Dakof GA, Parker K, et al. Multidimensional family therapy for adolescent drug abuse: results of a randomized clinical trial. Am J Drug Alcohol Abuse 2001;27(4):651–88.
18. Henggeler SW, Clingempeel WG, Brondino MJ, et al. Four-year follow-up of multisystemic therapy with substance-abusing and substance-dependent juvenile offenders. J Am Acad Child Adolesc Psychiatry 2002;41(7):868–74.
19. Azrin NH, Donohue B, Besalel VA, et al. Youth drug abuse treatment: a controlled outcome study. J Child Adolesc Subst Abuse 1994;3(3):1–16.
20. Azrin NH, McMahon PT, Donohue B, et al. Behavior therapy for drug abuse: a controlled treatment outcome study. Behav Res Ther 1994;32(8):857–66.
21. Krishnan-Sarin S, Duhig AM, McKee SA, et al. Contingency management for smoking cessation in adolescent smokers. Exp Clin Psychopharmacol 2006;14(3):306–10.
22. Cavallo DA, Cooney JL, Duhig AM, et al. Combining cognitive behavioral therapy with contingency management for smoking cessation in adolescent smokers: a preliminary comparison of two different CBT formats. Am J Addict 2007;16(6):468–74.
23. Reynolds B, Dallery J, Shroff P, et al. A web-based contingency management program with adolescent smokers. J Appl Behav Anal 2008;41(4):597–601.
24. Henggeler SW, Halliday-Boykins CA, Cunningham PB, et al. Juvenile drug court: enhancing outcomes by integrating evidence-based treatments. J Consult Clin Psychol 2006;74(1):42–54.
25. Cunningham PB, Donohue B, Randall J, et al. Integrating contingency management into multisystemic therapy. Charleston (SC): Family Services Research Center, Medical University of South Carolina; 2002.
26. Godley SH, Godley MD, Wright KL, et al. Contingent reinforcement of personal goal activities for adolescents with substance use disorders during post-residential continuing care. Am J Addict 2008;17(4):278–86.
27. Kamon JL, Budney AJ, Stanger C. A contingency management intervention for adolescent marijuana abuse and conduct problems. J Am Acad Child Adolesc Psychiatry 2005;44(6):513–21.
28. Stanger C, Budney AJ, Kamon J, et al. A randomized trial of contingency management for adolescent marijuana abuse and dependence. Drug Alcohol Depend 2009;105(3):240–7.

29. Budney AJ, Higgins ST, Radonovich KJ, et al. Adding voucher-based incentives to coping-skills and motivational enhancement improves outcomes during treatment for marijuana dependence. J Consult Clin Psychol 2000;68:1051–61.

30. Higgins ST, Budney AJ, Bickel WK, et al. Incentives improve outcome in outpatient behavioral treatment of cocaine dependence. Arch Gen Psychiatry 1994; 54:568–76.

31. Dishion TJ, Kavanagh K. Intervening in adolescent problem behavior: a family-centered approach. New York: Guilford Press; 2003.

32. Brook JS, Whiteman M, Finch S, et al. Aggression, intrapsychic distress, and drug use: antecedent and intervening processes. J Am Acad Child Adolesc Psychiatry 1995;34(8):1076–84.

33. Lynskey MT, Fergusson DM. Childhood conduct problems, attention deficit behaviors, and adolescent alcohol, tobacco, and illicit drug use. J Abnorm Child Psychol 1995;23(3):281–302.

34. Nye CL, Zucker RA, Fitzgerald HE. Early intervention in the path to alcohol problems through conduct problems: treatment involvement and child behavior change. J Consult Clin Psychol 1995;63(5):831–40.

35. Petry NM, Martin B, Cooney JL, et al. Give them prizes, and they will come: contingency management for treatment of alcohol dependence. J Consult Clin Psychol 2000;68:250–7.

36. Webb CPM, Scudder M, Kaminer Y, et al In: The motivational enhancement therapy and cognitive behavioral therapy for adolescent cannabis users, vol. 2. Rockville (MD): Center for Substance Abuse Treatment, Substance Abuse and Mental Health Services Administration; 2001.

37. Sampl S, Kadden RIn: Motivational enhancement therapy and cognitive behavioral therapy for adolescent cannabis users: 5 sessions, vol. 1. Rockville (MD): Center for Substance Abuse Treatment, Substance Abuse and Mental Health Services Administration; 2001.

38. Budney AJ, Moore BA, Rocha HL, et al. Clinical trial of abstinence-based vouchers and cognitive-behavioral therapy for cannabis dependence. J Consult Clin Psychol 2006;74(2):307–16.

39. Lussier J, Higgins S, Heil S, et al. Voucher-based reinforcement therapy for substance use disorders: a quantitative review. Addiction 2006;101:192–203.

40. Dishion TJ, Kavanagh K, Veltman M, et al. Family management curriculum V2.0: leader's guide. Eugene (OR): Child and Family Center Publications; 2003.

41. Randall J, Henggeler SW, Pickrel SG, et al. Psychiatric comorbidity and the 16-month trajectory of substance-abusing and substance-dependent juvenile offenders. J Am Acad Child Adolesc Psychiatry 1999;38:1118–24.

42. Young SE, Corley RP, Stallings MC, et al. Substance use, abuse and dependence in adolescents: prevalence, symptoms profiles and correlates. Drug Alcohol Depend 2002;68(3):309–22.

43. Lott DC, Jencius S. Effectiveness of very low-cost contingency management in a community adolescent treatment program. Drug Alcohol Depend 2009; 102(1–3):162–5.

44. Henggeler SW, Chapman JE, Rowland MD, et al. Statewide adoption and initial implementation of contingency management for substance-abusing adolescents. J Consult Clin Psychol 2008;76(4):556–67.

45. Hamilton J, Kellogg S, Killeen T, et al. Promoting awareness of motivational incentives (PAMI). Available at: http://pami.nattc.org/explore/priorityareas/science/blendinginitiative/pami/. Accessed September 29, 2009.

Multidimensional Family Therapy: Addressing Co-occurring Substance Abuse and Other Problems Among Adolescents with Comprehensive Family-based Treatment

Cynthia L. Rowe, PhD

KEYWORDS

- Adolescent substance abuse • Delinquency • Families
- Multidimensional Family Therapy • Co-occurring disorders

Adolescent substance abuse rarely occurs in isolation from other developmental and psychiatric problems. Studies with community-based, clinical, and juvenile justice samples document that adolescent substance abuse is frequently comorbid with a host of other psychiatric disorders, most commonly conduct disorder (CD), attention deficit-hyperactivity disorder (ADHD), depression, and posttraumatic stress disorder (PTSD).[1–5] Rates of co-occurring adolescent substance use and psychiatric disorders average 60% in community-based samples[6] and can range up to 80% or 90% in treatment and juvenile justice samples.[7–10] Several studies also show that treatment engagement and successful outcomes can be more difficult to achieve with adolescents who have co-occurring substance use and psychiatric disorders.[9,11–13] Many

Department of Epidemiology and Public Health, University of Miami Miller School of Medicine, Center for Treatment Research on Adolescent Drug Abuse, 1120 North West 14th Street, Suite 1014, Miami, FL 33136, USA
E-mail address: crowe@med.miami.edu

Child Adolesc Psychiatric Clin N Am 19 (2010) 563–576
doi:10.1016/j.chc.2010.03.008
childpsych.theclinics.com
1056-4993/10/$ – see front matter © 2010 Elsevier Inc. All rights reserved.

substance abusing youths with severe CD are at risk to progress to antisocial personality disorder and to experience chronic substance abuse, mental health, employment, health, and relationship difficulties into adulthood.[14,15]

Common factor or general deviance models are often invoked to explain the close association between substance use and psychiatric disorders, particularly externalizing problems such as CD.[2] As posited by Jessor and Jessor's[16] problem behavior theory, adolescent substance abuse tends to co-occur with a range of other disruptive behaviors that can have long-term consequences, including unsafe sexual practices, school failure, and social isolation, alienation, and conflict. The consistent clustering of these behaviors, and evidence that they can have reciprocal effects,[17] has led to the examination of shared risk factors that may explain a range of adolescent problems, such as early temperament and environmental vulnerabilities.[18,19] Given that common risk factors are known to contribute to substance abuse and other disorders in adolescence, addressing these vulnerabilities and promoting protective processes through targeted intervention may have broad and lasting effects.[20,21]

Family factors including parental rejection and family conflict, ineffective monitoring and parental discipline strategies, and compromised parental functioning resulting from substance abuse and mental health problems are among the strongest and most consistent predictors of adolescent problem behaviors such as substance abuse and CD.[22,23] Protective factors within the family can also buffer against the negative effects of risk factors such as deviant peer involvement.[24] Involved and supportive parenting was even found to ameliorate genetic risk for adolescent drug abuse in a recent study.[25] The consistent associations among family factors and adolescent problem behaviors, as well as strong empirical support for family-based interventions tested in several rigorously controlled trials in the past 2 decades,[26,27] has firmly established family involvement as a critical ingredient in the treatment of adolescent substance use disorders (SUDs).[28] Because family factors predict a range of problems in adolescence, including internalized distress and externalizing behaviors, intervening to change negative interactions and patterns within the family may also be critical in improving co-occurring disorders as well as teen substance abuse.

Although several treatments have been shown to reduce adolescent substance use,[26,27] many of these interventions focus on alleviating substance use alone rather than targeting multiple adolescent problem behaviors. In addition, with community programs and funding generally fragmented into substance abuse or mental health silos, progress in developing and implementing effective interventions for co-occurring disorders has been slow.[29,30] Clinical research that purposely excludes complex cases with multiple comorbidities has not helped matters. Thus there are few examples of broad-based interventions that simultaneously and effectively tackle substance abuse, related risky behaviors such as unsafe sexual practices, delinquency, psychiatric symptoms, and school problems among adolescents.[2] Given that substance abuse among teens tends to co-occur with, and may exacerbate (and be exacerbated by), other emotional and behavioral problems, interventions for this population must address multiple comorbidities.[28] Integrated interventions that simultaneously treat SUDs and co-occurring problems are frequently recommended,[3,5,31] but are rare in practice.

In recent guideline and review articles of co-occurring disorders for teens and adults, several experts call for interventions for substance abuse and mental health problems that are delivered in a truly integrated way rather than distinct treatments offered concurrently or consecutively.[5,31] For instance, American Academy of Child and Adolescent Psychiatry (AACAP) practice parameters for the treatment of adolescent substance abuse include thorough assessment of possible co-occurring disorders as well as systematic incorporation of pharmacologic agents and other psychosocial interventions that address psychiatric symptoms.[28] Similarly, in addition to multidimensional assessment of potential comorbidities, Kaminer and colleagues[3] recommend "simultaneous and coordinated implementation of psychiatric and substance abuse treatment services" in which psychotherapy targets the range of presenting symptoms and medications are used and closely monitored to reduce the debilitating symptoms of disorders such as depression. Although there seems to be consensus on the importance of such coordination and integration to reduce substance abuse and comorbid conditions among teens, there are few empirical studies of truly integrated approaches or detailed clinical protocols for how such a model can be delivered in practice.

This article reviews the evidence base for Multidimensional Family Therapy (MDFT),[32] a comprehensive treatment that targets change in the multiple domains of the teen's life that are known to influence the development and maintenance of substance abuse and other problems. Clinical effectiveness of MDFT has been shown in 5 completed clinical randomized controlled trials (RCTs) and with promising interim findings from the same number of ongoing RCTs.[33–37] The model is recognized as exemplary in independent reviews and is regularly listed as a best-practice model for teen drug abuse and delinquency.[27,38–44]

MDFT was recently included in a review of "a handful of research-supported integrated interventions that simultaneously address both mental health and substance use disorders."[2(p207)] In that review, Hawkins emphasizes the negative clinical, systems, and policy implications of separating mental health and substance abuse arbitrarily into different categories for funding and treatment purposes. "Both mental health and substance abuse disorders must be conceptualized as psychiatric conditions, with common developmental etiologies and trajectories," Hawkins[2(p215)] concludes; "In an adolescent with co-occurring disorders, both conditions must be considered primary and treated as such." Additional recommendations made in that review include reconceptualizing adolescent co-occurring disorders as chronic relapsing conditions potentially requiring multiple treatments, follow-up, and after care; greater attention and resources devoted to prevention and early intervention; simultaneous and integrated care plans for behavioral, emotional, and substance abuse disorders; and closer collaboration among agencies so that adolescents and families may access comprehensive quality services through any possible route, whether it be schools, courts, child welfare systems, mental health clinics, substance abuse treatment programs, or other social service agencies. The review concludes that additional research is needed to determine mechanisms and effects of treatment models with adolescents suffering from different types of co-occurring disorders.

This article describes a comprehensive family-based approach to treating adolescent substance abuse and related comorbid conditions. Following a discussion of the clinical approach, the article reviews findings supporting MDFT's ability to achieve reductions in adolescent substance abuse, as well as co-occurring problems including risky sexual behaviors, school problems, delinquency, and mental health symptoms. The conclusions present certain challenges and the need for additional research on this and similar models.

MDFT

MDFT is an integrative outpatient treatment that has blended family therapy, individual therapy, drug counseling, and multiple-systems oriented intervention approaches.[45] Interventions target the interconnected domains of adolescent development, and, within these contexts, the circumstances and processes known to create and/or continue dysfunction.[46,47] MDFT interventions work in 4 domains: changes in the adolescent (intrapersonal and relational development issues), the parent(s) (individual functioning of the parent as well as parenting), the family environment (family transactional patterns), and extrafamilial systems of influence on the adolescent and family (eg, working with schools, social service agencies, or the juvenile justice system). Early-stage interventions aim to develop multiple alliances with teens, parents, and influential members of extrafamilial systems, as well as motivating each to participate and change. Systematic and effective engagement strategies have paid off in high retention rates. For example, 87% of families completed 3 months of intensive outpatient MDFT compared with 59% in residential treatment, and 96% of young teens and families completed 4 months of MDFT compared with 78% in group therapy.[48] MDFT retained 97% of youths in treatment during detention stays compared with 65% of youths receiving services as usual (SAU) in detention; 87% percent of youths in MDFT were retained in outpatient treatment for 3 months following detention release, compared with only 23% of youths in SAU.[49]

MDFT is a treatment system and not a singular, one-size-fits-all approach.[50] It has been adapted and tested in various forms or versions according to target population and contextual characteristics in community-based clinical trials with samples of substance abusing teens demonstrating high rates of comorbid emotional and behavioral problems. Studies of MDFT have been conducted at sites across the United States and Europe, among diverse samples of adolescents (African American, Hispanic, and White youths aged 11–18 years) in urban, suburban, and rural settings, and youths of various socioeconomic backgrounds. These studies have primarily been conducted in community settings with masters-level nonresearch clinicians, increasing the transfer potential of the approach to standard clinical and juvenile justice settings. The model has been implemented successfully in substance abuse, mental health, and juvenile justice settings across the United States, Canada, and several European countries.

Several features of the MDFT model are hypothesized to increase its success with teens experiencing multiple problems. First, as recommended in virtually every review or practice guideline for co-occurring disorders, MDFT stage 1 work involves comprehensive, multidimensional assessment. Assessment in MDFT provides a therapeutic map, directing therapists where to intervene in the multiple domains of the adolescent's life. A comprehensive, multidimensional assessment process involves not only the identification of different problem areas, symptoms, and co-occurring disorders, but also risk and protective factors in all relevant domains, so that these factors can be targeted for change. Through a series of individual and family interviews, meetings with school, court, and other mental health professionals, and observations of directed family interactions, the therapist seeks to answer critical questions about functioning in each area of the adolescent's life. Assessment is based on empirically derived knowledge of the deficits of adolescent substance abusers and their life contexts as well as areas of strength, so as to provide a complete clinical picture of the unique combination of assets and weaknesses that the adolescent, family, and other systems bring to therapy. Assessment is an ongoing process throughout therapy, continually integrated with interventions to calibrate treatment planning and execution, and addressing what has not yet been sufficiently resolved.

Second, guided by this multidimensional assessment, the model addresses common root factors underlying a range of emotional and behavioral symptoms that co-occur with adolescent substance abuse, most importantly family relationship factors, parenting practices, family conflict and communication, and parental substance abuse. Because these shared factors have an influence on a range of negative developmental outcomes, the intensive work done in all domains of the therapy, but especially family sessions, alters the trajectories of these risk factors, promotes protective processes, and presumably improves adolescents' outcomes as well.

Third, the therapy mobilizes and actively coordinates the efforts of many different systems affecting the teen's life, including other mental health services and psychiatric consultation. A previous review of the model's integrative treatment development framework described the systematic way in which MDFT therapists collaborate with psychiatrists in the treatment of adolescents with comorbid substance abuse and psychiatric problems.[51] As with other components of MDFT, the therapists strive to integrate psychopharmacological interventions into the adolescent's overall treatment plan in a way that is consistent with MDFT theory and principles, and ensure that they are based on a comprehensive evaluation of the adolescent's functioning. MDFT therapists work in close collaboration with child/adolescent psychiatrists, encouraging the teen and family to participate actively in the close monitoring and integration of medication into the comprehensive treatment plan. The psychiatrist is integrated as an important member of the therapeutic team, and MDFT therapists may arrange conjoint phone calls or face-to-face visits with the family and psychiatrist to monitor symptoms, compliance issues, and the effectiveness of medications. Medications are presented to teens and families as being important in reducing the effect of symptoms, as well as improving the teen's functioning so that he or she is more effective in his or her efforts in MDFT, school, and home.

Fourth, this type of active collaboration and coordination of services is also critical in reducing school problems. School success and reconnection are among the most important areas of work in MDFT because they are critical in creating a prosocial trajectory for the teen. Work in this realm is one of the most direct ways to bolster protective factors for teens because it gives them a sense of accomplishment, a powerful success experience, a tangible product (a General Equivalency Diploma or high-school diploma), and new relationships with more positive peers and adult advocates and role models. MDFT therapists, with parents, work actively with school personnel to institute changes in this realm, including integration of special programs, tutoring, and vocational training. Tutoring and vocational training services have also been established within several MDFT teams so that these efforts can be truly integrated with the MDFT treatment.

Fifth, conduct problems and delinquency are addressed not only in ongoing individual and family sessions but also through intensive collaborative work with representatives from the juvenile justice system. Using the same principles of alliance building, regularity and consistency of contacts, and careful assessment and follow-through that characterize the therapist's work in all domains, these relationships are built on respect and mutual accountability for the adolescent's outcome. Therapists clarify with the probation officer (PO) the monitoring protocol (eg, weekly drug screens, meetings) and takes steps with the adolescent and family to abide by the PO's requests. The therapist offers an analysis of the teen and family that provides hope for change, helping the PO understand that the focus on family relationship dynamics will pay off in practical terms: in better parental monitoring and compliance with the terms of probation. Judges also must have adequate information on treatment to make informed decisions on the disposition of adolescent cases; not only an understanding of the theory and the science supporting MDFT's efficacy but also the basic structure and progress in therapy. POs and judges act on their experience with the teens and families, and therapists can help emphasize areas of progress and strengths that may elicit reasonableness from the system.

MDFT treatment incorporates specific protocols for addressing certain symptoms, such as depression and trauma, as well as high-risk behaviors. For example, a new module created as part of the Detention to Community (DTC) study (described later[49]) integrated multifamily groups within ongoing MDFT for the specific purpose of reducing high-risk sexual behaviors. Marvel and colleagues[52] described the process of developing and testing this new component of MDFT with juveniles recruited in detention and following release to the community. First, treatment developers designed the new human immunodeficiency virus (HIV)/sexually transmitted disease (STD) prevention multifamily groups focusing specifically on reducing sexual risk-taking behaviors; and second, the groups were integrated into ongoing adolescent, parent, and family sessions in MDFT. Multiple revisions, pilot testing, and a rigorous evaluation attest to the effectiveness of the family-based HIV prevention module.

EFFECTS OF MDFT ON ADOLESCENT SUBSTANCE USE

Previous reviews have shown MDFT's potential to reduce adolescent drug and alcohol use to a greater extent than a range of high-quality, closely monitored, active comparison interventions.[22,26,27,39,42] For instance, in the first randomized trial of MDFT conducted in the San Francisco Bay area in the mid-1980s, the model was compared with 2 manualized active treatments, Adolescent Group Therapy and Multifamily Educational Intervention, with 182 clinically referred drug and alcohol abusing adolescents.[34] The results revealed significant decreases in substance use and problem behaviors at termination for all treatments, with youths receiving MDFT showing significantly less substance use than the 2 comparison treatments. At the 1-year follow-up, MDFT youths again decreased their substance use to a greater extent than either of the other treatments. The second randomized trial compared MDFT with an empirically supported, individual-based adolescent treatment, Cognitive behavioral therapy (CBT),[36] with 224 primary male and African American adolescents referred to a drug treatment clinic in North Philadelphia. Youths who received MDFT showed more rapid decreases in psychological involvement with drugs through the 12-month follow-up. In addition, youths receiving MDFT continued to improve following treatment discharge, so that at the 6- and 12-month follow-up assessments, their psychological involvement with substances was lower than that of youths in CBT. A greater proportion of youths receiving MDFT (64% vs 44%) reported no or 1 occasion of drug use at the 12-month follow-up. A third randomized trial tested MDFT as an early intervention for 83 young minority adolescents (ages 11–15 years) referred for drug treatment in Miami.[35] MDFT youths showed greater decreases in marijuana and alcohol abuse than youths receiving a manualized CBT-based peer-group treatment. Youths in MDFT were more likely to abstain from drug use, report no problems associated with drug use, and decrease their delinquent behavior more rapidly than youths in group treatment over 12 months of follow-up.[37]

The Cannabis Youth Treatment (CYT) study, a rigorous 4-site clinical trial of 5 adolescent substance abuse treatment models,[33] showed the long-term sustainability of MDFT's effects on teens' substance use frequency and problems up to 30 months posttreatment.[53] This study also involved the first evaluation of adolescent drug treatment costs and benefits using standard economic methods, and found average weekly cost estimates of MDFT to compare favorably with cost parameters of standard outpatient adolescent treatment ($164 vs $365).[54] Benefit-cost analyses revealed that MDFT had a statistically significant baseline to 12-month reduction in drug use consequences and greater net benefits associated with reduced drug use consequences than a brief, inexpensive intervention (motivational enhancement therapy [MET]/cognitive behavioral therapy 5 [CBT5]) at 30-month follow-up.[53]

To summarize, MDFT reduces drug and alcohol between 41% and 66% from intake to completion, and treatment gains are consistently maintained up to 1-year follow-up.[34–37] Between 64% and 93% of adolescents receiving MDFT report abstinence from substance use at 1 year.[36,37] MDFT also reduces the severity of substance-related impairment 1 year after intake; 93% of young adolescents in MDFT reported no substance-related problems at 12-month follow-up.[37] The rigorous multisite CYT study also supports the sustainability of MDFT's effects and its positive benefit-cost ratio up to 30-month follow-up.[53]

The research evidence supporting MDFT's effects is strong in several respects. First, the studies have shown favorable outcomes for youths in MDFT in comparison with other state-of-the-art, well-articulated, and carefully monitored treatments. Second, the studies have recruited clinically referred samples with a range of problems, and the authors have achieved effects within community clinics, showing MDFT's effectiveness in real-world settings as well as its efficacy. Third, youths' and families' functioning in a range of domains have been shown to improve during treatment and to maintain gains following treatment. The following sections highlight findings from completed and ongoing studies that show MDFT's potential to address problem behaviors that frequently co-occur with substance abuse.

EFFECTS ON DELINQUENT BEHAVIORS AND AFFILIATION WITH DELINQUENT PEERS

Four trials showed that MDFT decreases delinquent behavior and affiliation with delinquent peers more than comparison treatments.[34,37,49,55] Hogue and colleagues[55] tested MDFT as a prevention approach with a sample of at-risk, inner-city young adolescents and their families in North Philadelphia. Study participants were early adolescents (mean age 12.5 years), predominantly girls (56%), African American (97%), and from low-income homes. Youths in MDFT showed greater gains than controls in decreasing involvement with antisocial peers over the course of the intervention. Although controls reported increased peer delinquency, MDFT subjects reduced peer delinquency.

In the randomized trial of MDFT with clinically referred young teens described earlier, official court records showed that MDFT clients were less likely to be arrested or placed on probation than youths in group-based CBT during the 12-month follow-up period.[35,37] Similar to results in the prevention trial, although youths in the peer-group treatment increased their affiliation with delinquent peers during the 12-month follow-up period, MDFT teens showed marked reductions in peer delinquency during this period.[37]

In a third randomized trial, MDFT was tested as a therapeutic and cost-effective outpatient alternative to residential treatment.[56] All teens had at least 1 comborbid psychiatric disorder in addition to an SUD and were referred for residential treatment. The average age was 15 (standard deviation [SD] = 1.07); and the sample was predominantly male (74%), Hispanic (67%), and almost all were juvenile-justice involved. Outcomes were assessed at intake and 2-, 4-, 12-, 18-, 24-, 36-, and 48-months follow-up. Consistent with hypotheses, from 2 to 18 months, youths in MDFT more rapidly decreased their self- and parent-reported aggressive behavior and self- and parent-reported delinquent activity than youths who received residential treatment. Residential treatment youths spent an average of 60 more days in controlled environments during the 18-month follow-up period than youths in MDFT, leading to an average of more than $35,000 greater economic costs per client for residential treatment. Preliminary analyses also reveal that the gains favoring MDFT achieved through the 18 months are maintained through 48 months for self- and parent-reported aggressive behavior and parent-reported delinquency.

In the DTC study, MDFT was tested in a 2-site National Institute of Drug Abuse Criminal Justice Drug Abuse Treatment Studies randomized trial as a cross-systems integrative model with youths while they were in detention and providing continuous services in MDFT after they were released.[49] Starting in detention, eligible youths were randomized to MDFT or Enhanced Services as Usual (ESAU). Adolescents and their caregivers were assessed at intake to detention, discharge from detention, and at 3, 6, and 9 months following release from detention. Participants (average age 15 years) were primarily men (82%) and African American (60%); 17% were white, non-Hispanic, and 22% were Hispanic. At intake, participants averaged 3.9 lifetime arrests (SD = 3.3), with 2.3 (SD = 2.1) in the last year. Youths receiving MDFT were detained for fewer days (following their original discharge from detention) than youths in SAU. At 1 site that was characterized by greater juvenile justice systems collaboration, MDFT youths received fewer punitive dispositions (eg, diversion, dropping charges, judicial warnings, as opposed to being placed on probation or committed to Department of Juvenile Justice Custody) than youths in SAU. The study is currently following participants at 18-, 24-, 36-, and 42-months follow-up to determine the long-term effects of the integrative MDFT-DTC model.

EFFECTS ON SCHOOL FUNCTIONING

MDFT clients show significantly greater improvement in school behaviors and grades than youths in comparison treatments. For instance, in the first trial of MDFT, MDFT clients improved their grades drastically from mainly failing grades at intake to most receiving passing grades at 12-month follow-up. Specifically, in MDFT, only 25% had a grade-point average of C or higher at intake, whereas 76% were passing at 12-month follow-up; in the family educational group, 36% were passing at intake compared with 40% at 12-month follow-up; and in peer-group therapy, 43% were passing at intake compared with 60% at 12-month follow-up.[34] In the randomized trial of MDFT with clinically referred young teens described earlier, MDFT clients not only showed more significant improvements in academic grades but also improved their conduct grades (or school behavior) to a greater extent than in peer-group therapy.[37] In the prevention study described earlier with at-risk, inner-city young adolescents, MDFT more significantly increased school bonding than the control condition.[55]

EFFECTS ON HIV/STD RISK BEHAVIORS

In the 2-site DTC randomized trial described earlier,[49] an integrated substance abuse treatment and HIV prevention intervention (MDFT-HIV) was developed, and then experimentally tested, specifically for juvenile detainees. All youths received a high-quality, but standard, HIV prevention in detention, and MDFT youths received family-based HIV/STD prevention[52] during the outpatient phase. Youths receiving MDFT engaged in fewer unprotected sex acts between intake and 9-month follow-up at both sites.

EFFECTS ON INTERNALIZING SYMPTOMS AND OUTCOME TRAJECTORIES OF YOUTHS WITH GREATER COMORBIDITY

In 2 of the studies described earlier, MDFT also showed greater effects on internalized distress, including depression and anxiety symptoms. In our early adolescent trial,

MDFT showed more significant effects on internalized distress between intake and 12-month follow-up than CBT peer-group treatment.[35,37] In addition, in the DTC study, MDFT was more effective in reducing self-reported internalizing symptoms among youths recruited in detention facilities than SAU.[49]

Another important line of investigation has examined trajectories of youths with greater severity of comorbid problems in 2 RCTs.[57] In the trial comparing MDFT with individually focused CBT, and in the DTC study, analyses supported the distinctiveness of 2 classes of substance use severity, characterized primarily by adolescents with higher and lower initial severity (higher severity class having greater psychiatric comorbidity). As hypothesized, in both studies, the 2 treatments (MDFT and CBT in study 1, and MDFT and ESAU in study 2) were similarly effective in the classes with fewer comorbid diagnoses, but MDFT was more effective for the class with greater overall severity and comorbidity. Results suggest that general therapy factors might be sufficient to understand outcomes for youths with less-severe drug use and less comorbidity. However, for more-severe drug users with greater psychiatric comorbidity, the results suggest specific treatment factors such as family-based, multiple-systems interventions may produce superior treatment outcomes.

An ongoing randomized trial set in Greater New Orleans tests MDFT as an integrative family-based approach to treating comorbid substance abuse and trauma symptoms among teens and families in the wake of Hurricane Katrina. This study has a treatment development component in which MDFT developers have systematically incorporated trauma-focused interventions within the model.[58] The approach is unique in that few trauma-focused interventions have been integrated within an empirically supported substance abuse program. In addition, few empirically based trauma interventions concurrently address the stress and coping of teens and their parents, or leverage the healing potential of the family as a larger unit. Participants were adolescents aged 13 to 17 years who had lived in a Greater New Orleans parish when Hurricane Katrina struck and were referred for drug treatment. Adolescents were randomized into standard group drug treatment or MDFT, both delivered within the same community-based treatment agency. Outcomes are assessed at intake, 2-, 4-, 6-, and 12-months follow-up.

Eighty adolescents and their parents participated in the trial. The average age of participants was 15.6 years (SD = 1.0) and the sample was predominantly male (87%) and juvenile-justice involved (65% had 1 or more arrests at intake). The sample was 29% African American; 49% white, non-Hispanic, 4% Hispanic, and 3% other. Participants were primarily marijuana users with 21% meeting Diagnostic and Statistical Manual IV (DSM-IV) diagnostic criteria for cannabis dependence and 43% meeting criteria for cannabis abuse (another 18% had alcohol abuse or dependence). A total of 68% met criteria for any SUD. Comorbid psychiatric diagnoses were also common among youths (78%): 30% had CD, 21% generalized anxiety disorder, 34% ADHD, and 18% major depressive disorder. Trauma symptoms were of particular interest given high rates of PTSD among youths in previous disaster studies. In addition to the disruptive experience and aftermath of Hurricane Katrina, 73% had experienced the death of a loved one, and 71% reported 1 or more significant traumatic life events (average life events = 2). According to youth reports on the Diagnostic Interview Schedule for Children, 29% had PTSD symptoms, and parents also reported high rates of youths' symptoms meeting criteria for PTSD (13%). Parents' own psychological symptoms were also high: 22% of parents scored in the clinical range on the Brief Symptom Inventory Global Severity Index; 41% were in the clinical range for depression; 45% for anxiety; 58% for somatization; 54% for obsessive-compulsive symptoms. According to youth and parent reports, 34% had a family member with an alcohol problem; 35% had a family member with a drug problem; and 45% had a family member with police/court involvement. Although outcome analyses are ongoing, the study has shown that an integrated substance abuse and trauma intervention could be delivered with youths and parents following a major disaster. In addition, community-based providers delivered the approach with fidelity and good retention rates.

SUMMARY

Given the difficulties inherent in treating substance abusing youths with multiple impairments (including school failure; family dysfunction; relationships with antisocial, drug using peers; co-existing psychiatric disorders; high-risk sexual behavior; and other problems), there is general agreement that interventions for these youths must be comprehensive and integrated.[59] Family-based approaches, such as MDFT, which target change in the multiple systems associated with development and maintenance of these problems, are among the most effective treatments for adolescent substance abuse and comorbid psychiatric symptoms.[22,26]

However, challenges remain in maximizing the effect of these treatments on the range of problems that co-occur with adolescent substance abuse. Despite the strong outcomes across many functional domains shown here, it is certainly difficult to address all of the related problems that some adolescents and families present with given 4 to 6 months of even the most intensive treatment. Some have advocated for a chronic-care model in which 1 treatment episode would set a foundation for ongoing services and booster sessions, but would not be considered a cure-all for the rest of the teen's development.[2] MDFT has not yet been tested as a continuing-care model; however, the model lends itself well to such an approach in practice.

Although certain features of the model are believed to explain MDFT's effects on multiple problems as outlined earlier, empirical research on mediators of such effects are only in beginning stages. Henderson and colleagues[60] recently found that changes in parental monitoring mediated reductions in adolescent substance use in MDFT. However, there is virtually no research examining mediators of co-occurring adolescent problems.

A new and important area of research involves the modeling of different emotional and behavioral symptoms and how these trajectories interact over time, which would also apply in critical ways to treatment outcomes. For instance, Hussong and colleagues[61] recently showed, using different growth curve models, that substance use in late adolescence plays a launching role on trajectories of antisocial behavior in young adulthood, as well as predicting increases at specific periods of time. This type of analysis, combined with parallel growth mixture modeling, has the potential to assist treatment researchers in understanding whether reductions in substance use drive decreases in other problem behaviors during and following treatment, or whether there are reciprocal effects. These and other studies represent great opportunities for further development of effective intervention for co-occurring adolescent problems.

ACKNOWLEDGMENTS

This research was made possible through funds from NIDA (grants P50 DA11328, 1U01 DA016193, Liddle, PI; DA021887, Rowe, PI) and CSAT (1KD1 TI11871, Liddle, PI), and the dedication and untiring work of Drs Howard Liddle and Gayle Dakof. Sincere thanks go to all of the families who participated in these studies.

REFERENCES

1. Couwenbergh C, van den Brink W, Zwart K, et al. Comorbid psychopathology in adolescents and young adults treated for substance use disorders. Eur Child Adolesc Psychiatry 2006;15:319–28.
2. Hawkins EH. A tale of two systems: co-occurring mental health and substance abuse disorders treatment for adolescents. Annu Rev Psychol 2009;60:197–227.
3. Kaminer Y, Connor DF, Curry JF. Treatment of comorbid adolescent cannabis use and major depressive disorder. Psychiatry 2008;5(9):34–9.
4. Kandel DB, Huang FY, Davies M. Comorbidity between patterns of substance use dependence and psychiatric syndromes. Drug Alcohol Depend 2001; 64(2):233–41.
5. Riggs P. Clinical approach to treatment of ADHD in adolescents with substance use disorders and conduct disorder. J Am Acad Child Adolesc Psychiatry 1998; 37:331–2.
6. Armstrong TD, Costello EJ. Community studies on adolescent substance use, abuse, or dependence and psychiatric comorbidity. J Consult Clin Psychol 2002;70(6):1224–39.
7. Chan YF, Dennis ML, Funk RR. Prevalence and comorbidity of major internalizing and externalizing problems among adolescents and adults presenting to substance abuse treatment. J Subst Abuse Treat 2008;34:14–24.
8. Robbins MS, Kumar S, Walker-Barnes C, et al. Ethnic differences in comorbidity among substance-abusing adolescents referred to outpatient therapy. J Am Acad Child Adolesc Psychiatry 2002;41(4):394–401.
9. Rowe CL, Liddle HA, Greenbaum PE, et al. Impact of psychiatric comorbidity on treatment of adolescent drug abusers. J Subst Abuse Treat 2004;26(2):129–40.
10. Vreugdenhil C, Van Den Brink W, Wouters LF, et al. Substance use, substance use disorders, and comorbidity patterns in a representative sample of incarcerated male Dutch adolescents. J Nerv Ment Dis 2003;191:372–8.
11. Cornelius JR, Maisto SA, Pollock NK, et al. Rapid relapse generally follows treatment for substance use disorders among adolescents. Addict Behav 2003;28(2):381–6.
12. Grella CE, Hser YI, Joshi V, et al. Drug treatment outcomes for adolescents with comorbid mental health and substance abuse disorders. J Nerv Ment Dis 2001; 189(6):384–92.
13. Riggs PDG, Whitmore EJ. Substance use disorders and disruptive behavior disorders. In: Hendren RL, editor. Disruptive behavior disorders in children and adolescent, vol. 18. 2nd edition. Washington, DC: American Psychiatric Press; 1999. p. 133–73.
14. Clingempeel WG, Britt SC, Henggeler SW. Beyond treatment effects: comorbid psychopathologies and long term outcomes among substance-abusing delinquents. Am J Orthop 2008;78(1):29–36.
15. Myers MG, Stewart DG, Brown SA. Progression from conduct disorder to antisocial personality disorder following treatment for adolescent substance abuse. Am J Psychiatry 1998;155:479–85.
16. Jessor R, Jessor SL. Problem behavior and psychosocial development: a longitudinal study of youth. New York: Academic Press; 1977.
17. D'Amico EJ, Edelen MO, Miles JN, et al. The longitudinal association between substance use and delinquency among high-risk youth. Drug Alcohol Depend 2008;93:85–92.
18. Reinherz HG, Giaconia RM, Hauf AM, et al. General and specific childhood risk factors for depression and drug disorders by early adulthood. J Am Acad Child Adolesc Psychiatry 2000;39(2):223–31.

19. Zucker RA, Donovan JE, Masten AS, et al. Early developmental processes and the continuity of risk for underage drinking and problem drinking. Pediatrics 2008;121:S252–72.

20. Glantz MD. Introduction to the special issue on the impact of child psychopathology interventions on subsequent substance abuse: pieces of the puzzle. J Consult Clin Psychol 2002;70(6):1203–6.

21. Spooner C, Hall W. Public policy and the prevention of substance abuse disorders. Curr Opin Psychiatry 2002;15:235–9.

22. Rowe CL, Liddle HA. Substance abuse. J Marital Fam Ther 2003;29(1): 97–120.

23. Skeer M, McCormick MC, Normand ST, et al. A prospective study of familial conflict, psychological stress and the development of substance use disorders in adolescence. Drug Alcohol Depend 2009;104(1–2):65–72.

24. Capaldi DM, Stoolmiller M, Kim HK, et al. Growth in alcohol use in at-risk adolescent boys: two-part random effects prediction models. Drug Alcohol Depend 2009;105:109–17.

25. Brody GH, Beach SR, Philibert RA, et al. Parenting moderates a genetic vulnerability factor in longitudinal increases in youths' substance use. J Consult Clin Psychol 2009;77(1):1–11.

26. Hogue A, Liddle HA. Family-based treatment for adolescent substance abuse: controlled trials and new horizons in services research. J Fam Ther 2009;31: 126–54.

27. Williams RJ, Chang SY. A comprehensive and comparative review of adolescent substance abuse and treatment outcome. Clin Psychol Sci Pract 2000;7(2): 138–66.

28. AACAP. Practice parameters for the assessment and treatment of children and adolescents with substance use disorders. J Am Acad Child Adolesc Psychiatry 2005;44(6):609–21.

29. Cleary M, Hunt G, Matheson S, et al. Psychosocial interventions for people with both severe mental illness and substance misuse. Cochrane Database Syst Rev 2008;(1):CD001088.

30. Hall W, Degenhardt L, Teesson M. Understanding comorbidity between substance use, anxiety, and affective disorders: broadening the research base. Addict Behav 2009;34:526–30.

31. Craig TK, Johnson S, McCrone P, et al. Integrated care for co-occurring disorders: psychiatric symptoms, social functioning, and service costs at 18 months. Psychiatr Serv 2008;59(3):276–82.

32. Liddle HA. Multidimensional family therapy for adolescent cannabis users. Cannabis Youth Treatment (CYT) manual series, vol 5. Rockville (MD): Center for Substance Abuse Treatment, Substance Abuse and Mental Health Services; 2002.

33. Dennis M, Godley SH, Diamond G, et al. Main findings of the Cannabis Youth Treatment (CYT) randomized field experiment. J Subst Abuse Treat 2004;27: 197–213.

34. Liddle HA, Dakof GA, Parker K, et al. Multidimensional family therapy for adolescent drug abuse: results of a randomized clinical trial. Am J Drug Alcohol Abuse 2001;27(4):651–88.

35. Liddle HA, Rowe CL, Dakof GA, et al. Early intervention for adolescent substance abuse: pretreatment to posttreatment outcomes of a randomized control trial comparing multidimensional family therapy and peer group treatment. J Psychoactive Drugs 2004;36:2–37.

36. Liddle HA, Dakof GA, Turner RM, et al. Treating adolescent drug abuse: a randomized trial comparing multidimensional family therapy and cognitive behavior therapy. Addiction 2008;103:1660–70.

37. Liddle HA, Rowe CL, Dakof GA, et al. Multidimensional family therapy for young adolescent substance abuse: twelve month outcomes of a randomized control trial. J Consult Clin Psychol 2009;77(1):12–25.

38. Austin AM, Macgowan MJ, Wagner EF. Effective family-based interventions for adolescents with substance use problems: a systematic review. Res Soc Work Pract 2005;15:67–83.

39. Becker SJ, Curry JF. Outpatient interventions for adolescent substance abuse: a quality of evidence review. J Consult Clin Psychol 2008;76(4):531–43.

40. Brannigan R, Schackman BR, Falco M, et al. The quality of highly regarded adolescent substance abuse treatment programs. Arch Pediatr Adolesc Med 2004;158(9):904–9.

41. Vaughn MG, Howard MO. Adolescent substance abuse treatment: a synthesis of controlled evaluations. Res Soc Work Pract 2004;14:325–35.

42. Waldron HB, Turner CW. Evidence-based psychosocial treatments for adolescent substance abuse. J Clin Child Adolesc Psychol 2008;37(1):238–61.

43. Drug Strategies. Treating teens: a guide to adolescent drug problems. Washington, DC: Drug Strategies; 2003.

44. Rigter H, Van Gageldonk A, Ketelaars T. Treatment and other interventions targeting drug use and addiction: state of the art 2004. Utrecht: National Drug Monitor; 2005.

45. Liddle HA. Theory development in a family-based therapy for adolescent drug abuse. J Clin Child Psychol 1999;28:521–37.

46. Bronfenbrenner U. Contexts of child rearing: problems and prospects. Am Psychol 1979;34(10):844–50.

47. Hawkins DJ, Catalano RF, Miller JY. Risk and protective factors for alcohol and other drug problems in adolescence and early adulthood: implications for substance abuse prevention. Psychol Bull 1992;112(1):64–105.

48. Dakof GA, Quille TJ, Tejeda MJ, et al. Enrolling and maintaining mothers of substance-exposed infants in drug abuse treatment. J Consult Clin Psychol 2003;71(4):764–72.

49. Liddle HA, Rowe CL, Dakof GA, et al. Effectiveness of cross-systems multidimensional family therapy for justice-involved youth. Presented at the APA 116th Annual Convention 2008; Boston.

50. Rowe CL, Liddle HA, Dakof GA, et al. Development and evolution of an evidence-based practice: multidimensional family therapy as treatment system. In: Collins F, Cohen L, editors. Pharmacology and treatment of substance abuse. New York (NY): Routledge/Taylor & Francis Group, Erlbaum; 2009. p. 441–63.

51. Rowe CL, Liddle HA, McClintic K, et al. Integrative treatment development: multidimensional family therapy for adolescent substance abuse. Integrative/eclectic therapies. In: Kaslow F, Lebow J, editors, Comprehensive handbook of psychotherapy, vol. 4. New York: John Wiley and Sons; 2002. p. 133–61.

52. Marvel F, Rowe CL, Colon L, et al. Multidimensional family therapy HIV/STD risk reduction intervention: an integrative family-based model for drug-involved offenders. Fam Process 2009;48:69–83.

53. Dennis M. Short (3–12 month) and long (30 month) term outcomes of the Cannabis Youth Treatment experiment. Adolescent substance abuse treatment Symposium. College on Problems of Drug Dependence Annual Conference 2003. Bal Harbor (FL).

54. French MT, Roebuck MC, Dennis M, et al. The economic cost of outpatient marijuana treatment for adolescents: findings from a multisite experiment. Addiction 2002;97(Suppl 1):S84–97.
55. Hogue AT, Liddle HA, Becker D, et al. Family-based prevention counseling for high-risk young adolescents: immediate outcomes. Am J Community Psychol 2002;30(1):1–22.
56. Liddle HA, Dakof GA. Controlled trial of a family-based alternative to residential drug treatment for co-morbid adolescent substance abusers: preliminary findings. College on Drug Dependence Annual Conference 2002. Quebec City, Canada.
57. Henderson CE, Dakof GA, Greenbaum P, et al. Effectiveness of multidimensional family therapy with higher-severity substance abusing adolescents: report from two randomized controlled trials. J Consult Clin Psychology, submitted for publication.
58. Rowe CL, Liddle HA. When the levee breaks: treating adolescents and families in the aftermath of Hurricane Katrina. J Marital Fam Ther 2008;34(2):132–48.
59. Rounds-Bryant JL, Kristiansen PL, Hubbard RL. Drug abuse treatment outcome study of adolescents: a comparison of client characteristics and pretreatment behaviors in three treatment modalities. Am J Drug Alcohol Abuse 1999;25: 573–91.
60. Henderson CE, Rowe CL, Dakof GA, et al. Parenting practices as mediators of treatment effects in an early intervention trial of multidimensional family therapy. Am J Drug Alcohol Abuse 2009;35:220–6.
61. Hussong AM, Curran PJ, Moffitt TE, et al. Testing turning points using latest growth curve models: competing models of substance abuse and desistance in young adulthood. In: Cohen P, editor. Applied data analytic techniques for turning points research. New York: Routledge/Taylor & Francis Group; 2008. p. 81–104.

From Assessment Reactivity to Aftercare for Adolescent Substance Abuse: Are We There Yet?

Yifrah Kaminer, MD, MBA[a],*, Mark Godley, PhD[b]

KEYWORDS

- Adolescent substance abuse • Assessment reactivity
- Aftercare • Continued care • Adaptive treatment

Significant progress has been made in the development of evidence-based practice treatment protocols for youth with alcohol and substance use disorders (AOSUD) in the last 20 years.[1] Most interventions have been provided in outpatient settings where more than 80% of youth are being treated.[2] The focus has been on several therapeutic approaches and modalities including family/community therapies, cognitive behavioral therapy (CBT), motivational interviewing (MI), and 12-step/fellowship meetings as reviewed in recent meta-analyses,[3,4] as well as integrated interventions reported in the benchmark Cannabis Youth Treatment (CYT) study.[5]

The purpose of this article is to address less developed areas of clinical research that are of great importance for better understanding the therapeutic process along the continuum of care in youth with AOSUD. These include the rationale, design, mechanisms of behavior change (MBCs), implementation, monitoring, and outcome-based modification of treatment continuum for youth with AOSUD. The specific objectives are: (1) present current knowledge pertaining to the pretreatment phase including the effect of baseline assessment on treatment outcome; (2) address potential MBCs in treatment; (3) discuss the importance of aftercare, also known as continued care, to prevent postintervention relapse; (4) consider how reconceptualization of therapeutic paradigms might advance the field, in particular treatment algorithm or adaptive treatment (AT) strategies addressing poor response to treatment.

---

[a] Department of Psychiatry, Alcohol Research Center, University of Connecticut Health Center, 263 Farmington Avenue, Farmington, CT 06030-2103, USA
[b] Chestnut Health Systems, 448 Wylie Drive, Normal, IL 61761, USA
* Corresponding author.
E-mail address: Kaminer@uchc.edu

Child Adolesc Psychiatric Clin N Am 19 (2010) 577–590
doi:10.1016/j.chc.2010.03.009
1056-4993/10/$ – see front matter © 2010 Elsevier Inc. All rights reserved.

childpsych.theclinics.com

YOUTH VERSUS ADULTS

Treated teens differ from their adult counterparts in length and severity of substance use, typical patterns and context of use, type of substance-related problems most often experienced, and source of referral to treatment.[6,7] Adolescent substance use and abuse should be evaluated in a developmental perspective. There are subgroups of adolescents who have not yet started drinking, or who have not yet reached the peak of the trajectory characterizing their drinking pattern. Therefore, any effort to reduce or eliminate drinking amounts to "swimming against the tide or current." Furthermore, youth are less motivated to change substance use, and often enter treatment because of external pressures.[8] This happens either as a suggested referral by a concerned parent, mental health clinician, school staff, or as a mandate initiated by the legal system.

An important question is "when does treatment begin and when does it end for adolescents"? Most clinicians who are not versed in the developmental perspective of youth treatment are likely to cut and paste from their experience with adult patients. That is, focus on a single or repeated treatment episode and determine that the goal is no less than abstinence. Only a limited proportion of adolescents, however, will achieve sobriety from alcohol or abstinence from substance abuse following a single episode of treatment. Some outpatient teens might be more appropriately considered continuing users, who did not have the opportunity for relapse because they either achieved only partial response (ie, harm reduction in terms of frequency, dosage, or transition from heavier to lighter drugs) or did not accomplish complete abstinence from use while in treatment.[6] (Relapse is referred to sometimes as an event; in that case it is more appropriate to define it as a lapse. Relapse is more commonly perceived as a process.) Even those who achieved abstinence are likely to relapse 3 to 6 months later[5,9] and will get in and out of abstinence repeatedly thereafter.[10]

Treatment of youth is not an event but a continued process. The extent of an optimal intervention continuum should include an assessment,[11] treatment, and continued care, which take into consideration the specific needs such as psychiatric comorbidity[12] and the response of the adolescent AOSUD and associated psychiatric comorbidity to treatment.[13]

PRETREATMENT FACTORS AND BASELINE ASSESSMENT REACTIVITY

Therapeutic changes may commence before treatment has begun. The contribution of pretreatment events, baseline assessment, and even an advice to change harmful behaviors, have been underestimated or mostly ignored in clinical practice regardless of empiric findings to the contrary.[14]

Sobell and colleagues[15] reported that some adults with problematic drinking stopped using alcohol by simply being exposed to an advertisement of a clinical trial. Others responded to advice by a clinician to stop smoking[16] or drinking[17] because it might be harmful to their health. More participants quit smoking in the month immediately preceding the research interview than had quit in the month following brief intervention.[16] According to the classic study by Edwards and colleagues[17] 2 groups of alcoholics received either 1 counseling session or several months of in- and outpatient treatment. One year later there was no significant differences in outcome between the 2 groups.

Although youth are not highly motivated for treatment, advice may be an effective brief intervention with older adolescent cannabis users in its own right.[18] Moreover, when fidelity of MI treatment provided to those randomized to the experimental condition was not high, it was not more effective than advice. Given the scarcity of resources for treatment and because only 10% to 15% of youth who need some form of intervention will eventually get it, further trials on the potential merit of advice for youth substance abusers are warranted.

Baseline Assessment Reactivity

Participants in treatment outcome studies undergo extensive assessment protocols to assess eligibility and to provide information before beginning therapy sessions. Participants might be exposed, therefore, to a professional who does not necessarily function as a therapist, such as a research assistant in a clinical trial or a nurse in an outpatient clinic setting. Such interactions might be effective in initiating change and reducing substance use although, a priori, they were not intended to be therapeutic. This change is defined as assessment reactivity.[19] In this case, assessment reactivity refers to a change of substance use status from positive to negative from baseline to the time of initiation of the first therapy session.

Kaminer and colleagues[20] conducted a study to examine if a change from positive to negative alcohol use from baseline assessment to the onset of the first session (ie, pretreatment phase) occurs in adolescents (ie, baseline assessment reactivity [BAR]), and compare what mediators differentiate BAR-positive and BAR-negative youths. Participants were 177 adolescents with alcohol use disorders (82% used additional substances) in 9 weekly group sessions of CBT. Self-reports for alcohol and urinalysis for drug use in the last 30 days before baseline assessment and immediately before the first session of treatment were obtained to determine BAR. For alcohol use 51.4% reported abstinence at the first session; 29% of those who were positive for other drugs at baseline assessment tested negative for drugs. The finding was highly significant. It was also reported that variables such as age, gender, criminal justice involvement, or waiting duration from baseline assessment to first session were not associated with BAR. The likelihood of manifesting BAR was significantly correlated with the level of readiness to change and with 3 of 8 subscales measuring self-efficacy. In this study, alcohol and substance use at first session predicted use at last session. Participants continued to improve from first to last session. That is, treatment outcome was not solely attributed to BAR.

These findings support the validity of BAR as a construct relevant to youth waiting for the initiation of treatment of AOSUD. For the second objective of the study, Epstein and colleagues,[19] who found that alcohol baseline assessment is therapeutic in adults, provide 3 possible explanations for observed changes in adults drinking before initiating treatment: "(1) decision making about changing drinking that is prompted by seeing an advertisement, (2) telling someone in the social network about a decision to seek help, resulting in a change in others' responses to drinking and abstinence, and (3) initiation of a therapeutic change process as a result of the assessment itself. For instance, realizing the extent and severity of one's drinking problems in the course of verbalizing them to another person. This possible explanation can be considered assessment reactivity."[19]

As in the study by Epstein and colleagues[19] it is possible that the assessment per se supported motivation to change. We do not know whether these youth would have changed their alcohol and substance use patterns based on sheer insight without the assessment as might happen with adults.[15] Based on our clinical experience this is unlikely to happen with youth.

Assessment reactivity was also reported in association with posttreatment follow-up assessments in adults.[21–23] No studies of assessment reactivity in youth during the posttreatment phase have been reported.

Clifford and Maisto[21] posit that the integration of self regulation processes, that is, the ability to modify one's behavior in response to changing environmental demands that is achieved through the integration of comparison processes and FRAMES (see next section) might explain the MBC of assessment reactivity.

In conclusion, it is important to identify assessment reactivity and separate it from treatment effects[20] because, "if change is indeed occurring prior to treatment proper and this initial change is not taken into account in interpreting outcome data, then positive findings may be misattributed to the experimental treatment rather than to the processes of change that began before treatment."[19] Therefore, it is recommended that BAR should be considered in any analysis targeting adolescent alcohol treatment outcomes.

MECHANISMS OF BEHAVIORAL CHANGE

In the search to identify the effective ingredients of successful therapy, 1 therapist characteristic in particular, accurate empathy, as defined by Carl Rogers,[24] has been shown to be a predictor of therapeutic success. Within the addiction field, the search for critical conditions that are necessary and sufficient to induce change has led to the identification of 6 critical elements[25]: (1) Feedback regarding personal risk or impairment; (2) emphasis on personal Responsibility for change; (3) clear Advice to change; (4) a Menu of alternative change options; (5) therapist's Empathy; and (6) facilitation of participant optimism about the potential to change and Self-efficacy. These 6 active ingredients of effective brief interventions are represented best by the acronym FRAMES. Therapeutic interventions containing some or all of these elements have been effective in initiating change and reducing alcohol use. Baseline and posttreatment assessments conducted by emphatic and caring research staff contain some or all of the components or active ingredients of FRAMES. Consequently, these interactions might be effective in initiating change and reducing substance use although, a priori, they were not intended to be therapeutic.

Despite prominent differences in theory, design, and methodology, the most recent studies using various treatment modalities in youth with AOSUD have reported remarkably similar outcomes.[3] Rates of adolescent relapse of substance involvement are comparable with those of adults during the first year after treatment completion.[6,26] About 60% of adolescents continued to vacillate in and out of recovery after discharge from 3-month treatment programs.[5,9,27] These findings point to the increased need to understand what (if any) are the specific differences between MBCs of therapeutic approaches that carry diverse names, have been distinguished by different ideologies, hypotheses, and technologies although they have produced similar outcomes.[5,9,28] Are there similar and/or nonspecific ingredients that these therapies share?

Most evidence-based treatments are also theory based, at least to some degree. However, recent meta-analyses examining the hypothesized mechanisms of action on which the interventions are based did not yield clear results.[29,30] These results apply to Alcoholics Anonymous,[31] CBT,[32] and MI.[33] Some theorists have argued that positive treatment effects are due primarily to what are referred to as general therapeutic factors, such as an empathic and caring therapist, and the structure and support provided by regularly scheduled treatment sessions over a prolonged period of time.[34,35] Three important mediators have been noted in the limited adolescent literature: self-efficacy,[36,37] coping skills acquisition and/or improvement,[28] and motivation or readiness to change.[38]

CBT hypothesizes that those who do not make progress in treatment or relapse lack or are deficient in the coping skills necessary to deal with life stressors and high-risk situations. Therefore, provision of these skills will increase self-efficacy or confidence in the ability to refrain from drug use.[28] Change in self-efficacy seems to be a partial mediator of treatment outcome in a large multicenter study for the treatment of cannabis use disorders in adults. Increase in self-efficacy before and after treatment was a more powerful predictor of decrease in drug use than was coping skills.[39] A later study by the same team reported that early abstinence seems to be important, to the extent that it increases self-efficacy.[40] Nevertheless, contrary to expectations, CBT in adults did not result in greater coping skills acquisition than did an MI comparison group. Similarly, in an adolescent treatment study self-efficacy was found to be directly correlated with treatment outcome even when controlling for drug-positive urine in treatment and regardless of therapeutic approach.[36] That is, regardless of the implementation of theory driven CBT, this approach did not produce higher levels of self-efficacy compared with interpersonal treatment.

No studies in adolescents with AOSUD have yet reported measurements of improved coping skills. One way of achieving this goal is an ongoing effort to compare data on self-efficacy generated by the Situational Confidence Questionnaire[41] with the youth Coping Skills Inventory.[42]

MI is an approach focusing on improved motivation to change in a nonconfrontational manner.[43] MI has been found efficacious in reducing alcohol use in college students. However, increased motivation or readiness to change does not seem to be the mechanism or mediator of behavior change.[44] Some studies in adults have indicated that MI does not lead to improved outcomes through the Stages of Change Theory[45] that drives the intervention.[46] Furthermore, clear operational definitions of commonly used terms such as motivation, readiness, and/or commitment to change or to engage in treatment are not available. These terms seem to overlap and are measured by different rating scales (Chung, Winters and Kaminer, personal correspondence, November 2009).

Several studies in youths emphasize the importance of readiness to change in predicting treatment outcomes. Increased motivation to change has been cited often as a predictor for positive outcome in the adult and youth literature. Subscales from the Stages of Change Readiness and Treatment Eagerness Scales (SOCRATES) have been found to predict the level of alcohol use at 1-year follow-up in treated youths.[47] Higher motivation to abstain predicted fewer days of marijuana use in adolescents.[48] Chung and Maisto[49] reported that there was a reciprocal association between motivation to change and substance use. Furthermore, most adolescents reported that substance abuse treatment helped to increase their readiness to change substance use behavior. MI was suggested to increase change talk, a construct describing more assertive statements about the wish to limit or stop using drugs that was associated with better outcomes in adults[50] and youth.[51] However, the mechanism that foster change talk in youth has not yet been identified. Chung[52] suggests investigating social network characteristics that might affect motivation to change.

In conclusion, it seems that improved self-efficacy and motivation to change are correlated with better outcomes in youth regardless of the chosen therapeutic approach.

AFTER/CONTINUED CARE FOR YOUTH AOSUD

Historically, aftercare referred to maintenance interventions (eg, group counseling, mutual aid meetings) following a successful course of an index biopsychosocial treatment for AOSUD. Step-down care (ie, referral to successively lower intensity treatment episodes) is the most common form of aftercare.[53,54] The step-down model with adolescents has not proved to be a common course for adolescents.[2] A more typical course is to for adolescents to either discontinue their acute care episode prematurely or experience relapse relatively soon after discharge without being involved in aftercare.[2,9,55] The American Society of Addiction Medicine (ASAM[56]) thus defined continuing care as flexible services that provide AOSUD patients the type of treatment needed at any given time. This definition of continuing care implies that for many, perhaps most, AOSUD is ongoing and prone to relapse in the same manner as other chronic diseases. Although the ASAM definition is well recognized in practice, even the best intended referrals are more likely to result in failure to show without assertive intercession by a clinician.[57]

Until recently almost all randomized clinical trials (RCTs) published on after/ continuing care were studies of adults whose inclusion in the trial required successful completion of their index treatment episode.[53,58] Reviews of these studies reveal a slight advantage for more structured, CBT-derivative interventions such as coping skills, specific relapse prevention skill training, sometimes combined with interpersonal counseling and/or attendance at 12-step meetings. A trend was noted for aftercare interventions with greater intensity and duration to perform better relative to controls.[53]

More recently, addiction treatment researchers have reported after/continuing care RCTs for adolescents with AOSUD. Godley and colleagues[59,60] reported on an assertive continuing care (ACC). This manualized approach[61] is a combination of community visits (home, school, other location), case management, and the Adolescent Community Reinforcement Approach (A-CRA[62]). The latter is an operant learning model that helps youth and caregivers learn how to restructure their environment (friends, social activities) to reinforce sobriety. A-CRA also uses elements of CBT to relabel or reappraise events, and to build competing skills to improve communication with caregivers and others, problem solving, anger management, and drinking/drug use peer refusal. In a recent clinical trial of this approach 183 adolescents discharged from residential treatment (only half successfully completed this treatment) were randomized to either ACC or usual continuing care (UCC).[63] In this study ACC included community visits, A-CRA, and case management services to help adolescents better comply with educational, juvenile justice, and other social systems in which they were involved. The UCC condition included a referral to attend an outpatient clinic (usually group psychoeducation and process counseling) and 12-step meetings. The active continuing care phase was limited to 3 months with an additional 6 months of follow-up. A large ACC effect was found for initiation of continuing care services (d = 1.07) and retention (d = 0.90). A main effect for more ACC participants to maintain total abstinence from cannabis use for the 9-month combined continuing care and follow-up phase was also found (d = .32). In this and a subsequent study[64] the clinical outcome was mediated in part by a measure of general continuing care adherence (GCCA) factors recommended by clinicians for good continuing care (eg, case coordination with probation officer, communication, relapse prevention skills, and so forth), improvements in the recovery environment, and decreased social risk.

Because most adolescents receive their index care episode in outpatient treatment, studies are needed to extend our understanding of after/continuing care following outpatient treatment. Burleson and Kaminer[65] established the acceptability and feasibility of a brief aftercare intervention involving a single face-to-face session to conduct a functional analysis of environmental contingencies supporting substance use followed by a series of 15-minute telephone calls at 2- to 3-week intervals to assess status of use, motivation to change, and then identify problem areas and provide skills guidelines to address problems. This intervention was later tested in an RCT where 177 adolescents with DSM IV alcohol use disorders, 80% of whom were also diagnosed with cannabis use disorders, completed 9 weekly in-person (IP) outpatient CBT sessions. Adolescents were then randomized to either a 5-session face-to-face booster course of CBT, a brief telephone condition, or no active aftercare condition (NA). At the end of the 3-month aftercare phase, the likelihood of relapse, days of alcohol use, and days of heavy alcohol use were significantly greater for the NA condition than the combined active aftercare conditions.[14] This significant relapse prevention outcome was moderated by gender with girls receiving active aftercare showing no significant relapse relative to girls in the NA condition. Active aftercare interventions, although effective in slowing the expected posttreatment relapse process for alcohol use, did not show lasting effects at 6-, 9-, and 12-month follow-ups.[66] This study provides experimental support that during the aftercare phase, active aftercare prevents relapse, and may be especially effective for girls. Postaftercare outcomes are still needed to assess long-term effectiveness of active aftercare. Similar to findings with adults[53] the brief telephone intervention was as effective as the IP aftercare intervention.

In another outpatient study, Godley and colleagues[67] conducted a 4-group randomized study (N = 320) of brief outpatient motivational enhancement training (MET) integrated with CBT[66] compared with a more intensive, individualized course of outpatient treatment. This latter intervention was also manual guided, and primarily delivered through behavioral/cognitive behavioral skill and process groups, and included family and individual sessions for treatment planning. These 2 conditions were crossed with either ACC (as described earlier) or no ACC. All participants were randomized to 1 of the 4 conditions and retained for follow-up and outcome analyses, including youth who failed to successfully complete the index outpatient treatment. An interesting feature of this study was that it contrasted a brief highly standardized evidence-based treatment (MET/CBT) with a less standardized, more intensive, and individualized length of stay approach, which is more characteristic of contemporary outpatient treatment practice. Differences in dosage were substantial but overall there was not a dose-response relationship in alcohol or substance use outcomes. However, at the 6- and 9-month follow-up there was a main effect for the more intensive outpatient plus ACC approach; but by the 12-month follow-up there were no condition main effects. Because the more intensive, individualized outpatient treatment combined with ACC resulted in the most extensive length of stay (M = 172 days) and demonstrated main effects until services were withdrawn (virtually all subjects were discharged by the 9-month follow-up), the results seem consistent with recommendations for extended care interventions with adults.[68]

FUTURE RESEARCH DIRECTIONS: EXTENDING CARE WITH ADAPTIVE TREATMENT

A decade ago researchers asserted that AOSUDs are better understood as a chronic relapsing illness requiring acute treatment and ongoing management strategies to prevent or reduce harm from relapse.[69–71] Subsequently, the limitations of short-term specific effects designs to evaluate addiction treatment were noted.[30,72] The traditional experimental designs for youth AOSUD have emphasized the comparison of standardized fixed interventions as the primary method for evaluating treatment efficacy. These fixed interventions tend to be brief and unresponsive to the considerable variation in patient response and changing environmental contexts. Most treatments studied in the addictions strive to deliver essentially the same intervention to all patients, regardless of how the patient is responding. Indeed, treatment research based on this approach has overlooked the most urgent challenges facing the field. These are the heterogeneity of adolescent response to treatment, the problem of poor response to treatment, and the need to provide ongoing monitoring, support, and reintervention to prevent or manage the likelihood of relapse.[3,73]

McKay[53] presented a series of key questions in treatment pertaining to what to do with patients who do not respond to an initial treatment episode. Should their initial treatment be switched to something else? If so, to what treatment? Or, should they receive another treatment to augment what they are already taking? In accordance with the stepped care approach,[44,74,75] patients are started at the lowest appropriate level of care, and then stepped up to more intensive treatment if warranted by poor initial response. This approach has the potential to increase rates of participation, as it may be more palatable to patients because it places a lower burden on them at the beginning of treatment. Stepped care may also increase cost-effectiveness and cost-benefit, because lower intensity treatments are also often less costly.[53] Adaptive or stepped care treatment algorithms have been developed and evaluated for several disorders, including depression and anxiety,[76–78] obesity, and eating disorders.[79,80]

In most cases, AT protocols contain separate algorithms for 2 main classes of patients: poor-responders (stepped up) and responders (stepped down). After an optimized adaptive algorithm is developed via the experimental method, it should be further tested against treatment as usual or some other control condition in an RCT. This step is needed to determine whether the algorithm in fact improves outcomes relative to standard care.[53,81–83]

According to an extensive review included in a book authored by McKay,[53] several elements are critical for the design of AT:

Tailoring variables are selected to assess key markers of progress that are going to be used to construct the adaptive algorithm. The most common approach is the outcome measure approach. In this approach, the therapist regularly assesses substance use during treatment, and uses that information to decide whether treatment should be continued as currently delivered or modified in some way. Using the outcome measure as a tailoring variable has several advantages. Most important, it gets around the issue of whether the tailoring variable is a good marker of progress and is in fact related to outcome.

Menu of clinical interventions. The key requirement here is that the clinical services in the menu are meaningfully different on at least 1 dimension, such as frequency, intensity, modality, content, theoretic orientation, and so forth. For an adaptive strategy to work, the treatment options must be different enough that failure in 1 treatment approach will not strongly predict failure in all the other possible approaches in the menu.[53]

Decision rules. In an adaptive protocol they link the tailoring variables and the menu of clinical intervention options into 1 algorithm. The finished algorithm reads like a series of if–then statements. The decision rules that link specific scores on tailoring variables to modifications in treatment are arrived at through 1 of 2 processes, either expert consensus or an experimental study. In this proposal the "if" is poor response and the "then" is assignment to adaptive treatment.

The adult literature on AT includes a total of 15 studies that yielded significant results in which adaptive procedures led to either better substance use outcomes or to equivalent outcomes in treatments with other advantages (eg, lower cost, lower patients burden, greater safety, and so forth), or produced algorithms that specified which patients would benefit most from what continuation treatments.[53,84] Practicing child and adolescent psychiatrists have developed algorithms to address the issue of nonresponse for depression, most notably the Texas algorithm by Hughes and colleagues.[85] However, adolescent substance abuse treatment which relies mostly on psychosocial interventions has not generated an empirically supported set of tailoring variables and decision rules specifying the intervention that is most likely to be effective in the face of initial nonresponse. The findings of AT in the adult literature and the dire needs of youth with AOSUD underscore the importance of extending AT to youth substance abuse treatment outcome research.

SUMMARY

Similar to the development of substance use disorder as a process and not as a sudden event, the undoing of the disorder is a multiphased lengthy process that may require several repeated interventions for the adolescent. Relapse should therefore be perceived as a process and not as an event.[86] The research of MBCs is in its infancy and Magill[29] noted that what we know about the treatment process to date is what we have chosen to measure and that evidence points to a common process of change. Consequently, continued research on other potential MBCs (in addition to self-efficacy, motivation/readiness to change,[87] and coping skills) is necessary. Further examination of the role of the therapist and their interactions with the clients in individual, family, and group interventions is warranted see article by Macgowan and Engle elsewhere in this issue for further exploration of this topic. This includes examination of specificity as well as the nonspecific components of treatment.

Extending care through adaptive treatment and management of adolescent AOSUD has yet to be studied for at least 12 months, following McKay's[68] findings of empiric support for interventions extending past 12 months. More recently, an adult study of quarterly recovery management checkups (RMC) and readmission to treatment (when clinically indicated) was superior to quarterly follow-up interviews.[88] A key to the value of RMC is the similarity of methodology used to locate patients in multiyear longitudinal studies. Future research to extend care and monitoring with adolescents should consider testing similar methods for long-term retention and testing of adaptive treatment algorithms.

Future strategies should also consider using communications technologies embraced by youth in contemporary society. Most youth today, including those receiving AOSUD treatment, have mobile phones. The brief telephone protocol[89,90] provides a flexible protocol that can be paired with assertive patient locating procedures. A short message service (SMS) texting version of the protocol could also be tested as many adolescents' increasingly prefer this mode of communication over voice. In 1 survey of treated youth more than 90% reported http://MySpace.com profiles[57] underscoring just how ubiquitous web-based social networking has become among adolescents. Future research on adaptive treatment of adolescents should be mated to tracking technologies that are clearly embraced by youth to increase the chances of long-term retention, monitoring, support, and when necessary, reintervention. The gap between clinical care and science persists in clinical care of youth. To promote delivery of evidence-based effective care a meta-systematic approach should be adopted.[91]

REFERENCES

1. Dennis ML, Kaminer Y. Introduction to special issue on advances in the assessment and treatment of adolescent substance use disorders. Am J Addict 2006; 15(Suppl 1):1–3.
2. Office of Applied Studies. Treatment episode data set (TEDS): 2002. Discharges from substance abuse treatment services. (DASIS series S-25, DHHS publication

no. (SMA) 04-3967). Rockville (MD): Substance Abuse and Mental Health Services Administration; 2005.

3. Waldron HB, Turner CW. Evidence-based psychological treatments for adolescent substance abuse. J Clin Child Adolesc Psychol 2008;37:238–61.

4. Becker SJ, Curry JF. Outpatient interventions for adolescent substance abuse: a quality of evidence review. J Consult Clin Psychol 2008;76(4):531–43.

5. Dennis ML, Godley SH, Diamond G, et al. Main findings of the cannabis youth treatment randomized field experiment. J Subst Abuse Treat 2004;27:197–213.

6. Chung T, Maisto SA. Review and reconsideration of relapse as a change point in clinical course in treated adolescents. Clin Psychol Rev 2006;26:149–61.

7. Chung T, Martin C. Adolescent substance use and substance use disorders: prevalence and clinical course. In: Kaminer Y, Winters KC, editors. Clinical manual of adolescent substance abuse treatment. Washington DC: American Psychiatric Association; 2010, in press.

8. Battjes RJ, Gordon MS, O'Grady KE, et al. Factors that predict adolescent motivation for substance abuse treatment. J Subst Abuse Treat 2003;24:221–32.

9. Brown SA, Vik PN, Creamer V. Characteristics of relapse following adolescent substance abuse treatment. Addict Behav 1989;14:291–300.

10. Winters K, Stinchfield R, Latimer WW, et al. Internalizing and externalizing behaviors and their association with the treatment of adolescents with substance use disorder. J Subst Abuse Treat 2008;35:269–78.

11. Winters K, Kaminer Y. Screening and assessing adolescent substance use disorders in clinical population. J Am Acad Child Adolesc Psychiatry 2008;47:740–4.

12. Kaminer Y, Bukstein O, editors. Adolescent substance abuse: dual diagnosis and high risk behaviors. New York: Routledge/Taylor & Francis; 2008, in press.

13. Hawke JM, Kaminer Y, Burleson J, et al. Stability of comorbid psychiatric diagnoses among youths in treatment and aftercare for alcohol use disorders. Subst Abuse 2008;29(2):33–42.

14. Kaminer Y, Burleson J, Burke R. Efficacy of outpatient aftercare for adolescents with alcohol use disorders: a randomized controlled study. J Am Acad Child Adolesc Psychiatry 2008;47(12):1405–12.

15. Sobell LC, Agrawla S, Sobell MB, et al. Responding to an advertisement: a critical event in promoting self-change of drinking behavior. Poster Presented at the 37th Annual Meeting of the Association for the Advancement of Behavior Therapy. Boston, November 20–23, 2003.

16. Russell MA, Wilson C, Taylor C, et al. Effect of general practitioner's advice against smoking. BMJ 1979;6184:231–5.

17. Edwards G, Orford J, Egert S, et al. Alcoholism: a controlled trial of treatment and advice. J Stud Alcohol 1977;38:1004–31.

18. McCambridge J, Slym RL, Strang J. Randomized controlled trial of motivational interviewing compared with drug information and advice for early intervention among 16 to 19 years old weekly or more frequently cannabis users. Addiction 2008;103:1809–18.

19. Epstein EE, Drapkin ML, Yusko DA, et al. Is alcohol assessment therapeutic? Pretreatment change in drinking among alcohol-dependent women? J Stud Alcohol 2005;66:369–78.

20. Kaminer Y, Burleson JA, Burke R. Can assessment reactivity predict treatment outcome among adolescents with alcohol and other substance use disorders. Subst Abuse 2008;29(2):63–70.

21. Clifford PR, Maisto SA. Subject reactivity effects and alcohol treatment outcome research. J Stud Alcohol 2000;61:787–93.

22. Clifford PR, Maisto SA, Franzke LH, et al. Alcohol treatment research follow-up interviews and drinking behaviors. J Stud Alcohol 2000;61:736–43.
23. Clifford PR, Maisto SA, Davis CM. Alcohol treatment research assessment exposure subject reactivity effects: part I. Alcohol use and related consequences. J Stud Alcohol Drugs 2007;68:519–28.
24. Rogers CR. The necessary and sufficient conditions of therapeutic personality change. J Consult Psychol 1957;21:95–103.
25. Miller WR, Sanchez V. Motivating young adults for treatment and lifestyle change. In: Howard G, Nathan P, editors. Alcohol use and misuse by young adults. Notre Dame (IN): University of Notre Dame Press; 1994. p. 51–81.
26. Williams RJ, Chang SY. A assertive and comparative review of adolescent substance abuse treatment outcome. Clin Psychol Sci Pract 2000;7:138–66.
27. Kaminer Y, Burleson J, Goldberger R. Psychotherapies for adolescent substance abusers: short-and long-term outcomes. J Nerv Ment Dis 2002;190:737–45.
28. Waldron H, Kaminer Y. On the learning curve: cognitive behavioral therapies for adolescent substance abuse. Addiction 2004;99(Suppl 2):93–105.
29. Magill M. Treatment mechanisms: shifting evaluation priorities in alcoholism research. Brown Univ Dig Addict Theory Appl 2009;9:8.
30. Morgenstern J, McKay JR. Rethinking the paradigms that inform behavioral treatment research for substance use disorders. Addiction 2007;102:1377–89.
31. Kelly JF, Magill M, Stout RL. How do people recover from alcohol dependence? A systematic review of the research on mechanisms of behavior change in alcoholic anonymous. Addict Res Theory 2009;17:236–59.
32. Morgenstern J, Longabaugh R. Cognitive-behavioral treatment for alcohol dependence: a review of evidence for its hypothesized mechanisms of action. Addiction 2000;95:1475–90.
33. Apodaca TR, Longabaugh R. Mechanisms of change in motivational interviewing: a review and preliminary evaluation of the evidence. Addiction 2009;104: 705–15.
34. Baskin TW, Tierney SC, Minami T, et al. Establishing specificity in psychotherapy: meta-analysis of structural equivalence of placebo controls. J Consult Clin Psychol 2003;71:973–9.
35. Wampold BE. The great psychotherapy debate: models, methods, and findings. Mahwah (NJ): Lawrence Erlbaum Associates; 2001.
36. Burleson J, Kaminer Y. Adolescent substance use disorders: self-efficacy as a predictor of relapse. Addict Behav 2005;20:1751–64.
37. Moss HB, Kirisci L, Mezzich AC. Psychiatric comorbidity and self-efficacy to resist heavy drinking in alcoholic and nonalcoholic adolescents. Am J Addict 1994;3:204–12.
38. O'Leary TT, Monti PM. Motivational enhancement and other brief interventions for adolescent substance abuse: foundations, applications and evaluations. Addiction 2004;99(Suppl 2):63–75.
39. Litt MD, Kadden RM, Cooney NL, et al. Coping skills and treatment outcomes in cognitive-behavioral and interactional group therapy for alcoholism. J Consult Clin Psychol 2003;71:118–28.
40. Litt MD, Kadden RM, Kabela-Cormier E, et al. Coping skills training and contingency management treatments for marijuana dependence: exploring mechanisms of behavior change. Addiction 2008;103:638–48.
41. Kirisci L, Moss HB, Tarter RE. Psychometric evaluation of the situational confidence questionnaire in adolescents: fitting a graded item response model. Addict Behav 1996;21:303–17.

42. Moos RH. Coping response inventory CRI-youth form professional manual. Odessa (FL): Psychological Assessment Resources; 1993.
43. Miller WR, Rollnick S. Motivational interviewing: preparing people for change. 2nd edition. New York: Guilford Press; 2002.
44. Borsari B, O'Leary Tevyaw T, Barnett NP, et al. Stepped care for mandated college students: a pilot study. Am J Addict 2007;16:131–7.
45. Prochaska JO, DiClemente CC, Norcross JC. In search of how people change: application to addictive behaviors. Am Psychol 1992;47:1102–14.
46. Stotts AL, DeLaune KA, Schmitz JM, et al. Impact of motivational intervention on mechanisms of change in low-income pregnant smokers. Addict Behav 2004;29: 1649–57.
47. Maisto SA, Chung TA, Cornelius JR, et al. Factor structure of the SOCRATES in a clinical sample of adolescents. Psychol Addict Behav 2003;17:98–107.
48. King KM, Chung T, Maisto SA. Treated adolescents'; thoughts about abstinence snare the return to marijuana use. J Consult Clin Psychol 2009;77:554–65.
49. Chung T, Maisto SA. What I got from treatment: predictors of treatment content received and association of treatment content with 6-month outcomes. J Subst Abuse Treat 2009;37:171–81.
50. Moyers TB, Martin T, Christopher PJ, et al. Client language as a mediator of motivational interviewing efficacy: where is the evidence? Alcohol Clin Exp Res 2007; 31:40s–7s.
51. Baer J, Beadnell B, Garrett S, et al. Adolescent change language within a brief motivational intervention and substance use outcomes. Psychol Addict Behav 2008;22:570–5.
52. Chung T. What factors influence and maintain motivation to change. Brown Univ Dig Addict Theory Appl 2009;10:8.
53. MacKay JR. Treating substance use disorders with adaptive continuing care. Washington, DC: American Psychological Association Press; 2009.
54. Jainchill N. Therapeutic communities for adolescents: the same and not the same. In: De Leon G, editor. Community as method: therapeutic communities for special populations and special settings. Westport (CT): Praeger; 1997. p. 161–78.
55. Godley SH, Godley MD, Dennis ML. The assertive aftercare protocol for adolescent substance abusers. In: Wagner E, Waldron H, editors. Innovations in adolescent substance abuse interventions. New York: Elsevier Science; 2001. p. 311–29.
56. American Society of Addiction Medicine (ASAM). Patient placement criteria for the treatment of substance-related disorders. 2nd edition. Chevy Chase (MD): American Society of Addiction Medicine; 2001.
57. Godley MD, Godley SH. Assertive continuing care for adolescents. In: Kelly J, White W, editors. Addiction recovery management: theory, science and practice. New York: Springer Science; in press.
58. McKay JR. The role of continuing care in outpatient alcohol treatment programs. In: Galanter M, editor, Recent developments in alcoholism: services research in the era of managed care, vol. 15. New York: Kluwer Academic; 2001. p. 357–72.
59. Godley MD, Godley SH, Dennis ML, et al. Preliminary outcomes from the assertive continuing care experiment for adolescents discharged from residential treatment. J Subst Abuse Treat 2002;23:21–32.
60. Godley MD, Godley SH, Dennis MI, et al. The effectiveness of assertive continuing care on continuing care linkage, adherence, and abstinence following residential treatment. Addiction 2007;102:81–92.

61. Godley SH, Godley MD, Karvinen T, et al. The assertive continuing care protocol: a clinician's manual for working with adolescents after residential treatment of alcohol and other substance use disorders. 2nd edition. Bloomington (IL): Lighthouse Institute; 2006.

62. Godley SH, Meyers RJ, Smith JE, et al. (DHHS publication no. (SMA) 01-3489)In: The adolescent community reinforcement approach (ACRA) for adolescent cannabis users, cannabis youth treatment manual series, vol. 4. Rockville (MD): Center for Substance Abuse Treatment, Substance Abuse and Mental Health Services Administration; 2001.

63. Godley SH, Risberg RA, Adams L, et al. Chestnut Health System's Bloomington outpatient and intensive outpatient treatment manual. Bloomington (IL): Lighthouse Institute; 2003. Available at: http://www.chestnut.org/LI/bookstore/blurbs/Manuals/ATM/ATM105-CHS-Bloomington.html. Accessed January 19, 2010.

64. Garner BR, Godley MD, Godley SH, et al. The impact of continuing care adherence on environmental risks, substance use, and substance-related problems following adolescent residential treatment. Psychol Addict Behav 2007;21(4):488–97.

65. Burleson JA, Kaminer Y. Aftercare for adolescent alcohol use disorder: feasibility and acceptability of a phone intervention. Am J Addict 2007;16:202–5.

66. Burleson J, Kaminer Y. Outcomes at twelve-month follow-up of aftercare for adolescents with alcohol use disorders. Presented at Annual Meeting of the Research Society on Alcoholism. San Diego (CA), June 26–30, 2009.

67. Godley SH, Garner BR, Passetti LL, et al. Adolescent outpatient treatment and continuing care: main findings from a randomized clinical trial. Drug Alcohol Depend, in press.

68. McKay JR. Is there a case for extended interventions for alcohol and drug use disorders? Addiction 2005;100:1594–610.

69. Boyle MG, White WL, Loveland D, et al. The behavioral health recovery management project: project summary and concept. Available at: http://www.bhrm.org; 2000. Accessed January 19, 2010.

70. McLellan AT, Lewis DC, O'Brien CP, et al. Drug dependence, a chronic medical illness: implications for treatment, insurance, and outcomes evaluation. JAMA 2000;284:1689–95.

71. White W, Boyle M, Loveland D. Addiction as chronic disease: from rhetoric to clinical application. Alcoholism Treat Quart 2002;20(3/4):107–30.

72. McLellan AT, McKay JR, Forman R, et al. Reconsidering the evaluation of addiction treatment: from retrospective follow-up to concurrent recovery monitoring. Addiction 2005;100(4):447–58.

73. Dennis ML, Scott CK. Managing addiction as a chronic condition. Addict Sci Clin Pract 2007;4(1):45–55.

74. Breslin FC, Sobell MB, Sobell LC, et al. Problem drinkers: evaluation of a stepped-care approach. J Subst Abuse 1999;10:217–32.

75. Sobell MB, Sobell LC. Stepped care as a heuristic approach to the treatment of alcohol problems. J Consult Clin Psychol 2000;68:573–9.

76. Fava M, Rush AJ, Wisniewski SR, et al. A comparison of mirtazapine and nortriptyline following two consecutive failed medication treatments for depressed outpatients: a STAR*D report. Am J Psychiatry 2006;163:1161–72.

77. Scogin FR, Hanson A, Welsh D. Self-administered treatment in stepped-care models of depression treatment. J Clin Psychol 2003;59:341–9.

78. Otto MW, Pollack MH, Maki KM. Empirically supported treatments for panic disorder: costs, benefits, and stepped care. J Consult Clin Psychol 2000;68:556–63.

79. Carels RA, Darby L, Cacciapaglia HM, et al. Applying a stepped-care approach to the treatment of obesity. J Psychosom Res 2005;59:375–83.

80. Wilson GT, Vitousek KM, Loeb KL. Stepped care treatment for eating disorders. J Consult Clin Psychol 2000;68:564–72.

81. Collins LM, Murphy SA, Bierman KL. A conceptual framework for adaptive preventive interventions. Prev Sci 2004;5:185–96.

82. Lavori PW, Dawson R. Dynamic treatment regimes: practical design considerations. Clin Trials 2004;1:9–20.

83. Murphy SA, Lynch KG, McKay JR, et al. Developing adaptive treatment strategies in substance abuse research. Drug Alcohol Depend 2007;88:S24–30.

84. Collins LM, Murphy SA, Strecher V. The multiphase optimization strategy (MOST) and the sequential multiple assignment randomized trial (SMART): new methods for more potent eHealth interventions. Am J Prev Med 2007;32:112–8.

85. Hughes CW, Emslie GJ, Crismon ML, et al. Texas children's medication algorithm project: update on medication treatment of childhood major depression. J Am Acad Child Adolesc Psychiatry 2007;46:667–86.

86. Miller WR. What is relapse? Fifty ways to leave the wagon. Addiction 1996;91: S15–27.

87. Borsari B, Murphy JG, Carey KB. Readiness to change in brief motivational interventions: a requisite condition for drinking reduction? Addict Behav 2009;34: 232–5.

88. Scott CK, Dennis ML. Results from two randomized clinical trials evaluating the impact of quarterly recovery management checkups with adult chronic substance users. Addiction 2009;104:959–71.

89. Kaminer Y, Napolitano C. Dial for therapy: aftercare for adolescent substance use disorders. J Am Acad Child Adolesc Psychiatry 2004;43:171–4.

90. Kaminer Y, Napolitano C. Brief telephone continuing care therapy for adolescents. Center City (MN): Hazelden; 2010.

91. Kazak AE, Hoagwood K, Weisz JR, et al. A meta-systems approach to evidence-based practice for children and adolescents. Am Psychol 2010;65(2):85–97.

Pharmacotherapies for Adolescent Substance Use Disorders

Deborah R. Simkin, MD[a],*, Severin Grenoble, MD[b]

KEYWORDS

- Adolescent • Substance use disorders • Pharmacotherapies
- Developmental issues • Neurobiology

PHARMACOTHERAPY IN ADOLESCENT SUBSTANCE ABUSERS

Reports on pharmacotherapy of substance use disorders (SUD) have been published mostly in adults. This article focuses on adolescents less than 19 years of age. However, it is extended to young adults (aged 18–24 years) because there is increasing evidence that the adolescent brain does not reach maturity until the mid 20s.[1–3]

A successful initial treatment plan includes potential pharmacotherapies as part of a comprehensive biopsychosocial approach. This approach includes psychosocial interventions, such as motivational enhancement therapy; cognitive behavioral therapy (CBT); and various family/community therapies with attention to patient-treatment matching.[4] Treatment plans should integrate the assessment and treatment of any comorbid psychiatric disorder, such as major depressive disorder or social anxiety disorder, that might be independent of substance use and that continues to persist after substance discontinuation.[5,6] Likewise, learning disorders must be addressed.[7–9]

Understanding the risks and benefits of pharmacotherapy by the adolescent, family, referral source, and public is necessary for treatment initiation, engagement, adherence, and successful outcomes.[10]

PHARMACOTHERAPY

Similar to adults, the pharmacotherapies for adolescent substance use disorders may be broadly categorized by the following mechanisms of action: aversion, craving

Dr Simkin is the corresponding author who will receive reprints and proofs.
[a] Division of Child and Adolescent Psychiatry, Department of Psychiatry, University South Alabama College of Medicine, AL, USA
[b] Department of Psychiatry, University South Alabama College of Medicine, AL, USA
* Corresponding author. 4641 Gulfstarr Drive Suite 106, Destin, FL 32541.
E-mail address: Deb62288@aol.com

Child Adolesc Psychiatric Clin N Am 19 (2010) 591–608
doi:10.1016/j.chc.2010.03.010
1056-4993/10/$ – see front matter © 2010 Elsevier Inc. All rights reserved.
childpsych.theclinics.com

reduction, substitution, detoxification, and treatment of comorbid psychiatric disorders.[10–12] The main reason for the paucity of pharmacotherapy research for adolescents with SUD is associated with the fact that although drug dependence may develop in adolescence it is most commonly developed or diagnosed in early adulthood.[13–15] Therefore, most pharmacologic research has focused on adults with SUD.

Pharmacotherapy for youth diagnosed with substance dependence has been practiced with caution because of concerns regarding the impact of drug interactions with medications on the developing brain and the hope that substance abusers will cease using when they mature in their early 20s. This belief is based on the growing literature regarding the maturation of the prefrontal cortex (PFC) that leads to improved executive brain functions and reduces the potential for impulsive decision making.[16] However, maturation alone cannot fully explain the considerable number of young adults who quit substance abuse without treatment. This outcome is more likely a combination of biopsychosocial variables, such as protective factors, later onset of use, and genetic predisposition. Adolescent substance-abuse patterns are different from adults. For example, youth are most likely to binge on alcohol only during weekends. This pattern does not require detoxification.[17]

In the following sections, the pharmacotherapies using aversion, detoxification, anti-craving, and substitution are reviewed. Research on interventions for substances of abuse are discussed under each section. When appropriate, relevant studies in the adult literature are referenced, but the generalizability to adolescents, although maybe appropriate in some cases, should remain cautioned. A detailed discussion on treatment of comorbid psychiatric and substance use disorders in adolescents and agents of prevention are not discussed in this article.

AVERSION AGENTS

The goal of aversion therapy is to reduce alcohol or drug use through the development of unpleasant responses following the consumption of the abused substance. Only disulfiram (Antabuse) for alcohol dependence strictly applies to this category. Several studies have been published with positive results using other forms of aversion therapy in alcohol and cocaine-dependent adults.[18–23] Given the small number of subjects, lack of treatment randomization, and possible bias in such studies, evidence-based conclusions cannot be reached and may not be applicable for adolescents with substance use disorders.

Alcohol

Disulfiram is the only US Food and Drug Administration (FDA)-approved aversive agent for alcohol dependence. It acts as an inhibitor of the liver enzyme acetaldehyde dehydrogenase, resulting in an accumulation of acetaldehyde (a toxic by-product with adverse effects) when consumed with alcohol. These adverse effects may last up to 2 weeks with alcohol consumption after disulfiram is discontinued. Rare but serious adverse reactions have been reported, including arrhythmias, respiratory depression, toxic hepatitis, seizures, and death. The issue of medication compliance is directly correlated to efficacy using disulfiram in alcohol-dependent adults.[24] Given these findings, disulfiram may only be appropriate for adolescents who are medically healthy and highly motivated to achieve and maintain sobriety.

Only two known studies have been published to date on disulfiram treatment in adolescents. A double-blind, randomized, controlled trial compared disulfiram (200 mg daily) to placebo in 49 alcohol-dependent adolescents (aged 16–19 years). Time to first occurrence of relapse was the primary outcome measure, and cumulative abstinence duration was the secondary outcome measure. The investigators did not report the compliance rates, but at 90 days the proportion of subjects who remained abstinent was statistically higher in the disulfiram group compared with placebo ($P = .0063$). Also, the mean cumulative abstinence duration was statistically greater in the disulfiram group versus placebo (68.5 [standard deviation (SD) 37.5] vs 29.7 [SD 19.0] days; $P = .012$). The most common reason for study withdrawal was relapse in both groups, and occasional diarrhea was the only adverse effect reported more frequently in the disulfiram group.[25] A case report was published studying disulfiram (200 mg daily) in two alcohol-dependent adolescents. One subject had comorbid dysthymic disorder and remained abstinent for 4 months, whereas the other subject had comorbid major depressive disorder and oppositional defiant disorder and was never compliant with treatment.[26]

ANTI-CRAVING AGENTS

The goal of this class of agents is to assist in craving and withdrawal reduction, and therefore help prevent relapse.

Alcohol

The FDA approved acamprosate in 2004 for the treatment of alcohol dependence in adults. Although the exact mechanism of action is not completely understood, in vitro and in vivo studies suggest that it restores the central balance between glutamate and the γ aminobutyric acid (GABA) that are disrupted by prolonged alcohol exposure. When drug-associated drug cues are recognized, there is a profound activation of the PFC and glutamatergic drive to the core of nucleus accumbens (NAc). Drug craving occurs in this scenario. Thus, acamprosate may play a role in decreasing cravings by restoring glutamate and GABA imbalance and influencing the role that the PFC and the core of the NAc plays after chronic substance use.[27–30]

Only one study of acamprosate has been studied in the treatment of adolescents. A double-blind, randomized, controlled trial compared acamprosate (1332 mg daily) to placebo in 26 alcohol-dependent adolescents (aged 16–19 years). Time to first occurrence of relapse was the primary outcome measure, and cumulative abstinence duration was the secondary outcome measure. The authors observed (at 90 days) that the proportion of subjects who remained abstinent was statistically higher in the acamprosate group compared with the placebo group (7 of 13 vs 2 of 13; $P = .0076$). Also, the mean cumulative abstinence duration was statistically greater in the acamprosate group versus placebo (79.8 [SD 37.5] vs 32.8 [SD 19.0] days; $P = .012$). The most common reason for study withdrawal was relapse in both groups. The drug was well tolerated with no significant differences in adverse effects between the two groups.[31] Given that this medication requires three times daily dosing, outpatient compliance may only be practical in highly motivated adolescents. However, it may be a better choice than naltrexone, which is less expensive.

The FDA approved oral naltrexone in 1994 for the treatment of alcohol dependence in adults. As a pure μ-opioid antagonist, it is thought to restore central balance of the endogenous opioid system that is disrupted by prolonged alcohol exposure. This restoration is thought to occur by blocking opioid peptides produced by the influence of alcohol on the arcuate nucleus, which influences the ventral tegmentum and the nucleus accumbens.[32,33] Only three known studies have been published to date on oral naltrexone treatment in adolescents. A 6-week, open-label trial was conducted with oral naltrexone (50 mg daily) in five alcohol-dependent adolescents (aged 16.8 years ± 3.11); including two subjects with comorbid conduct disorder and three subjects with comorbid oppositional defiant disorder. At the end of 6 weeks, the average drinks per day decreased by an average reduction of 7.61 standard drinks from 8.94 to 1.33 (P = .0049) with a statistically significant reduction in craving also reported. Adverse effects were minimal, although two subjects reported nausea.[34] A case report included a 17-year-old adolescent with a 6-year history of daily drinking treated with oral naltrexone (50 mg daily) for alcohol dependence who remained abstinent during the 30-day treatment phase.[35] Another case report included two alcohol-dependent adolescents (aged 16 and 18 years) treated with oral naltrexone (50 mg daily) for 12 weeks. One subject remained abstinent for 26 weeks, whereas the other subject reported a marked decrease in the number of drinking days and amount of alcohol consumed. Both subjects reported a decrease in alcohol craving. No adverse effects from naltrexone were observed.[36]

The FDA approved long-acting injectable naltrexone in 2006 for the treatment of alcohol dependence in adults. Given once every 4 weeks as an intramuscular injection, medication compliance issues are mitigated compared with once daily oral naltrexone. No systemic data exist on the use of long-acting injectable naltrexone in alcohol-dependent adolescents. A case report of an adolescent girl diagnosed with alcohol dependence was observed to remain abstinent for more than 12 months while receiving once-monthly naltrexone injections. A self report from the subject of decreased craving was the reason the adolescent felt she no longer sought the use of alcohol. Four years later, the adolescent is still alcohol free (Simkin and colleagues unpublished data, 2010).

Only one known study has been published to date on ondansetron treatment in adolescents, although ondansetron has shown positive preliminary results in several small studies in alcohol-dependent young adults with early onset alcohol disorders, defined as before 25 years of age.[37–41] Ondansetron is a highly specific and selective serotonin 5-HT$_3$ receptor antagonist, and it is not shown to have activity at other known serotonin receptors and has low affinity for dopamine receptors. The exact mechanism for its anti-craving properties is not completely understood but it may attenuate the rewarding effects of ethanol or of ethanol-conditioned cues (eg, the operant environment).[42] An 8-week, prospective, open-label study of ondansetron (4 mcg/kg twice daily) was conducted in 12 alcohol-dependent adolescents (aged 14–20 years). Intent-to-treat analyses showed a significant within-group decrease (improvement) for drinks/drinking per day (t = -3.10, df = 11, P = .01), and decrease in drinks per day (t = -2.01, df=11, P = .06) and higher percentage of days abstinent (t = 1.45, df = 11, P = .18). No subjects discontinued because of adverse effects. The investigators suggested that one mechanism by which ondansetron diminishes drinking in adolescents with alcohol dependence is through a reduction in cravings as measured by the Adolescent Obsessive-Compulsive Drinking Scale (A-OCDS). Results showed that "irresistibility" and total scores as measured by the A-OCDS were correlated significantly with drinking indices (drinks/day, percent days abstinent) at the end of treatment, and that "irresistibility" and total A-OCDS scores decreased significantly by the end of treatment.[43,44]

The anti-craving properties of several other agents, including topiramate [45,46] and baclofen,[47] are currently being explored and have shown positive preliminary results in several small studies in alcohol-dependent adults, presumably because of their central effect on central GABA receptors. Studies with antidepressants, including selective serotonin reuptake inhibitors, in alcohol-dependent adults have yielded mixed results regarding cessation of alcohol use.[48,49] There are no systemic data on the use of these agents in the treatment of alcohol-dependent adolescents with or without comorbidity.

Marijuana

Currently, there are no FDA-approved medications for marijuana dependence in adults. To date, no systemic pharmacologic studies have been conducted in either adults or adolescents. Recent advances have correlated the endocannabinoid system (ECS) with drug addiction and alcoholism,[50] and have implicated the role of the ECS in the development of tolerance to alcohol.[51] Evidence points to the possibility that pharmacologic management of the ECS might not only block the direct reinforcing effect of cannabis, opioids, nicotine and ethanol but also may prevent the relapse to various drugs of abuse, including opioids, cocaine, nicotine, alcohol, and amphetamine.[52]

Only one known study has been published to date on divalproex in marijuana-dependent adolescents. A 5-week, open-label trial was conducted with divalproex (1000 mg daily) in eight adolescents with marijuana abuse and dependence who also reported frequent mood irritability and temper outbursts. At the end of the 5-week trial, all subjects showed a significant improvement in marijuana use (P<.007), although this was measured only by self-report.[53,54] Whether this effect was caused by anti-craving effects or improving mood lability is unclear.

The anti-craving properties of several agents, including buspirone, entacapone, mirtazapine, and oral Tetrahydrocannabinol (THC), and the experimental anti-obesity agent rimonabant, are currently being explored and have shown positive preliminary results in several small studies in cannabis-dependent adults.[55-58] No studies have been done on adolescents.

Cocaine

Currently, there are no FDA-approved medications for cocaine dependence in adults. To date, no systemic pharmacologic studies have been conducted in either adults or adolescents. Several classes of medications have shown promise in pilot studies in cocaine-dependent adults to reduce withdrawal, such as beta-blockers, and to reduce craving, including antidepressants, anticonvulsants, baclofen, naltrexone, disulfiram, N-acetylcysteine, modafinil, and ondansetron. However, overall the results appear mixed and no medication has emerged as consistently effective.[59-65]

Antipsychotics have also been studied in a limited number of trials for cocaine dependence in adults, including olanzapine and risperidone, although neither has been proven more effective than placebo, whereas an earlier open-label trial with flupenthixol decanoate reported positive results.[66-68] A promising new development still in human trials includes human cocaine vaccine (TA-CD) vaccine for treatment of cocaine dependence.[69,70]

Only two known studies have been published to date on desipramine in cocaine-dependent adolescents. In a detailed case report, one adolescent was treated for cocaine craving, depression, and attention-deficit hyperactivity disorder with desipramine on an inpatient adolescent unit. At 6-months follow-up, continued abstinence and improvement in other life domains were observed.[71] Another case report included two cocaine-dependent adolescents treated with desipramine. One subject reported symptom improvement at 30 days, whereas the other subject was never compliant with treatment.[72]

Nicotine

In an study of adults who smoked at least 10 cigarettes a day for 6 months and who were motivated to quit, one of six treatment conditions were used: nicotine lozenge, nicotine patch, sustained-release bupropion, nicotine patch plus nicotine lozenge, bupropion plus nicotine lozenge, or placebo. Although the nicotine lozenge, bupropion, and bupropion plus lozenge produced effects that were comparable with those reported in previous research, the nicotine patch plus lozenge produced the greatest benefit relative to placebo for smoking cessation at the 6-month post quit date.[73] In another adult study involving older cigarette smokers (aged 50 years or older), participants completed a 12-week treatment that included group counseling, nicotine replacement therapy (NRT), and group counseling. The groups, independent of smoking status, were assigned randomly to follow up conditions: (1) standard treatment (ST; no further treatment); (2) extended NRT (E-NRT; 40 weeks of nicotine gum availability); (3) extended cognitive behavioral therapy (E-CBT; 11 cognitive behavioral sessions over a 40-week period); or (4) E-CBT plus E-NRT (E-combined; 11 cognitive behavioral sessions plus 40 weeks nicotine gum availability). The E-CBT condition produced high cigarette abstinence rates that were maintained throughout the 2-year study period (week 24 [58%]; 52 [55%]; 64 [55%]; and 104 [55%]), and was significantly more effective than E-NRT and ST across that period. No other treatment condition was significantly different to ST. No effects for gender were found. In this study, extended cognitive behavioral treatments produced high and stable cigarette abstinence rates for men and women. NRT did not add to the efficacy of extended CBT. Research is needed to determine if these results can be replicated in a sample with a greater range of ages, and improved upon with the addition of medications other than NRT.[74]

Nicotine use in adolescents remains high. *The Cochrane Database of Systematic Reviews* conducted a search of published randomized, controlled trials, cluster-randomized controlled trials, and controlled trials on the pharmacologic treatments for tobacco cessation in young people aged less than 20 years. In two relevant studies with nicotine replacement and bupropion, neither of these pharmacologic interventions achieved statistically significant results, although both studies were small in size with a low power to detect an effect.[75] In an update of this *Cochrane Database of Systemic Reviews*,[76] three studies were discussed. One study investigated the effectiveness of nicotine replacement therapy in patch form or gum to placebo, one tested bupropion as an adjunct to NRT, and one tested bupropion alone in two dosages (150 mg or 300 mg). In the first two studies no effect size was detected. In the study involving the two doses of bupropion, both interventions did not have a persistent effect (6 months or longer) for either of the doses tried. This latter study suggested that in the short term, one may see a decrease in nicotine use but the effect does not continue long term. Perhaps longer-term benefits would be reached by using the previously mentioned studies based on adults.

A randomized, open-label trial was conducted using nicotine patch, nicotine gum, and an added placebo control. At the end of the treatment study, 49.4% of the participants (n = 41/83) had reduced smoking by at least 50%, but there were no significant differences among treatment groups.[77]

In July of 2009, the FDA announced that the previously approved anti-craving agents bupropion and varenicline for tobacco dependence must carry a boxed warning that the use of these medications has been associated with serious mental health events, including changes in behavior, hostility, agitation, depressed mood, suicidality, and attempted suicide. Given this recent warning, further studies may be needed because of safety concerns in adolescents.

Opioids

Only two known studies have been published to date on anti-craving agents in opioid-dependent adolescents. An observational study conducted by a chart review examined antidepressant treatment patterns in adolescents in a New York City methadone maintenance treatment program (MMTP). The goal of the study was to investigate demographic and clinical characteristics that were associated with prescribing patterns and whether antidepressant use was associated with sobriety. Antidepressant treatment was significantly associated with gender, education, marital status, and relapse. However, after controlling for demographic and clinical characteristics, antidepressant treatment was not significantly associated with a reduction in risk for relapse.[78]

AGENTS OF SUBSTITUTION

The goal of substitution therapy allows the patients' drug of choice to be replaced with the supervised administration of a related medication, whereby shifting control of addiction back to the patients and clinicians. Agents of substitution are usually used to replace addictive substances with another substance that prevents withdrawal. However, continued use should occur under supervision to prevent functional impairment, such as lethargy, cognitive decline, so forth, and misuse of the drug or use of other illicit drugs.

Alcohol

As previously mentioned, long-term use of benzodiazepines poses an obvious risk for cross addiction and is generally not recommended for alcohol substitution in either adults or adolescents.

Marijuana

A limited number of studies with oral THC in marijuana-using adults have reported positive results for reducing marijuana withdrawal symptoms. However, oral THC has not demonstrated efficacy for maintaining cannabis abstinence in adults.[56] There is no systemic data on oral THC for substitution treatment in marijuana-dependent adolescents.

Cocaine

No systemic data exist on medications for substitution treatment in either cocaine-dependent adults or adolescents. There have been a limited number of studies in cocaine-dependent adults using various dopamine repletion strategies with mixed results for direct and indirect dopaminergic medications, such as levodopa, bromocriptine, amantadine, and mazindol.[79–83] In a limited number of trials, promising results for various stimulants have been reported for cocaine dependence in adults, including methylphenidate,[84,85] dextroamphetamine,[86–88] and methamphetamine.[89] An obvious risk for abuse and dependence is related to stimulant medications and should only be administered with strict monitoring.

Opioids

Currently, there are five FDA-approved medications for opioid dependence in adults. These include oral methadone (approved in 1972); oral naltrexone (1984); oral levo-α-acetylmethadol (1993); sublingual buprenorphine (2002); and sublingual combination buprenorphine-naloxone (2002). Long-acting injectable naltrexone, although it may be used off-label, is only currently FDA-approved for alcohol dependence. Methadone is a full μ-opioid agonist and also binds to the glutamatergic NMDA (N-methyl-D-aspartate) receptor, and thus acts as a receptor antagonist against glutamate transmission, which may be one mechanism by which methadone decreases craving for opioids and has less tolerance. Levo-α-acetylmethadol (LAAM) is similar to methadone, but has a longer duration of action and therefore may be administered three times per week versus once daily for opioid substitution treatment. Buprenorphine is a partial μ-opioid agonist, and in standard doses it acts similar to other μ-opioid agonists, such as morphine or heroin, but at high doses it can act as an antagonist and precipitate withdrawal symptoms. In a 4:1 combination with naloxone (pure μ-opioid antagonist), this formulation is intended to discourage intravenous abuse of buprenorphine.

No systemic data exist on methadone treatment in opioid-dependent adolescents. In the United States according to the Panino State Methadone Maintenance Treatment Guidelines (1992), methadone treatment is currently allowed for those younger than 18 years of age only if they have relapsed to opioid use following two attempts at medication taper or short-term rehabilitation.[11,31,69,90,91] However, methadone maintenance and not opioid detoxification remains the treatment of choice for pregnant adolescents given risks and benefits to the fetus.[92] Also, there is no systemic data on buprenorphine or buprenorphine-naloxone treatment in opioid-dependent adolescents. In the United States, both treatments are FDA-approved only for patients aged 16 years and older citing a lack of data on efficacy and safety in younger adolescents.[93] Likewise, there is no systemic data on either oral naltrexone or LAAM treatment in opioid-dependent adolescents.

The Cochrane Database of Systematic Reviews examined all randomized and controlled clinical trials comparing any maintenance pharmacologic intervention for opioid dependence alone or associated with psychosocial intervention with no intervention, placebo, and other pharmacologic intervention, including pharmacologic detoxification or psychosocial intervention in adolescents (aged 13–18 years). Two trials involving 187 participants were included. One study compared methadone with LAAM for maintenance treatment lasting 16 weeks after which subjects were detoxified. The other study compared 12-week maintenance treatment with buprenorphine-naloxone to 2-week detoxification treatment with buprenorphine-naloxone.[94,95] No meta-analysis was performed because the two studies assessed different comparisons. In a study by Woody and colleagues[95] the investigators concluded that maintenance treatment seems more efficacious in retaining patients in treatment, but not in reducing patients with positive urines by toxicology at the end of the study. However, self-reported opioid use at 1-year follow-up favored the maintenance group even if both groups continued to report high levels of opioid use. More subjects in the maintenance group were enrolled in other addiction treatments at 12-months follow-up.[96]

A literature search of pharmacologic treatment studies for heroin-using youth was conducted searching Medline and Psychinfo and revealed only seven non-controlled trials (six with methadone maintenance, and one with oral naloxone) that were then independently reviewed.[97–104] All reported favorable results, although the largest treatment study found that methadone maintenance had the highest retention rate, and subsequently time in treatment was the major factor in outcome variables.[90,105] The reader should be aware that some of these studies[97,100–104] were done in the 1970s and did not reveal the better outcomes seen in more recent studies, such as the Woody and colleagues[95] study (2008), the Minnozzi and colleagues[96] study (2009) and the two Hopfer and colleagues[90,105] studies (2002 and 2000). Reasons for some of these differences will be discussed later.

An observational study involving 153 heroin-dependent adolescents (mean age of 17.4 years) compared therapeutic detoxification to methadone maintenance treatment. Out of 59 detoxified subjects, 41 subjects remained drug free, 12 subjects resumed methadone maintenance, 3 subjects were again abusing substances, 2 subjects died presumably of heroin overdose, and 1 subject was lost to follow-up.[102]

An open-label, nonrandomized trial involving 5407 subjects aged 19 years and younger (897 daily opioid users, 1276 daily opioid plus other illicit drug users, 903 less than daily opioid users plus other illicit drug users, 2329 non-opioid users of other illicit drugs) compared four treatment modalities: therapeutic detoxification, methadone maintenance, therapeutic community, and outpatient abstinence based. Results revealed retention of opioid users was greatest in the methadone-maintenance group. All treatment modalities were associated with a large reduction in opioid use and time in treatment was the major factor in every modality in outcome variables, such as opioid use, time spent in productive activities, and employment. In a follow-up study 4 to 6 years later, methadone-maintenance treatment was associated with a substantial reduction in opioid use, but did poorly when considering non-opioid use, alcohol problems, employment, or productive activities. Youth in therapeutic communities had superior outcomes compared with methadone maintenance when considering all opioid use, other substance use, and employment. Youth in abstinence-based treatment did well, but the number of pretreatment opioid users was low. The number of youth in therapeutic detoxification was too small to analyze.[104]

Several other observational studies have also reported favorable results with methadone-maintenance treatment in opioid-dependent adolescents in longer retention time in treatment and subsequently less opioid use.[106,107]

An observational study compared methadone, buprenorphine, and symptomatic (non-opioid) medication only in retention time and reentry into treatment in 61 heroin-dependent adolescents (aged 14–17 years; 61% female) in Australia. The first episode of treatment was methadone maintenance in 20 subjects, buprenorphine in 25 subjects, and symptomatic medication only in 15 subjects. One subject underwent assessment only. These 61 subjects had a total of 112 episodes of treatment. Results revealed subjects treated with methadone had significantly longer retention in first-treatment episode than subjects treated with buprenorphine (mean 354 vs 58 days, p50.01 by Cox regression) and missed fewer days in the first month of treatment (mean 3 vs 8 days, p50.05 by t-test). Subsequent reentry for further treatment occurred in 25% of subjects treated with methadone, 60% of subjects treated with buprenorphine, and 60% of subjects treated with symptomatic medication only. Also, time to reentry after first episode of buprenorphine treatment was significantly shorter than after methadone treatment.[106]

An observational study examined the impact of methadone-maintenance treatment in 147 adolescent and young adult opiate-dependent subjects (aged 15–23 years) admitted over a 6-year period during their first year in the program. Retention in treatment was the primary outcome variable, and at 12 months 48% were still in treatment. Among subjects who stayed in treatment for 1 year, there was a significant reduction in heroin use, a trend toward a reduction in cocaine use, and no significant impact on benzodiazepine use. No adverse effects were reported.[107]

DETOXIFICATION

Medications for detoxification usually provide relief (eg, clonidine for opioid) during withdrawal.

Opioids

The Cochrane Database of Systematic Reviews examined all randomized and controlled clinical trials comparing any detoxification pharmacologic intervention for opioid dependence alone or associated with psychosocial intervention as treatment with no intervention, placebo, other pharmacologic intervention or psychosocial intervention in adolescents (aged 13–18 years). One trial involving 36 participants was included comparing buprenorphine with clonidine for detoxification.[91] No difference was found for drop out (relative risk [RR] 0.45 [95% confidence interval (CI): 0.20 –1.04]) or acceptability of treatment withdrawal score weighted mean difference (3.97 [95% CI -1.38, 9.32]). However, more participants in the buprenorphine group initiated oral naltrexone treatment post-detoxification (RR 11.00 [95% CI 1.58, 76.55]).[108]

A double-blind, randomized, controlled trial was conducted with 36 self-referred adolescents (aged 13–18 years) with opioid dependence assigned to a 28-day outpatient medication-assisted withdrawal treatment with 18 subjects assigned to oral buprenorphine condition (dosage based on weight and self-reported heroin use at intake; 6 mg/day versus 8 mg/day, then decreased by 2 mg every 7 days) and 18 subjects to a transdermal clonidine condition, with participants in both groups receiving identical placebo matching and in combination with behavioral therapy. Post-detoxification, all subjects were offered the opportunity for continued treatment with oral naltrexone. Results favored the buprenorphine condition, including retention time in treatment (72% vs 39%; P<.05) and overall opioid negative urinalysis (64% vs 32%; P = .01). However, opioid negative urinalysis for those retained in treatment only independent of the larger attrition in the clonidine condition was not significant (78% buprenorphine vs 81% clonidine condition). Likewise, positive urinalysis for non-opioid drugs, drug-related HIV risk behavior, ease of withdrawal, and psychomotor impairment were similar for both groups. At the end of the 4-week treatment period, a significantly greater number of subjects in the buprenorphine condition (61% vs 5%) initiated treatment with oral naltrexone, although follow-up analysis was not performed.[91]

Only two other known studies have been published to date on buprenorphine detoxification in opioid-dependent adolescents in the United States. An open-label, non-randomized trial compared buprenorphine versus methadone to determine which medication is better for detoxification treatment in 93 opioid-dependent adolescents on an inpatient unit in Germany. A nonrandom assignment included 42 subjects in the buprenorphine group and 51 subjects in the methadone group with roughly equal characteristics (age, gender, sociodemographic status, age of initiation of drug consumption, and duration of opioid intake). The observed results included 38.1% of the buprenorphine subjects versus 23.5% of the methadone subjects finished detoxification successfully, although this was not statistically significant. No adverse effects or differences between the two agents were observed.[109] A prospective, randomized follow-up trial examined the outcomes at 1, 3 and 6 months after an outpatient 3-day detoxification with buprenorphine (2–4 mg sublingual or 0.3 mg intramuscular per day) in 123 heroin-dependent young adults (aged 18–25 years; mean age 21.8 years; 56% male; 95% Caucasian). Participants were randomly assigned to receive either of two buprenorphine dose schedules: standard or high dose (2 mg vs 4 mg sublingual or 0.3 mg vs 0.6 mg intramuscular). Also, subjects were allowed to receive buprenorphine up to twice a day, but the second administration was only the standard dose. By self-report, 37% of the total sample were not currently using heroin at 1 month, 32% at 3 months, and 29% at 6 months, and 6.7%, 10.1%, and 11.8% had an opioid-negative urine test at 1, 3, and 6 months, respectively. There was a significant reduction from the baseline in mean Addiction Severity Index drug-use composite score and the mean number of days of heroin and cocaine use during the past 30 days, which was sustained over the three follow-up points (P<.01). Engagement in aftercare was generally poor. No adverse effects were reported.[110]

A double-blind, randomized trial compared LAAM versus methadone in 35 heroin-dependent adolescents (aged 16 to 21 years) for a 16-week detoxification period; 14 subjects were assigned LAAM and 21 subjects were assigned methadone. Results revealed no clinically significant differences in either treatment group, including opioid-positive urinalysis, positive urinalysis for non-prescribed drugs, and ease of withdrawal. Also, other outcome measures were similar between the two groups, including physical and emotional reactions, performance in individual and group therapy, academics, athletics, employment, community and home involvement, and toxic reactions.[94]

A multicenter, randomized, controlled trial was conducted with 152 self-referred opioid-dependent adolescents (aged 15–21 years) assigned to either 2-week detoxification or 12-week maintenance treatment. Eighty adolescents were assigned to buprenorphine-naloxone and 2-weeks detoxification (up to 14 mg/day and then tapered to day 14), and 74 adolescents were assigned to buprenorphine-naloxone and 12-weeks maintenance with subsequent detoxification (up to 24 mg/day for 9 weeks and then tapered to week 12), both in combination with behavioral therapy. Opioid-positive urinalysis at weeks 4, 8, and 12 was more prevalent amongst subjects in the shorter 2-week group compared with the longer 12-week treatment group (41/80 subjects in the 2-week group and 49/74 subjects in the 12-week group provided urine samples through weeks 12): week 4 (61% vs 26%; $P<.001$); week 8 (54% vs 23%; $P = .001$); and week 12 (51% vs 43%; $P = .18$). Retention time in treatment also favored the longer 12-week condition (70% vs 20.5%; $P<.001$). Likewise, during weeks 1 through 12, subjects in the 12-week group reported less opioid use ($P<.001$); less injecting ($P = .01$); less marijuana use ($P = .001$); less cocaine use ($P = .001$); and less non-study addiction treatment ($P<.001$). However, the two groups did not differ in rates of self-reported alcohol use during the study period ($P = .42$). In follow-up analysis at 12 months, the difference between the groups was not statistically significant in regards to self-reported opioid use in the past month with reported relapse of 72% in the 2-week group versus 53% in the 12-week group.[95]

Alcohol

The efficacy and safety of benzodiazepines for treatment of alcohol-withdrawal syndrome in adults is well established and used. Long-term use of benzodiazepines poses an obvious risk for cross addiction and may contribute to opioid toxicity symptoms reported in association with methadone and buprenorphine consumption.[111] There is no systemic data on the use of benzodiazepines in the treatment of alcohol-dependent adolescents. For uncomplicated alcohol withdrawal without a history of seizures, oral propranolol or clonidine may be administered in a monitored setting and used in adolescents for detoxification, as is the common practice in adults.[112]

SUMMARY

Overall, there is a paucity of high-quality, evidence-based studies for pharmacotherapy of adolescent substance use disorders. Although case reports and uncontrolled studies may suggest future directions of research, controlled studies are needed to evaluate medication effectiveness, potential for abuse, possible interactions with other medications, and factors related to patient compliance. A systematic assessment of outpatient adolescents with substance use disorders reported that 25% of these subjects were noncompliant with their prescribed medication and 8% of these subjects had abused their prescribed medication or had diverted it to others.[113]

Additionally, further studies are required to address issues of safety and tolerability given the unknown and potentially adverse interaction between psychotropic medications and psychoactive substances.[114] Such an example has been documented in a case report of drug-induced delirium between tricyclic antidepressants and marijuana.[115] As a consequence, no firm recommendations are currently available, such as when to initiate treatment and which agent in particular confers the greatest benefit and least risk profile for a given psychoactive substance of abuse. An extrapolation from the adult literature may also guide future directions in research, but the generalizability to adolescents is cautioned. For strictly short-term detoxification from various substances, such as alcohol, benzodiazepines, barbiturates, and opioids, it may be reasonable to assume that the same closely followed protocols in adults would also be applicable to adolescents, as long as consent for such treatment is obtained.[112]

In cannot be overemphasized how important it is to perform a complete biopsychosocial evaluation followed by a corresponding comprehensive treatment plan that addresses a multidimensional approach with a multidisciplinary team, including the necessary pharmacotherapies integrated with psychosocial intervention that meet the adolescents therapeutic needs. The clinician should confirm that the family, adolescent, and referral source understand the potential side effects, drug interactions with other psychotropic drugs and substances of abuse, and difficult situations that may occur when compliance becomes an issue.[10] Appropriate plans should also be discussed in the event of a life threatening or serious adverse event.[114,116] Finally, the interested reader is referred to additional most recent reviews of pharmacotherapies for adolescent SUD.[10,17]

REFERENCES

1. Baird A, Fugelsang J, Bennett C. What you were thinking: an fMRI study of adolescent decision-making. Poster Presentation at the Cognitive Neuroscience Conference. New York, April, 2005.
2. Casey BJ, Getz S, Galvan A. The adolescent brain. Dev Rev 2008;28(1):62–77.
3. Luna B, Sweeney JA. The emergence of collaborative brain function: FMRI studies of the development of response inhibition. Ann N Y Acad Sci 2004; 1021:296–309.
4. Dennis M, Godley SH, Diamond G, et al. The cannabis youth treatment (CYT) study: main findings from two randomized trials. J Subst Abuse Treat 2004; 27(3):197–213.
5. Ambrosini PJ, Bianchi MD, Rabinovich H, et al. Antidepressant treatments in children and adolescents. I. Affective disorders. J Am Acad Child Adolesc Psychiatry 1993;32(1):1.
6. Ambrosini PJ, Bianchi MD, Rabinovich H, et al. Antidepressant treatments in children and adolescents: II. Anxiety, physical, and behavioral disorders. J Am Acad Child Adolesc Psychiatry 1993;32(3):483–93.
7. Hops H, Davis B, Lewin LM. The development of alcohol and other substance use: a gender study of family and peer context. J Stud Alcohol Suppl 1999; 13:22–31.
8. Simkin D. Adolescent substance abuse. In: Sadock B, Sadock V, editors, Comprehensive textbook of psychiatry, vol. 2. 8th edition. Philadelphia (PA): Lippincott Williams and Wilkins; 2004. p. 3470–90.
9. Tapert SF, Baratta MV, Abrantes AM, et al. Attention dysfunction predicts substance involvement in community youths. J Am Acad Child Adolesc Psychiatry 2002;41(6):680–6.

10. Kaminer Y, Marsch LA. Pharmacotherapy of adolescent substance use disorders. In: Kaminer Y, Winters K, editors. Clinical manual of adolescent substance abuse treatment. Washington, DC: American Psychiatric Publishing Inc; 2010. p. 205–34.
11. Waxmonsky JG, Wilens TE. Pharmacotherapy of adolescent substance use disorders: a review of the literature. J Child Adolesc Psychopharmacol 2005; 15(5):810–25.
12. Kaminer Y. Pharmacotherapy for adolescents with psychoactive substance abuse disorders. In: Adolescent drug abuse: clinical assessment and therapeutic interventions. NIDA Res Monogr 1995;156:291–394.
13. Schuckit MA, Daeppen JB, Tipp JE, et al. The clinical course of alcohol-related problems in alcohol dependent and nonalcohol dependent drinking women and men. J Stud Alcohol 1998;59(5):581–90.
14. DeWit DJ, Adlaf EM, Offord DR, et al. Age at first alcohol use: a risk factor for the development of alcohol disorders. Am J Psychiatry 2000;157(5):745–50.
15. von Diemen L, Bassani DG, Fuchs SC, et al. Impulsivity, age of first alcohol use and substance use disorders among male adolescents: a population based case-control study. Addiction 2008;103(7):1198–205.
16. Hasin DS, Grant B, Endicott J. The natural history of alcohol abuse: implications for definitions of alcohol use disorders. Am J Psychiatry 1990;147(11):1537–41.
17. Upahdyaya H, Deas D. Pharmacological interventions for adolescent substance use disorders. In: Kaminer Y, Bukstein O, editors. Adolescent substance abuse: psychiatric comorbidity and high-risk behaviors. New York: Routledge; 2008. p. 145–62.
18. Smith JW, Frawley PJ. Long-term abstinence from alcohol in patients receiving aversion therapy as part of a multimodal inpatient program. J Subst Abuse Treat 1990;7(2):77–82.
19. Smith JW, Frawley PJ, Polissar L. Six- and twelve-month abstinence rates in inpatient alcoholics treated with aversion therapy compared with matched inpatients from a treatment registry. Alcohol Clin Exp Res 1991;15(5):862–70.
20. Smith JW, Frawley PJ. Treatment outcome of 600 chemically dependent patients treated in a multimodal inpatient program including aversion therapy and pentothal interviews. J Subst Abuse Treat 1993;10(4):359–69.
21. Smith JW, Frawley PJ, Polissar NL. Six- and twelve-month abstinence rates in inpatient alcoholics treated with either faradic aversion or chemical aversion compared with matched inpatients from a treatment registry. J Addict Dis 1997;16(1):5–24.
22. Frawley PJ, Smith JW. Chemical aversion therapy in the treatment of cocaine dependence as part of a multimodal treatment program: treatment outcome. J Subst Abuse Treat 1990;7(1):21–9.
23. Frawley PJ, Smith JW. One-year follow-up after multimodal inpatient treatment for cocaine and methamphetamine dependencies. J Subst Abuse Treat 1992; 9(4):271–86.
24. Fuller RK, Branchey L, Brightwell DR, et al. Disulfiram treatment of alcoholism. A Veterans Administration cooperative study. JAMA 1986;256(11):1449–55.
25. Niederhofer H, Staffen W. Comparison of disulfiram and placebo in treatment of alcohol dependence of adolescents. Drug Alcohol Rev 2003;22(3):295–7.
26. Myers WC, Donahue JE, Goldstein MR. Disulfiram for alcohol use disorders in adolescents. J Am Acad Child Adolesc Psychiatry 1994;33(4):484–9.
27. Kalivas PW, Volkow ND. The neural basis of addiction: a pathology of motivation and choice. Am J Psychiatry 2005;162(8):1403–13.

28. Koob GF. The neurobiology of addiction: a neuroadaptational view relevant for diagnosis. Addiction 2006;101(Suppl 1):23–30.

29. Nestler EJ. Is there a common molecular pathway for addiction? Nat Neurosci 2005;8(11):1445–9.

30. Nestler EJ. Molecular neurobiology of addiction. Am J Addict 2001;10(3):201–17.

31. Niederhofer H, Staffen W. Acamprosate and its efficacy in treating alcohol dependent adolescents. Eur Child Adolesc Psychiatry 2003;12(3):144–8.

32. Sanchis-Segura C, Grisel JE, Olive MF, et al. Role of the endogenous opioid system on the neuropsychopharmacological effects of ethanol: new insights about an old question. Alcohol Clin Exp Res 2005;29(8):1522–7.

33. Mendez M, Morales-Mulia M. Role of mu and delta opioid receptors in alcohol drinking behaviour. Curr Drug Abuse Rev 2008;1(2):239–52.

34. Deas D, May MP, Randall C, et al. Naltrexone treatment of adolescent alcoholics: an open-label pilot study. J Child Adolesc Psychopharmacol 2005;15(5):723–8.

35. Wold M, Kaminer Y. Naltrexone for alcohol abuse. J Am Acad Child Adolesc Psychiatry 1997;36(1):6–7.

36. Lifrak PD, Alterman AI, O'Brien CP, et al. Naltrexone for alcoholic adolescents. Am J Psychiatry 1997;154(3):439–41.

37. Johnson BA, Roache JD, Javors MA, et al. Ondansetron for reduction of drinking among biologically predisposed alcoholic patients: a randomized controlled trial. JAMA 2000;284(8):963–71.

38. Johnson BA, Roache JD, Ait-Daoud N, et al. Ondansetron reduces the craving of biologically predisposed alcoholics. Psychopharmacology (Berl) 2002;160(4):408–13.

39. Johnson BA, Ait-Daoud N, Ma JZ, et al. Ondansetron reduces mood disturbance among biologically predisposed, alcohol-dependent individuals. Alcohol Clin Exp Res 2003;27(11):1773–9.

40. Kranzler HR, Pierucci-Lagha A, Feinn R, et al. Effects of ondansetron in early-versus late-onset alcoholics: a prospective, open-label study. Alcohol Clin Exp Res 2003;27(7):1150–5.

41. Sellers EM, Toneatto T, Romach MK, et al. Clinical efficacy of the 5-HT3 antagonist ondansetron in alcohol abuse and dependence. Alcohol Clin Exp Res 1994;18(4):879–85.

42. Middaugh LD, Kelley BM, Groseclose CH, et al. Delta-opioid and 5-HT3 receptor antagonist effects on ethanol reward and discrimination in C57BL/6 mice. Pharmacol Biochem Behav 2000;65(1):145–54.

43. Dawes MA, Johnson BA, Ait-Daoud N, et al. A prospective, open-label trial of ondansetron in adolescents with alcohol dependence. Addict Behav 2005;30(6):1077–85.

44. Dawes MA, Johnson BA, Ma JZ, et al. Reductions in and relations between "craving" and drinking in a prospective, open-label trial of ondansetron in adolescents with alcohol dependence. Addict Behav 2005;30(9):1630–7.

45. Johnson BA, Ait-Daoud N, Bowden CL, et al. Oral topiramate for treatment of alcohol dependence: a randomised controlled trial. Lancet 2003;361(9370):1677–85.

46. Kenna GA, Lomastro TL, Schiesl A, et al. Review of topiramate: an antiepileptic for the treatment of alcohol dependence. Curr Drug Abuse Rev 2009;2(2):135–42.

47. Addolorato G, Caputo F, Capristo E, et al. Baclofen efficacy in reducing alcohol craving and intake: a preliminary double-blind randomized controlled study. Alcohol Alcohol 2002;37(5):504–8.

48. Gastfriend DR, Elman I, Solhkhah R. Pharmacotherapy of substance abuse and dependence. In: Dunner DL, Rosenbaum JF, editors. The psychiatric clinics of North America annual of drug therapy. Philadelphia (PA): W.B. Saunders Company; 1998. p. 211–29.

49. Naranjo CA, Kadlec KE, Sanhueza P, et al. Fluoxetine differentially alters alcohol intake and other consummatory behaviors in problem drinkers. Clin Pharmacol Ther 1990;47(4):490–8.

50. Mouslech Z, Valla V. Endocannabinoid system: an overview of its potential in current medical practice. Neuro Endocrinol Lett 2009;30(2):153–79.

51. Basavarajappa BS, Hungund BL. Role of the endocannabinoid system in the development of tolerance to alcohol. Alcohol Alcohol 2005;40(1):15–24.

52. Parolaro D, Rubino T. The role of the endogenous cannabinoid system in drug addiction. Drug News Perspect 2008;21(3):149–57.

53. Donovan SJ. Divalproex sodium for use with conduct disordered adolescent marijuana users: letter to the editor. Am J Addict 1996;5:181.

54. Donovan SJ, Susser ES, Nunes EV, et al. Divalproex treatment of disruptive adolescents: a report of 10 cases. J Clin Psychiatry 1997;58(1):12–5.

55. Benyamina A, Lecacheux M, Blecha L, et al. Pharmacotherapy and psychotherapy in cannabis withdrawal and dependence. Expert Rev Neurother 2008; 8(3):479–91.

56. Huestis MA, Gorelick DA, Heishman SJ, et al. Blockade of effects of smoked marijuana by the CB1-selective cannabinoid receptor antagonist SR141716. Arch Gen Psychiatry 2001;58(4):322–8.

57. Huestis MA, Boyd SJ, Heishman SJ, et al. Single and multiple doses of rimonabant antagonize acute effects of smoked cannabis in male cannabis users. Psychopharmacology (Berl) 2007;194(4):505–15.

58. Shafa R, Abdolmaleky S, Yaquili C, et al. COMT- Inhibitors may be a promising tool in treatment of marijuana addiction. In: Poster abstracts from the AAP 19th annual meeting and symposium: poster 3. Am J Addict 2009;18(4):321–31.

59. Johnson BA, Roache JD, Ait-Daoud N, et al. A preliminary randomized, double-blind, placebo-controlled study of the safety and efficacy of ondansetron in the treatment of cocaine dependence. Drug Alcohol Depend 2006;84(3):256–63.

60. Mardikian PN, LaRowe SD, Hedden S, et al. An open-label trial of N-acetylcysteine for the treatment of cocaine dependence: a pilot study. Prog Neuropsychopharmacol Biol Psychiatry 2007;31(2):389–94.

61. Minozzi S, Amato L, Davoli M, et al. Anticonvulsants for cocaine dependence. Cochrane Database Syst Rev 2008;16(2):CD006754.

62. Myrick H, Henderson S, Brady KT, et al. Divalproex loading in the treatment of cocaine dependence. J Psychoactive Drugs 2001;33(3):283–7.

63. Silva de Lima M, Farrell M. Antidepressants for cocaine dependence. Cochrane Database Syst Rev 2007;3:CD002950.

64. Pettinati HM, Kampman KM, Lynch KG, et al. A double blind, placebo-controlled trial that combines disulfiram and naltrexone for treating co-occurring cocaine and alcohol dependence. Addict Behav 2008;33(5):651–67.

65. Schmitz JM, Stotts AL, Rhoades HM, et al. Naltrexone and relapse prevention treatment for cocaine-dependent patients. Addict Behav 2001;26(2):167–80.

66. Gawin FH, Allen D, Humblestone B. Outpatient treatment of 'crack' cocaine smoking with flupenthixol decanoate. A preliminary report. Arch Gen Psychiatry 1989;46(4):322–5.

67. Kampman KM, Pettinati H, Lynch KG, et al. A pilot trial of olanzapine for the treatment of cocaine dependence. Drug Alcohol Depend 2003;70(3):265–73.

68. Reid MS, Casadonte P, Baker S, et al. A placebo-controlled screening trial of olanzapine, valproate, and coenzyme Q10/L-carnitine for the treatment of cocaine dependence. Addiction 2005;100(Suppl 1):43–57.
69. Kosten TR, Biegel D. Therapeutic vaccines for substance dependence. Expert Rev Vaccines 2002;1(3):363–71.
70. Martell BA, Mitchell E, Poling J, et al. Vaccine pharmacotherapy for the treatment of cocaine dependence. Biol Psychiatry 2005;58(2):158–64.
71. Kaminer Y. Desipramine facilitation of cocaine abstinence in an adolescent. J Am Acad Child Adolesc Psychiatry 1992;31(2):312–7.
72. Kaminer Y. Cocaine craving. J Am Acad Child Adolesc Psychiatry 1994;33(4):592.
73. Piper ME, Smith SS, Schlam TR, et al. A randomized placebo-controlled clinical trial of 5 smoking cessation pharmacotherapies. Arch Gen Psychiatry 2009;66(11):1253–62.
74. Hall SM, Humfleet GL, Munoz RF, et al. Extended treatment of older cigarette smokers. Addiction 2009;104(6):1043–52.
75. Grimshaw GM, Stanton A. Tobacco cessation interventions for young people. Cochrane Database Syst Rev 2006;18(4):CD003289.
76. Grimson G, Stanton A. Tobacco cessation interventions for young people. [review]. Cochrane Database Syst Rev 2010;1:CD003289. DOI:10.1002/14651858.CD003289 pub 4.
77. Hanson K, Zylla E, Allen S, et al. Cigarette reduction: an intervention for adolescent smokers. Drug Alcohol Depend 2008;95(1–2):164–8.
78. Galarneau DW, Teres JJ, Leon AC, et al. Antidepressant treatment patterns in a novel methadone maintenance clinic targeting young adults an observational study. J Addict Dis 2006;25(2):47–52.
79. Meyer RE. New pharmacotherapies for cocaine dependence. revisited. Arch Gen Psychiatry 1992;49(11):900–4.
80. Mooney ME, Schmitz JM, Moeller FG, et al. Safety, tolerability and efficacy of levodopa-carbidopa treatment for cocaine dependence: two double-blind, randomized, clinical trials. Drug Alcohol Depend 2007;88(2–3):214–23.
81. Schmitz JM, Mooney ME, Moeller FG, et al. Levodopa pharmacotherapy for cocaine dependence: choosing the optimal behavioral therapy platform. Drug Alcohol Depend 2008;94(1–3):142–50.
82. Shoptaw S, Watson DW, Reiber C, et al. Randomized controlled pilot trial of cabergoline, hydergine and levodopa/carbidopa: Los Angeles Cocaine Rapid Efficacy Screening Trial (CREST). Addiction 2005;100(Suppl 1):78–90.
83. Wolfsohn R, Sanfilipo M, Angrist B. A placebo-controlled trial of L-dopa/carbidopa in early cocaine abstinence. Neuropsychopharmacology 1993;9(1):49–53.
84. Levin FR, Evans SM, McDowell DM, et al. Methylphenidate treatment for cocaine abusers with adult attention-deficit/hyperactivity disorder: a pilot study. J Clin Psychiatry 1998;59(6):300–5.
85. Levin FR, Evans SM, Brooks DJ, et al. Treatment of cocaine dependent treatment seekers with adult ADHD: double-blind comparison of methylphenidate and placebo. Drug Alcohol Depend 2007;87(1):20–9.
86. Grabowski J, Rhoades H, Schmitz J, et al. Dextroamphetamine for cocaine-dependence treatment: a double-blind randomized clinical trial. J Clin Psychopharmacol 2001;21(5):522–6.
87. Grabowski J, Rhoades H, Stotts A, et al. Agonist-like or antagonist-like treatment for cocaine dependence with methadone for heroin dependence: two double-blind randomized clinical trials. Neuropsychopharmacology 2004;29(5):969–81.

88. Shearer J, Wodak A, van Beek I, et al. Pilot randomized double blind placebo-controlled study of dexamphetamine for cocaine dependence. Addiction 2003; 98(8):1137–41.

89. Mooney ME, Herin DV, Schmitz JM, et al. Effects of oral methamphetamine on cocaine use: a randomized, double-blind, placebo-controlled trial. Drug Alcohol Depend 2009;101(1–2):34–41.

90. Hopfer CJ, Mikulich SK, Crowley TJ. Heroin use among adolescents in treatment for substance use disorders. J Am Acad Child Adolesc Psychiatry 2000;39(10): 1316–23.

91. Marsch LA. Treatment of adolescents. In: Strain EC, Stitzer ML, editors. The treatment of opioid dependence. Baltimore (MD): Johns Hopkins University Press; 2005. p. 497–707.

92. Finnegan LP, Kandall SR. Maternal and neonatal effects of alcohol and drugs. In: Lowinson JH, Ruiz P, Millman RB, et al, editors. Substance abuse comprehensive textbook. Baltimore (MD): Williams & Williams; 1992. p. 628–56.

93. Fiellin DA. Treatment of adolescent opioid dependence: no quick fix. JAMA 2008;300(17):2057–9.

94. Lehmann WX. The use of 1-alpha-acetyl-methadol (LAAM) as compared to methadone in the maintenance and detoxification of young heroin addicts. 1973 [proceedings]. NIDA Res Monogr 1976;8:82–3.

95. Woody GE, Poole SA, Subramaniam G, et al. Extended vs short-term buprenorphine-naloxone for treatment of opioid-addicted youth: a randomized trial. JAMA 2008;300(17):2003–11.

96. Minozzi S, Amato L, Davoli M. Maintenance treatments for opiate dependent adolescent. Cochrane Database Syst Rev 2009;15(2):CD007210.

97. Pierson PS, Rapkin RM, Kleber HD. Naloxone in the treatment of the young heroin abuser. Am J Drug Alcohol Abuse 1974;1(2):243–52.

98. Crome IB, Christian J, Green C. Tip of the national iceberg? Profile of adolescent patients prescribed methadone in an innovative community drug service. Drugs: Education, Prevention, Policy 1998;5(2):195–7.

99. Crome IB, Christian J, Green C. The development of a unique designated community drug service for adolescents: policy, prevention and education implications. Drugs: Education, Prevention, Policy 2000;7(1):87–108.

100. DeAngelis GG, Lehmann WX. Adolescents and short term, low dose methadone maintenance. Int J Addict 1973;8(5):853–63.

101. Lloyd RA, Katon RN, DuPont RL. Evolution of a treatment approach for young heroin addicts. Comparison of three treatment modalities. Int J Addict 1974; 9(2):229–39.

102. Millman RB, Khuri ET, Nyswander ME. Therapeutic detoxification of adolescent heroin addicts. Ann N Y Acad Sci 1978;311:153–64.

103. Rosenberg CM, Patch VD. Methadone use in adolescent heroin addicts. JAMA 1972;220(7):991–3.

104. Sells SB, Simpson DD. Evaluation of treatment outcome for youths in the drug abuse reporting program (DARP): a follow-up study. In: Beschner GM, Friedman AS, editors. Youth drug abuse: problems, issues and treatment. Lanham (MD): Lexington Books; 1979. p. 571–622.

105. Hopfer CJ, Khuri E, Crowley TJ, et al. Adolescent heroin use: a review of the descriptive and treatment literature. J Subst Abuse Treat 2002;23(3):231–7.

106. Bell J, Mutch C. Treatment retention in adolescent patients treated with methadone or buprenorphine for opioid dependence: a file review. Drug Alcohol Rev 2006;25(2):167–71.

107. Kellogg S, Melia D, Khuri E, et al. Adolescent and young adult heroin patients: drug use and success in methadone maintenance treatment. J Addict Dis 2006; 25(3):15–25.

108. Minozzi S, Amato L, Davoli M, et al. Detoxification treatments for opiate dependent adolescents [review]. Cochrane Database Syst Rev 2009;2:CD006749.

109. Ebner R, Schreiber W, Zierer C. [Buprenorphine or methadone for detoxification of young opioid addicts?]. Psychiatr Prax 2004;31(Suppl 1):S108–10. [in German].

110. Gandhi DH, Jaffe JH, McNary S, et al. Short-term outcomes after brief ambulatory opioid detoxification with buprenorphine in young heroin users. Addiction 2003;98(4):453–62.

111. Nielsen S, Dietze P, Lee N, et al. Concurrent buprenorphine and benzodiazepines use and self-reported opioid toxicity in opioid substitution treatment. Addiction 2007;102(4):616–22.

112. Kaminer Y. Adolescent substance abuse: a comprehensive guide to theory and practice. New York: Plenum Press; 1994.

113. Wilens TE, Biederman J, Abrantes AM, et al. Clinical characteristics of psychiatrically referred adolescent outpatients with substance use disorder. J Am Acad Child Adolesc Psychiatry 1997;36(7):941–7.

114. Bukstein OG, Bernet W, Arnold V, et al. Practice parameter for the assessment and treatment of children and adolescents with substance use disorders. J Am Acad Child Adolesc Psychiatry 2005;44(6):609–21.

115. Wilens TE, Biederman J, Spencer TJ. Case study: adverse effects of smoking marijuana while receiving tricyclic antidepressants. J Am Acad Child Adolesc Psychiatry 1997;36(1):45–8.

116. Kaminer Y, Goldberg P, Connor D. Psychotropic medications and substances of abuse interactions in youth. Subst Abuse 2010;31:53–7.

Management of the Adolescent with Substance Use Disorders and Comorbid Psychopathology

Oscar G. Bukstein, MD, MPH*, Michelle S. Horner, DO

KEYWORDS

• Adolescents • Substance use disorders • SUD
• Psychiatric comorbidity • Dual diagnosis • Treatment

Substance use by adolescents is a critical problem in modern Western society due to the common use of psychoactive substances by youth. Understanding the consequences that result, the development of pathology related to substance use (substance use disorders; SUDs), and the persistence of such problems into adulthood is critical to delivering effective interventions. Among the issues that clinicians need to consider are risk factors for the development and the persistence of SUDs and obstacles to optimal intervention. Foremost among these issues is psychiatric comorbidity. In this article, the authors discuss the importance of comorbidity in clinical populations of adolescents with SUDs and other psychiatric disorders (including considerations to be taken in the assessment and treatment of psychiatric-SUD comorbidity), conduct a review of evidenced-based interventions and recommendations, and provide suggestions for the direction of future research.

Comorbidity refers to the coexistence of two or more diagnosable mental health disorders and in this case, two diagnosable entities in the realm of substance abuse and mental illness with each meeting *Diagnostic and Statistical Manual of Mental Disorders* (Fourth Edition, Text Revision) (DSM-IV-TR) criteria.[1] For children and adolescents, comorbidity has been used interchangeably with the term dual

---

This work was supported by: O.G.B.: 5 R01 MH077676-02 (NIMH); DA020036-05S1 & DA016631-03 (NIDA); M.S.H.: T32 MH018951.

Western Psychiatric Institute and Clinic, University of Pittsburgh School of Medicine, 3811 O'Hara Street, Pittsburgh, PA 15213, USA
* Corresponding author.
E-mail address: buksteinog@upmc.edu

diagnosis, although in many cases there are more than two diagnoses. For a detailed review of specific disorders and program development, please refer to a recent book by Kaminer and Bukstein.[2]

THE IMPORTANCE OF COMORBIDITY

In both community surveys of adolescents with SUDs and samples of adolescents in addictions treatment, the majority have a co-occurring nonsubstance-related psychiatric disorder.[3] More than half of adolescents in addictions treatment with co-occurring mental illness have three or more co-occurring psychiatric disorders.[4] The most commonly comorbid psychiatric disorders among youth in addictions treatment include conduct problems, attention deficit/hyperactivity disorder (ADHD), mood disorders (eg, depression), and trauma-related symptoms.[5] In a study examining the prevalence of self-reported substance use and mental health problems,[6] the pattern of comorbidity from 4930 adolescents admitted to substance abuse treatment in multisite studies was about one-third of adolescents endorsing depressive symptoms in the year before entering substance abuse treatment. Approximately half of adolescents younger than 15 years of age had ADHD and half met criteria for conduct disorder (CD). The co-occurrence of manifesting both internalizing and externalizing behaviors was more than 40% of adolescents. Among substance dependent adolescents younger than 15, about 90% had at least one mental health problem in the past year, with 69.2% having at least one internalizing problem and 81.3% having at least one externalizing problem. Adolescents with substance dependence had a fivefold elevated likelihood of having an internalizing problem compared with those who were not dependent. The most prevalent comorbid disorders in adolescents younger than 15 were CD (74.2%; odds ratio [OR] = 3.4), ADHD (63.6%, OR = 3.0), depression (52.7%, OR = 5.6), anxiety (24.6%, OR = 4.6), and traumatic distress (50.6%, OR = 2.9).

Comorbid psychopathology may precede, exacerbate, or follow the onset of heavy substance use. A review of adolescent community surveys found that childhood mental illness generally predicted earlier initiation of substance use and SUD onset, particularly in relation to CD.[7] The early symptoms of most psychiatric disorders, excluding depression, generally had an onset prior to the onset of substance use; full criteria for a nonsubstance psychiatric disorder was typically met prior to SUD onset in adolescence.[8]

Among treated adolescents, comorbid psychopathology generally predicted early return to substance use, particularly conduct problems[9] and major depression.[10] Co-occurring psychopathology also generally predicted a more persistent course of substance involvement over one year of follow-up.[5] Rather than type of diagnosis, the total number of psychiatric symptoms may predict relapse risk.[11] A four-year study of treated youth found that the majority (61%) of adolescents with CD at the time of treatment met criteria for antisocial personality disorder at follow-up, and that these individuals had higher levels of drug involvement over follow-up compared with those without antisocial personality disorder.[12] In one study of adolescents in substance abuse treatment, youth without co-occurring disorders showed the best long-term outcomes and those with co-occurring externalizing disorders recovered more slowly; those with co-occurring externalizing and internalizing disorders had the worst outcomes.[13] Youth with co-occurring disorders are more likely to relapse after treatment,[5] and relapse usually occurs more quickly than for youth with SUDs only.[14]

As comorbidity has an influence on the development and persistence of SUDs and related behaviors, clinicians should recognize the importance of identifying comorbid disorders in assessment and targeting them for intervention as part of a comprehensive and preferably integrated treatment plan.

ASSESSMENT

In the face of problems in one or more domains of adolescent functioning, clinicians and educational professionals who work with youth often need to screen for multiple problems and the need for more comprehensive evaluation of those problems with a positive screen. At the very least, screening during a psychiatric evaluation involves determination that there is a reasonable possibility that problems with substance use exist and that the adolescents may meet criteria for a SUD. A positive screen for a SUD subsequently requires more detailed, extensive questions including asking about substance use, quantity and frequency, the presence of adverse consequences of use, and the adolescent's attitude toward use. Substance use is one of several domains of adolescent functioning. These domains include substance use and related behaviors, psychiatric/behavioral, family, social/peer, school/vocational, recreational/leisure, and medical. Assessment of each domain is necessary to determine overall functioning as well as the effects of impairments in each domain on functioning in other domains (eg, the effect of substance use on the impairment of behavioral and emotional symptoms, and vice versa).

To supplement interview information, clinicians may use a variety of structured interviews and rating scales with established psychometric properties for screening and more comprehensive assessments. Several screening and assessment instruments include both substance use–related and psychiatric symptom items, thus providing a more comprehensive examination of symptoms and functioning (see Winters and Kaminer[15]). The result of this assessment is a diagnostic summary that identifies the adolescent's treatment needs and potentially, targets for intervention. An integrative treatment plan is developed to target multidimensional areas of dysfunction, which includes psychiatric comorbidity.

CAN SUBSTANCE USE DISORDERS AND PSYCHIATRIC TREATMENTS COEXIST?

The integrative treatment of SUDs and psychiatric disorders offers significant challenges (see Libby and Riggs[16]). Traditional behavioral health treatment in the United States revolves around separate and often disconnected systems of treatment for SUDs and other psychiatric disorders. In the past, conceptualizations of illness and corresponding treatment philosophies were profoundly different. The educational backgrounds, training experiences, and licensing requirements often varied widely between mental health and substance abuse treatment communities. Only recently have significant cross-training opportunities emerged in training programs,[17] as well as incentives and resources for seeking them out once students have become practitioners. There are no widely accepted models for specialist certification regarding co-occurring disorders, and becoming dually certified or licensed in each system may be a burden beyond the feasibility of most clinicians. As a result, few providers at the local level are knowledgeable in the treating co-occurring disorders.

Differences in training and philosophy have historically contributed to a lack of consensus with treatment planning, creating difficulties with coordination and collaboration across systems. Unfortunately, this parallels the frequent poor communication and coordination between behavioral health care systems and other child-serving agencies, such as education, child welfare, juvenile justice, and medical health care. This situation is especially problematic for youth with co-occurring disorders because of the multiple systems served by these youths. Having different funding streams and administrative requirements further impedes cross-system collaboration and the development of integrated treatment services.

There is often debate surrounding which disorder to treat first in adolescents with co-occurring disorders. Mental health systems may be unwilling to provide services until substance use has stopped or is controlled. Similarly, the substance abuse system may resist treating clients with active psychiatric symptoms or those who are on psychotropic medications. Neither system traditionally has the knowledge, experience, or capacity to provide integrated treatment. Previously "dual treatment" involved either serial treatment episodes or parallel interventions in each of the two systems.

To develop a more integrated conceptual framework for intervention with comorbid disorders to aid in understanding co-occurring conditions and the level of coordination needed between service systems poised to address them, the basis of treatment should be the severity of impairments rather than diagnosis.[18] The model recommends moving toward integration as the severity of the co-occurring disorder increases, and it delineates a continuum of care based on provider behavior that spans minimal coordination, consultation, collaboration, and integration.[19] Levels along this continuum include (1) minimal coordination, (2) consultation: an informal exchange of clinical information, (3) collaboration: a more structured arrangement involving regular, planned communication, often based on contractual agreements between systems or providers, and (4) integration. The final, and perhaps most desirable level of care, is integration. Integration refers to the development of a single treatment plan that addresses both mental health and SUDs. Both disorders should be considered primary and treated as such.[20] Because many adolescents with co-occurring disorders do not recognize their substance use as a problem, integrated services may offer an opportunity to engage and motivate youth in treatment while offering additional supportive services.[21]

According to the Substance Abuse and Mental Health Services Administration (SAMHSA), integrated care includes at a minimum providing integrated screening, assessment, treatment planning, treatment delivery, and continuing care.[22] An examination of these various evidence-based practices reveals a paucity of interventions developed to concurrently treat mental health and substance abuse disorders in adolescents. The existing integrated practices consist of two general approaches. The first is treatment planning and care coordination, which helps create a system of care in which individual services are provided to best meet the needs of each adolescent and his or her family. The second approach includes evidenced-based interventions that concurrently address both psychiatric and substance abuse disorders.

The numerous needs of youth with comorbid disorders often extend beyond the treatment of SUDs, behavioral, and emotional problems to include school and other environmental obstacles as well as services directly targeting the comorbid disorders. The use of intensive case management and wraparound services that help facilitate a more coordinated treatment approach with or without more integrated intervention programs is often warranted. In *intensive case management*, specially trained professionals assess and coordinate the supports and services necessary to help individuals with serious mental illness live in the community.[22] For adolescents with co-occurring disorders, this may include developing and monitoring a comprehensive service plan, providing support services to the client and his or her family, and providing crisis intervention and advocacy services as needed. *Wraparound* is a model of care coordination for children and youth with mental health problems who are also involved with one or more other systems (eg, child welfare, juvenile justice, special education).[23]

Wraparound requires a team-based planning process through which families, formal supports, and natural supports combine to develop, monitor, and evaluate an individualized plan. While this can improve coordination of SUDs and psychiatric treatment, it does not necessitate integrated treatment.

ARE THERE TREATMENTS FOR COMORBID DISORDERS?

Adolescents with co-occurring disorders often fail to receive effective treatment, if any. Although both mental health disorders and SUDs are considered psychiatric conditions and are contained in the DSM-IV,[24] there has been a divergence in how SUDs are assessed and treated. Many of the obstacles to treatment for either psychiatric disorders or SUDs such as stigma, resistance, family stressors, or familial psychopathology are often compounded in cases of comorbidity.

SPECIFIC INTERVENTION MODELS

Despite the current focus on evidence-based practices, very few psychosocial interventions have been developed and evaluated specifically for adolescents with co-occurring disorders. Clinical trials often suffer from difficulties engaging youth in treatment, poor attendance and compliance with treatment, and high rates of early termination.[25,26] While this is true for adolescents with SUDs or psychiatric disorders, it is especially true for the multiply-impaired comorbid patient. Despite these difficulties, a few effective and promising outpatient treatment models have emerged that, while directed at either SUDs or psychiatric disorders, could be considered integrated models as they often target problems shared by youth with either SUDs or psychiatric disorders. These interventions include cognitive-behavioral therapy (CBT), motivational interviewing and enhancement, and family therapies. Several attributes characterize these interventions as appropriate for SUD-psychiatric comorbidity, including targeting multiple behaviors across the spectrum of comorbid problems. For example, CBT incorporates a variety of interventions aimed at present-focused, goal-directed behavior change. Core strategies include identifying and challenging irrational and maladaptive thoughts and patterns, cognitive restructuring, and learning more functional skills through modeling and role-play exercises. From a cognitive-behavioral point of view, substance use is a learned behavior that is initiated and maintained by an interplay of cognitive processes, environmental factors, and behavioral reinforcement. Treatment often involves a focus on self-monitoring, identifying and changing reinforcement contingencies, coping skills training, and relapse prevention. Cognitive-behavioral interventions are well supported in the treatment of both adolescent psychiatric disorders[27–29] and SUDs.[30,31] Although few studies have examined the effectiveness of CBT for the treatment of adolescent co-occurring disorders, it is believed that they would likely be helpful, especially for youth with comorbid depression and substance abuse.[32]

A form of CBT, dialectic behavior therapy (DBT), has been adapted and used with a variety of adolescent treatment populations including inpatient[33,34] and outpatient[33] suicidal youth, young adolescents with oppositional defiant disorder,[35] and incarcerated juvenile offenders.[36] DBT's focus on emotional validation and acceptance coupled with skills training makes it applicable to adolescents with co-occurring conditions who often have mood dysregulation. The many successful adaptations of DBT to various treatment settings and populations demonstrate that it may be an effective intervention for youth with complicated and severe emotional and behavioral problems.

Similarly, motivational enhancement therapy interventions are often coupled with CBT, especially with adolescents.[37] Motivational interviewing (MI)[38] is a nonconfrontational, client-directed intervention that emphasizes an empathetic nonjudgmental stance, developing discrepancy, avoiding argumentation, rolling with resistance, and supporting self-efficacy for change. MI-based interventions have been found to be effective in reducing substance use among adolescents presenting to an emergency department[37] and among college students.[39–41] For youth with co-occurring disorders, MI/motivational enhancement treatment (MET) alone is likely insufficient to effect change.[42] However, it has been suggested that motivational enhancement interventions may be helpful with this population in increasing treatment engagement and retention, motivation to change, and goal setting, and may be very useful when combined with other interventions such as CBT.[4] The nonconfrontational stance of MI and its ability to be used with individuals in a wide range of readiness-to-change states may make MI particularly attractive to adolescents in their desire for autonomy.[41,43] The five-session MET/cognitive-behavioral therapy (MET/CBT5), developed for use in the Cannabis Youth Treatment Study (CYTS), consists of two individual MET sessions followed by three sessions of group CBT. Although there was little difference in clinical outcomes based on treatment condition in the CYTS, when treatment costs were combined with clinical outcomes, MET/CBT5 was found to be one of the most cost-effective interventions studied.[4,43]

Although various family-based therapies for adolescent co-occurring disorders may differ in terms of strategies and techniques, they share certain common elements. All emphasize the systemic and contextual nature of adolescent problem behavior, focus on the important role parents and caregivers play in youth treatment and outcomes, and use engagement, communication, and various behavioral techniques for achieving change in both the index adolescents and his or her family.[44] Research shows that compared with control conditions, family-based therapies often have better success than individual-targeted interventions in engaging and retaining families in treatment, reducing youth substance use, increasing school attendance and performance, and improving family functioning.[45–48]

Several types of family therapy deserve mention, as they target problems across the SUD-psychiatric divide and have received recognition from several organizations recognizing evidence-based practice. Family behavior therapy (FBT) has demonstrated increases in treatment retention and reductions in suicidal behavior, psychiatric hospitalization, substance abuse, anger, serious adolescent substance use, and associated behavioral problems.[47,49] FBT is recognized as a scientifically based approach to drug treatment by the National Institute on Drug Abuse (NIDA).[50] The theory underlying FBT draws heavily on the community reinforcement approach, and the model employs multiple evidence-based techniques such as behavioral contracting, stimulus control, urge control, and communication skills training.[45]

Multidimensional family therapy (MDFT) was developed as a family-based treatment for adolescents with substance use and related emotional and behavioral problems.[31] MDFT is a comprehensive approach that targets multiple domains of risk, protection, and functioning within the youth, his or her family, and community. Interventions concentrate on the individual problems, strengths, and goals of the adolescent, as well as focusing on parent issues, parenting and family relationships, and extrafamilial influences.[31] See the article by Cynthia L. Rowe elsewhere in this issue for further exploration of this topic.

Multisystemic therapy (MST) was developed as a family- and community-based treatment approach for youth with co-occurring substance abuse and antisocial behavior.[51,52] MST is based on a social ecology theory that suggests adolescent antisocial behavior is multidetermined and linked to variables of the individual and his or her family, peer group, school, and community. Interventions are developed in conjunction with the family with the explicit goal of structuring the youth's environment to promote healthier, less risky behavior. MST services are usually intense, short term (average of 4–6 months), and offered in the youth's natural environment, such as at home or school. MST draws heavily on strategies and techniques found in cognitive-behavioral, behavioral, and family therapies and often uses other specific interventions under the umbrella of MST. However, it differs by offering more intensive and direct interactions with the youth and his or her environment and by providing services outside of traditional care settings.[52] MST was related to posttreatment reductions in self-report of alcohol and drug use.[53] Follow-up studies show improvements in family and peer relations and a decrease in out-of-home placements,[53,54] decreases in psychiatric symptomatology and substance-related arrests at four-year follow-up,[53] and a decrease in rearrests and days incarcerated at the 14-year follow-up.[55] In a subsequent randomized trial of MST with substance-abusing and delinquent youth, adolescents in the MST condition had decreased alcohol and drug use, criminal activity, and number of out-of-home placement days post treatment,[54] although these results were not maintained at the six-month or four-year follow-up, and outcomes regarding criminal activity, substance use, and mental health functioning were not as good as earlier studies.[55]

Recently, several attempts at developing integrated treatments for adolescents with SUDs and depression, posttraumatic stress disorder, bipolar disorder, and suicidal behavior have provided models for both investigators and clinicians.[56–59] Among the challenges faced in the development and delivery of these interventions are choosing a group versus individual or family format, the use of urine drug screens and the level of confidentiality, minimal motivation, and selection of target-specific behaviors and cognitions. Adolescents with comorbid SUDs and psychopathology are among the most difficult youth to work with due to their combination of internalizing and externalizing symptoms and higher impairment, multiple risk factors across family, individual, social/peer, and community domains, and poor insight and motivation. Attempts to integrate these needs and targets under a single paradigm that simplifies treatment focus on the following: (1) psychoeducation, (2) problem solving, (3) decrease avoidance/increase positive social involvement, (4) motivation, and (5) family (communication and problem solving). There is an increased emphasis on motivational enhancement as key element of intervention (both with parents and adolescents) and on the development and enhancement of coping skills, relapse prevention, self-efficacy expectations, and awareness of high risk situations. The use of urine drug screens assures monitoring and discussion of substance use.

In addition, attention to training and supervision is mandatory in the administration of integrated treatments. Interventions that are developed should be practical in terms of the time and level of training involved, the possibility of adequate supervision, and the realistic expectations regarding the amount of time the adolescent and his or her family can devote to treatment.

PHARMACOTHERAPY

Although several family-based, behavioral, and cognitive-behavioral interventions have been shown to have efficacy in the treatment of adolescent SUDs, there is a paucity of controlled treatment outcome research evaluating the effectiveness of pharmacotherapies in the combined or integrated treatment of psychiatric comorbidity and SUDs.[60] The limited pharmacotherapy research using well-controlled studies is confined to two areas: mood disorders (including major depressive disorder/bipolar disorder), and ADHD. Surprisingly, despite high present and lifetime rates of anxiety disorders, at present, there are no published large scale controlled trials treating comorbid anxiety disorders and SUDs in adolescents.

One small study (n = 22) supported the safety and efficacy of lithium carbonate for bipolar disorder in adolescents with concurrent SUD.[61] Another controlled trial evaluated the safety and efficacy of fluoxetine versus placebo in 126 adolescents with DSM-IV diagnoses of major depressive disorder (MDD), CD, and SUD.[62] Adolescents in both medication groups received weekly, individual, manualized CBT for their SUD during the 16-week trial. The study also evaluated the impact of pharmacotherapy for depression on change in drug use, substance treatment compliance, and retention. Results showed that fluoxetine had a good safety profile and demonstrated superior efficacy (0.78 effect size) to placebo for depression, despite nonabstinence in the majority of study participants. Most adolescents also decreased their drug use, about five to seven days per month on average. However, only about 10% of the sample achieved sustained abstinence of at least one month, and there was no difference between fluoxetine and placebo treatment in change in drug use. Because rates of depression remission were unexpectedly high in both the fluoxetine + CBT (75%) and the placebo + CBT (64%) treatment groups, but rates of abstinence were relatively low, researchers concluded that most cases of depression did not remit due to abstinence. However, the limitations of the study design did not allow more definitive conclusions to be drawn about the temporal relationships or directionality of change in depression and change in substance use. Researchers also speculated that CBT most likely contributed to the higher than expected depression response rates despite its primary focus on the treatment of SUD. More definitive conclusions about the contribution of CBT to depression response rates cannot be made because all study participants received the manualized CBT as outpatient treatment for SUD during the medication trial, and there was no comparison group without CBT. Post hoc analyses indicated that remission of depression was a stronger predictor of change in drug use than medication treatment. Those whose depression remitted, regardless of medication assignment, significantly decreased their drug use, whereas nonremitters' drug use did not decrease from baseline levels of use despite similar rates of treatment compliance and retention.

In two other placebo-controlled studies of fluoxetine in adolescents with MDD with alcohol use disorders and SUDs, respectively,[63,64] no differences were noted between the fluoxetine and placebo groups either on depression or drug use outcomes. Thirty-four subjects ages 12 to 17 years (mean age 16.5 years) with either a current MDD or a depressive disorder and a comorbid SUD were randomized to receive either fluoxetine or placebo in a single-site, 8-week double-blind, placebo-controlled study.[64] The primary outcome analysis was a random effects mixed model for repeated measurements of Children's Depression Rating Scale—Revised (CDRS-R) scores compared between treatment groups across time. Based on the results of an interim futility analysis performed after 34 patients were randomized, study enrollment was halted. Overall, both patients who received fluoxetine or placebo had a reduction in CDRS-R scores. However, there was no significant difference in mean change in CDRS-R total score in those subjects treated with fluoxetine versus those who received placebo, and no significant difference in rates of positive urine drug toxicology results between treatment groups at any post-randomization visit. In this study, subjects did not receive concurrent psychotherapy. Cornelius and colleagues,[63] examined the depressive symptoms and the drinking habits of 50 subjects ages 15–20 years old with comorbid major depression (MDD) and alcohol use disorder (AUD) in an acute phase

(12-week) randomized efficacy study of fluoxetine versus placebo. All participants in both treatment groups also received intensive manual-based CBT and MET. Although fluoxetine was well tolerated in this treatment population, no significant group-by-time interactions were noted for any depression-related or drinking-related outcome variables. Subjects in both the fluoxetine group and the placebo group showed significant within-group improvement in both depressive symptoms and level of alcohol consumption. End-of-study levels of depression and drinking were low in both treatment groups.

In summary, comorbid depression with SUDs in adolescents may remit without antidepressant pharmacotherapy or abstinence, in the context of individual outpatient CBT for SUDs (but not precluding the use of CBT for depression). However, if depression does not remit, their drug use may not decrease even if they continue with substance treatment. Thus, in dually diagnosed adolescents, if depression does not seem to be improving early in the course of substance treatment (eg, within the first several weeks of treatment) it appears to be safe, efficacious, and reasonable to initiate a serotonin reuptake inhibitor (fluoxetine), with careful monitoring, even if not yet abstinent, because ongoing depression may prevent further improvements in substance use.

For ADHD, three controlled trials have been published, including two by Riggs and colleagues.[65–67] In the first study, the authors evaluated the safety and efficacy of pemoline (a schedule-IV psychostimulant) for ADHD in 69 out-of-treatment adolescents with active SUD.[66] Results showed that pemoline had a good safety profile and a comparable effect size to that reported for ADHD in adolescents without a SUD, despite nonabstinence in most study participants. However, in the absence of specific behavioral treatment for SUD, pharmacotherapy for ADHD had no impact on drug use, which did not significantly decrease in either treatment group. Another study followed 16 male adolescents (mean age 17.5 years) with ADHD for six weeks using a crossover design in which half of the sample received active medication for three weeks while the other half received placebo. After three weeks, the groups were switched. The main outcome measures for ADHD were the parent report of ADHD symptoms and the Clinician Global Impression of Severity (CGI-S). The main outcome measure for substance use was the number of days of drug or alcohol use in the past week. Results showed a greater improvement in SNAP-IV scores (the primary ADHD outcome) and in CGI-S scores with active medication, compared with placebo. There was no between-group difference in substance use change. In a recently completed double-blind placebo-controlled study of OROS methylphenidate (MPH) in youth with ADHD and a nonopiate SUD, Riggs[67] administered CBT treatment for SUD to all subjects. Results showed that both groups improved on ADHD and SUD measures, although there were no differences in adolescent reports of ADHD symptoms or substance use (number of days used in past month). However, the OROS MPH group had lower ADHD scores than the placebo group on parent report. There were few significant adverse events.

Overall, these results suggest that pharmacologic treatment in comorbid adolescents (eg, with SUDs and MDD or ADHD) may result in improvements in the psychiatric target but will have little, if any, effect on the substance use, especially without concurrent and specific therapy for the SUD. However, there appears to be little medical risk or increase in adverse effects to treatment, and no evidence of abuse or diversion.

SAFETY AND DIVERSION ISSUES

None of the aforementioned controlled studies have identified significant safety issues. Despite few of the subjects showing abstinence for substance use, there were few serious adverse events. Some commonly used pharmacologic agents, such as stimulants, have inherent abuse potential.[60,68] The risk of diversion or misuse of a therapeutic agent by the adolescent, his or her peer group, or family members should prompt a thorough assessment of the risk of this outcome (eg, history of abuse of the specific or other potentially abusable agents, family/parental history of substance abuse or antisocial behavior). Often, parental or adult supervision of medication administration can alleviate concerns about potential abuse. The clinician should also consider alternative agents to psychostimulants, such as atomoxetine or bupropion, which do not have abuse potential.[68] The long-acting stimulant preparations (eg, OROS methylphenidate, mixed amphetamine salts extended release, or lisdexamfetamine dimesylate) may offer less potential for abuse or diversion due to their form of administration, reduced level of reinforcement due to more gradual and longer time to maximum plasma concentration, and the ability to more easily monitor and supervise once-a-day dosing. Many anxiety symptoms or disorders in adolescents can be treated successfully with psychosocial methods such as behavior therapy. If pharmacotherapy is required, the use of selective serotonin reuptake inhibitors, tricyclic antidepressants, or buspirone is preferred over the use of benzodiazepines.

RECOMMENDATIONS

The Practice Parameter for the Assessment and Treatment of Children and Adolescents with Substance Use Disorders from the American Academy of Child and Adolescent Psychiatry[24] set consideration of SUD-psychiatric comorbidity as a minimum standard. Adolescents with SUDs should receive a thorough evaluation for comorbid psychiatric disorders and, conversely, adolescents with psychiatric disorders should receive assessment for possible SUDs. Furthermore, comorbid disorders should be appropriately treated. As previously discussed, for severe presentations this involves integration of treatment modalities rather than merely serial or concurrent treatment. However, acute stabilization of moderate to severe substance use problems or more severe psychiatric presentations involving suicidal behavior and/or psychosis may need to precede integrated treatment approaches.

Critical elements of integrated treatment appear to be attention to motivation, family involvement, and the development of cognitive/behavioral skills. Recent emerging research and experience suggest that pharmacotherapy can be used safely and effectively in adolescents with SUDs,[60] although not all studies have been consistently positive. However, pharmacotherapy has its limits, and all adolescents will need treatment targeting their substance use and related behaviors.

FUTURE RESEARCH

There are many more questions about assessment and intervention with adolescents having SUD-psychiatric comorbidity. Given the prevalence and presumed importance of SUD-psychiatric comorbidity, a rigorous research agenda is suggested.[69] This agenda includes: (1) clinical trials of both pharmacologic agents and psychosocial interventions, alone and in concert, to enhance our understanding of the separate and combined effects of behavioral interventions and pharmacotherapy; (2) developing and testing medications that have the potential to directly target both SUDs and psychiatric comorbidity through amelioration of the presumed underlying neurobiological (eg, brain reward) dysfunction; (3) evaluation of the neurobiological/HPA axis, neuroimaging, or other relevant biomarker responses to both pharmacotherapy and behavioral/psychotherapy treatment modalities; and (4) effectiveness studies and efforts at evaluating and improving technology transfer of efficacious intervention to community treatment providers. These efforts will involve the further testing of existing agents and psychosocial interventions as well as development of novel agents. Finally, longer follow-up periods will be needed to identify the potential long-term effects of interventions.

REFERENCES

1. American Psychiatric Association. Diagnostic and statistical manual of mental disorders: fourth edition-text revision (DSM-IV-TR). Washington, DC: American Psychiatric Association; 2000.
2. Kaminer Y, Bukstein OG. Adolescent substance abuse: psychiatric comorbidity and high-risk behaviors. New York: Routledge/Taylor & Francis Group; 2008.
3. Hser YI, Grella CE, Hubbard RL, et al. An evaluation of drug treatments for adolescents in 4 US cities. Arch Gen Psychiatry 2001;58(7):689–95.
4. Dennis M, Godley SH, Diamond G, et al. The Cannabis Youth Treatment (CYT) study: main findings from two randomized trials. J Subst Abuse Treat 2004; 27(3):197–213.
5. Grella CE, Hser YI, Joshi V, et al. Drug treatment outcomes for adolescents with comorbid mental and substance use disorders. J Nerv Ment Dis 2001;189(6): 384–92.
6. Chan YF, Dennis ML, Funk RR. Prevalence and comorbidity of major internalizing and externalizing problems among adolescents and adults presenting to substance abuse treatment. J Subst Abuse Treat 2008;34(1):14–24.
7. Armstrong TD, Costello E. Community studies on adolescent substance use, abuse, or dependence and psychiatric comorbidity. J Consult Clin Psychol 2002;70(6):1224–39.
8. Costello EJ, Erkanli A, Federman E, et al. Development of psychiatric comorbidity with substance abuse in adolescents: effects of timing and sex. J Clin Child Psychol 1999;28(3):298–311.
9. Brown SA, Gleghorn A, Schuckit MA, et al. Conduct disorder among adolescent alcohol and drug abusers. J Stud Alcohol 1996;57(3):314–24.
10. Cornelius JR, Maisto SA, Martin CS, et al. Major depression associated with earlier alcohol relapse in treated teens with AUD. Addict Behav 2004;29(5): 1035–8.
11. McCarthy DM, Tomlinson KL, Anderson KG, et al. Relapse in alcohol- and drug-disordered adolescents with comorbid psychopathology: changes in psychiatric symptoms. Psychol Addict Behav 2005;19(1):28–34.
12. Myers MG, Brown SA, Mott MA. Preadolescent conduct disorder behaviors predict relapse and progression of addiction for adolescent alcohol and drug abusers. Alcohol Clin Exp Res 1995;19(6):1528–36.
13. Rowe CL, Liddle HA, Greenbaum PE, et al. Impact of psychiatric comorbidity on treatment of adolescent drug abusers. J Subst Abuse Treat 2004;26(2):129–40.
14. Tomlinson KL, Brown SA, Abrantes A. Psychiatric comorbidity and substance use treatment outcomes of adolescents. Psychol Addict Behav 2004;18:160–9.
15. Winters KC, Kaminer Y. Screening and assessing adolescent substance use disorders in clinical populations. J Am Acad Child Adolesc Psychiatry 2008; 47(7):740–4.
16. Bukstein OG, Bernet W, Arnold V, et al. Practice parameter for the assessment and treatment of children and adolescents with substance use disorders. J Am Acad Child Adolesc Psychiatry 2005;44(6):609–21.

17. Libby A, Riggs PD. Integrated substance use and mental health services for adolescents: challenges and opportunities. In: Kaminer Y, Bukstein OG, editors. Adolescent substance abuse: psychiatric comorbidity and high-risk behaviors. New York: Routledge/Taylor & Francis Group; 2008. p. 435–52.

18. Drake RE, Essock SM, Shaner A, et al. Implementing dual diagnosis services for clients with severe mental illness. Psychiatr Serv 2001;52(4):469–76.

19. Hawkins EH. A tale of two systems: co-occurring mental health and substance abuse disorders treatment for adolescents. Annu Rev Psychol 2009;60:197–227.

20. Cent Ment Health Services. Mental health care for youth: a national assessment, annual/final progress report. Rockville (MD): Subst Abuse Ment Health Serv Admin; January 2001–December 2001.

21. Drake RE, McLaughlin P, Pepper B, et al. Dual diagnosis of major mental illness and substance disorder: an overview. New Dir Ment Health Serv 1991;50:3–12.

22. Drake RE, Mercer-McFadden C, Mueser KT, et al. Review of integrated mental health and substance abuse treatment for patients with dual disorders. Schizophr Bull 1998;24(4):589–608.

23. U.S. Dep Health Human Serv. Report to Congress on the prevention and treatment of co-occurring substance abuse and mental disorders. Rockville (MD): Subst Abuse Ment Health Serv Admin; 2002.

24. Burchard JD, Bruns EJ, Burchard SN. The wraparound approach. In: Burns BJ, Hoagwood K, editors. Community treatment for youth: evidence-based interventions for severe emotional and behavioral disorders. New York: Oxford Univ. Press; 2002. p. 69–90.

25. Donohue B, Azrin NH, Lawson H, et al. Improving initial session attendance of substance abusing and conduct disordered adolescents: a controlled study. J Child Adolesc Subst Abuse 1998;8(1):1–13.

26. Wise BK, Cuffe SP, Fischer T. Dual diagnosis and successful participation of adolescents in substance abuse treatment. J Subst Abuse Treat 2001;21(3):161–5.

27. Barrett PM, Shortt AL, Wescombe K. Examining the social validity of the FRIENDS treatment program for anxious children. Behav Change 2001;18(2):63–77.

28. Kazdin AE. Conduct disorder. In: Verhulst FC, Koot HM, editors. The epidemiology of child and adolescent psychopathology. New York: Oxford University Press; 1995. p. 258–90.

29. Rohde P, Lewinsohn PM, Seeley JR. Response of depressed adolescents to cognitive-behavioral treatment: do differences in initial severity clarify the comparison of treatments? J Consult Clin Psychol 1994;62(4):851–4.

30. Kaminer Y, Burleson JA, Blitz C, et al. Psychotherapies for adolescent substance abusers: a pilot study. J Nerv Ment Dis 1998;186(11):684–90.

31. Liddle HA. Treating adolescent substance abuse using Multidimensional Family Therapy. In: Weisz J, Kazdin A, editors. Evidence-based psychotherapies for children and adolescents. 2nd edition. New York (NY): Guilford Press; 2009. p. 416–34.

32. Waldron HB, Kaminer Y. On the learning curve: the emerging evidence supporting cognitive-behavioral therapies for adolescent substance abuse. Addiction 2004;99:93–105.

33. Katz LY, Gunasekara S, Miller AL. Dialectical behavior therapy for inpatient and outpatient parasuicidal adolescents. In: Flaherty LT, editor, Adolescent psychiatry: developmental and clinical studies, vol. 26. New York: The Analytic Press/Taylor & Francis Group; 2002. p. 161–78.

34. Sunseri PA. Preliminary outcomes on the use of dialectical behavior therapy to reduce hospitalization among adolescents in residential care. Residential Treat Child Youth 2004;21:59–76.

35. Nelson-Gray RO, Keane SP, Hurst RM, et al. A modified DBT skills training program for oppositional defiant adolescents: promising preliminary findings. Behav Res Ther 2006;44(12):1811–20.

36. Trupin EW, Stewart DG, Beach B, et al. Effectiveness of a dialectical behaviour therapy program for incarcerated female juvenile offenders. Child Adolesc Ment Health 2002;7(3):121–7.

37. Monti PM, Colby SM, Barnett NP, et al. Brief intervention for harm reduction with alcohol-positive older adolescents in a hospital emergency department. J Consult Clin Psychol 1999;67(6):989–94.

38. Miller WR, Rollnick S. Motivational interviewing: preparing people for change. 2nd edition. New York: Guilford Press; 2002.

39. Baer JS, Marlatt GA, Kivlahan DR, et al. An experimental test of three methods of alcohol risk reduction with young adults. J Consult Clin Psychol 1992;60(6):974–9.

40. Marlatt GA, Baer JS, Kivlahan DR, et al. Screening and brief intervention for high-risk college student drinkers: results from a 2-year follow-up assessment. J Consult Clin Psychol 1998;66(4):604–15.

41. Tevyaw TO, Monti PM. Motivational enhancement and other brief interventions for adolescent substance abuse: foundations, applications and evaluations. Addiction 2004;99(Suppl 2):63–75.

42. Myers MG, Brown SA, Tate S, et al. Toward brief interventions for adolescents with substance abuse and comorbid psychiatric problems. In: Monti PM, Colby SM, O'Leary TA, editors. Adolescents, alcohol, and substance abuse: reaching teens through brief interventions. New York: Guilford Press; 2001. p. 275–96.

43. Compton WM, Pringle B. Services research on adolescent drug treatment. Commentary on "The Cannabis Youth Treatment (CYT) study: main findings from two randomized trials". J Subst Abuse Treat 2004;27(3):195–6.

44. Azrin NH, Donohue B, Teichner GA, et al. A controlled evaluation and description of individual-cognitive problem solving and family-behavior therapies in dually-diagnosed conduct-disordered and substance-dependent youth. J Child Adolesc Subst Abuse 2001;11(1):1–43.

45. Henggeler SW, Borduin CM, Melton GB, et al. Effects of multisystemic therapy on drug use and abuse in serious juvenile offenders: a progress report from two outcome studies. Fam Dynam Addiction Q 1991;1(3):40–51.

46. Liddle HA, Dakof GA. A randomized controlled trial of intensive outpatient, family-based therapy vs residential drug treatment for comorbid adolescent drug abusers. Drug Alcohol Depend 2002;66:S103.

47. Donohue B, Azrin N. Family behavior therapy. In: Wagner E, Waldron H, editors. Innovations in adolescent substance abuse interventions. New York: Pergamon; 2001. p. 205–37.

48. Szapocznik J, Kurtines WM, Foote FH, et al. Conjoint versus one-person family therapy: some evidence for the effectiveness of conducting family therapy through one person. J Consult Clin Psychol 1983;51(6):889–99.

49. Hogue A, Dauber S, Samuolis J, et al. Treatment techniques and outcomes in multidimensional family therapy for adolescent behavior problems. J Fam Psychol 2006;20(4):535–43.

50. National Institute on Drug Abuse (NIDA). Principles of drug addiction treatment: a research-based guide. Nat. Inst. Health Publ. No. 99–4180. Bethesda (MD): National Institute on Drug Abuse (NIDA); 1999.

51. Henggeler SW, Melton GB, Smith LA. Family preservation using multisystemic therapy: an effective alternative to incarcerating serious juvenile offenders. J Consult Clin Psychol 1992;60(6):953–61.

52. Henggeler S, Schoenwald S, Borduin C, et al. Multisystemic treatment of antisocial behavior in children and adolescents. New York: Guilford; 1998.

53. Borduin CM, Mann BJ, Cone LT, et al. Multisystemic treatment of serious juvenile offenders: long-term prevention of criminality and violence. J Consult Clin Psychol 1995;63(4):569–78.

54. Henggeler SW, Pickrel SG, Brondino MJ. Multisystemic treatment of substance-abusing and dependent delinquents: outcomes, treatment fidelity, and transportability. Ment Health Serv Res 1999;1(3):171–84.

55. Schaeffer CM, Borduin CM. Long-term follow-up to a randomized clinical trial of multisystemic therapy with serious and violent juvenile offenders. J Consult Clin Psychol 2005;73(3):445–53.

56. Fortuna L, Porche M. Cognitive behavioral treatment of adolescents with co-existing posttraumatic stress disorder and substance use disorders. In: Scientific Proceedings of the 56th Annual Meeting of the American Academy of Child and Adolescent Psychiatry. Honolulu (HI), October 29, 2009. p. 82–3.

57. Goldstein B, Goldstein T, Milkowitz D. Family-focused treatment for adolescents with bipolar disorder and substance use disorders. In: Scientific Proceedings of the 56th Annual Meeting of the American Academy of Child and Adolescent Psychiatry. Honolulu (HI), October 29, 2009. p. 83.

58. Goldston D, Esposito-Smythers C, Curry J. Psychosocial treatment of suicidal adolescents with substance use disorders. In: Scientific Proceedings of the 56th Annual Meeting of the American Academy of Child and Adolescent Psychiatry. Honolulu (HI), October 29, 2009. p. 83.

59. Curry J, Wells K. Clinical dilemmas in psychosocial treatment of depressed, substance abusing adolescents. In: Scientific Proceedings of the 56th Annual Meeting of the American Academy of Child and Adolescent Psychiatry. Honolulu (HI), October 29, 2009. p. 82.

60. Waxmonsky JG, Wilens TE. Pharmacotherapy of adolescent substance use disorders: a review of the literature. J Child Adolesc Psychopharmacol 2005;15(5):810–25.

61. Geller B, Cooper TB, Sun K, et al. Double-blind and placebo-controlled study of lithium for adolescent bipolar disorders with secondary substance dependency. J Am Acad Child Adolesc Psychiatry 1998;37(2):171–8.

62. Riggs PD, Mikulich-Gilbertson SK, Davies RD, et al. A randomized controlled trial of fluoxetine and cognitive behavioral therapy in adolescents with major depression, behavior problems, and substance use disorders. Arch Pediatr Adolesc Med 2007;161(11):1026–34.

63. Cornelius JR, Bukstein OG, Wood DS, et al. Double-blind placebo-controlled trial of fluoxetine in adolescents with comorbid major depression and an alcohol use disorder. Addict Behav 2009;34(10):905–9.

64. Findling RL, Pagano ME, McNamara NK, et al. The short-term safety and efficacy of fluoxetine in depressed adolescents with alcohol and cannabis use disorders: a pilot randomized placebo-controlled trial. Child Adolesc Psychiatry Ment Health 2009;3(1):11.

65. Szobot CM, Rohde LA, Katz B, et al. A randomized crossover clinical study showing that methylphenidate-SODAS improves attention-deficit/hyperactivity disorder symptoms in adolescents with substance use disorder. Braz J Med Biol Res 2008;41(3):250–7.

66. Riggs PD, Hall SK, Mikulich-Gilbertson SK, et al. A randomized controlled trial of pemoline for attention-deficit/hyperactivity disorder in substance-abusing adolescents. J Am Acad Child Adolesc Psychiatry 2004;43(4):420–9.

67. Riggs P. Multi-site study of OROS-MPH for ADHD in substance-abusing adolescents. In: Scientific Proceedings of the 56th Annual Meeting of the American Academy of Child and Adolescent Psychiatry. Honolulu (HI), October 30, 2009. p. 94–5.
68. Bukstein O. Substance use disorders in adolescents with attention-deficit/hyperactivity disorder. Adolesc Med State Art Rev 2008;19(2):242–53, viii.
69. Riggs P, Levin F, Green AI, et al. Comorbid psychiatric and substance abuse disorders: recent treatment research. Subst Abus 2008;29(3):51–63.

Non–Substance-Addictive Behaviors in Youth: Pathological Gambling and Problematic Internet Use

Christina Brezing, MD[a],*, Jeffrey L. Derevensky, PhD[b],
Marc N. Potenza, MD, PhD[c,d]

KEYWORDS

- Adolescence • Gambling • Internet • Computer use
- Treatment • Prevention

Funding Sources and Disclosures: This work was supported by the National Institutes of Health (NIH) grants R01 DA019039, R01 RL1 AA017539, P50 DA09241, P50 DA016556, UL1 DE19586, NIH Roadmap for Medical Research/Common Fund, the Office of Research on Women's Health, and a Center of Excellence on Gambling Research Award from the National Center for Responsible Gaming and its affiliated Institute for Research on Gambling Disorders. The contents of the manuscript are solely the responsibility of the authors and do not necessarily represent the official views of any of the funding agencies. Dr Potenza has received financial support or compensation for the following: M.N.P. consults for and is an advisor to Boehringer Ingelheim; has consulted for and has financial interests in Somaxon; has received research support from the National Institutes of Health, Veterans Administration, Mohegan Sun Casino, the National Center for Responsible Gaming and its affiliated Institute for Research on Gambling Disorders, and Forest Laboratories, Ortho-Mc-Neil, Oy-Control/Biotie and Glaxo-SmithKline pharmaceuticals; has participated in surveys, mailings or telephone consultations related to drug addiction, impulse control disorders or other health topics; has consulted for law offices and the federal public defender's office in issues related to impulse control disorders; provides clinical care in the Connecticut Department of Mental Health and Addiction Services Problem Gambling Services Program; has performed grant reviews for the National Institutes of Health and other agencies; has given academic lectures in grand rounds, CME events and other clinical or scientific venues; and has generated books or book chapters for publishers of mental health texts.
Dr Derevensky has received research support from the Social Sciences Humanities Research Council in Canada, Ministry of Health and Social Services, Quebec, Nova Scotia Gaming Corporation, Ontario Problem Gambling Research Center, and has consulted to a number of government bodies internationally. He has also performed research reviews for groups in Europe, North America, Asia, Australia, New Zealand, and South Africa.
[a] University of Florida College of Medicine, 2255 NW 16th Terrace, Gainesville, FL 32605, USA
[b] International Centre for Youth Gambling, Problems and High Risk Behaviors, McGill University, 3724 McTavish Street, Montreal, Quebec H3A 1Y2, Canada
[c] Department of Psychiatry, Yale University School of Medicine, Connecticut Mental Health Center, 34 Park Street, New Haven, CT 06519, USA
[d] Department of Child Study Center, Yale University School of Medicine, Connecticut Mental Health Center, 34 Park Street, New Haven, CT 06519, USA
* Corresponding author.
E-mail address: cbrezing@ufl.edu

Child Adolesc Psychiatric Clin N Am 19 (2010) 625–641
doi:10.1016/j.chc.2010.03.012
1056-4993/10/$ – see front matter © 2010 Elsevier Inc. All rights reserved.

Despite differences with respect to their respective histories, gambling and Internet use may share similarities with respect to representing 2 behaviors in which adolescents routinely participate. This article reviews youth participation in gambling and Internet use, describes when such participation may become problematic, and summarizes current prevention and treatment strategies for pathological gambling (PG) and problematic Internet use (PIU) in youth.

DEFINITIONS

Gambling and Internet use exist as a spectrum of behaviors ranging from abstinence to recreational participation to problematic engagement, with the extreme end including the disorders of PG and PIU. How PG and PIU are defined in adolescents has significant implications for prevalence estimates in this group. At present, there exists variability across studies that measure the prevalence of these disorders in youth, with differences in how these problems are defined and measured being thought to contribute to the observed variability. There exist formal diagnostic criteria for PG in the *Diagnostic and Statistical Manual of Mental Disorders* (Fourth Edition, Text Revised) (DSM-IV-TR) that states an individual with PG must have at least 5 inclusionary criteria reflective of impaired control over gambling behaviors that are associated with significant life disruption and/or negative psychosocial impact (American Psychiatric Association). PG typically involves strong motivations to engage in gambling, with elements of withdrawal and craving representing similarities with substance dependence reflected in the diagnostic criteria for the disorders. Researchers have proposed several subtypes of problem gambling based on a pathways model that identifies individuals as behaviorally conditioned, emotionally vulnerable, or antisocial impulsive.[1] These proposed adult-based definitions may not necessarily apply to adolescents with PG given the differences between adolescents and adults. As adults and adolescents have different roles and life experiences, PG may present and impact these groups in different ways.[2] A recent study attempting to validate this model with adolescents yielded some mixed results.[3]

Arguably the most commonly used definition of PIU is based on the DSM-IV-TR definition of PG. The following definition suggests that PIU shares many features with impulse control disorders and substance dependence; PIU reflects impaired control over the "use of the Internet that leads to significant psychosocial and functional impairments, and this pattern of use is not better accounted for by a primary psychiatric disorder such as mania or the physiological effects of a substance."[4,5] It is important to distinguish PIU from normal Internet use, other Axis I disorders, and compulsive-impulsive behaviors.[6] This process may prove difficult, however, as PIU may involve online gambling, Internet-enabled sexual behavior, and online gaming—behaviors that exist on a spectrum from innocuous to pathological and may themselves constitute impulse control disorders. For this reason, some have described the Internet as an "electronic needle" that provides an anonymous, socially connected, novel medium[7] to allow participation in impulse control disorders. It has been proposed that PIU may be subtyped based on specific behaviors forming the focus of the PIU,[8] although systematic studies describing potential differences in the clinical characteristics of individuals with PIU segregated by these behaviors are currently lacking. There exist clinical characteristics that all forms of PIU seem to share, which help to identify them as one general disorder with different manifestations. These characteristics were developed from observations largely derived from case reports of individuals with PIU, and the extent to which they represent generalizable clinically meaningful criteria warrants further investigation. The clinical characteristics include time spent on Internet exceeding 35 hours per week and longer than initially intended and planned, time distortion, compulsive behaviors, unsuccessful attempts with cessation or controlling use, deception about extent of use, use of the Internet behavior to cope or escape problems, and preoccupation with the Internet when offline.[5,6,9,10] These PIU behaviors have been proposed to be representative of a "technological addiction" and fall under the larger category of "behavioral" addictions, which has been proposed to include PG.[11,12] However, disorders considered "behavioral" or non-substance addictions are currently categorized in the DSM-IV-TR as impulse control disorders not elsewhere classified. The DSM-IV-TR does not currently define specific diagnostic criteria for PIU, but the disorder can be diagnosed as an impulse control disorder not otherwise specified.

FORMS OF PG AND PIU AND THEIR ADDICTIVE POTENTIALS

Adolescents engage in multiple forms of regulated and nonregulated gambling including scratchcards, bets with friends, sports betting, lottery purchases, and poker playing. The forms of gambling in which individuals participate may often be dependent on the individual's gender, age, cultural and ethnic background, availability, and accessibility. It has been proposed that forms of gambling that are continuous in nature and require an element of skill may have a stronger association with PG,[13] although others have proposed that nonstrategic forms of gambling such as electronic gambling (slot) machines may be more "addictive."[14] Some individuals have proposed that features of electronic gambling machines (potential for rapid gambling, relatively high event frequencies, intermittent reinforcement schedules) as well as ancillary features (sounds, music, and lights) may keep people, especially adolescents, entertained and engaged.[13,15,16] The fact that many of these machines incorporate video game technology may add to their appeal. However, a growing body of data does not uniformly indicate that specific forms of gambling have greater addictive potential, including among adolescents.[14,17] Although many regulated forms of gambling legally restrict minors from participation, adolescents often acknowledge gambling on both regulated and nonregulated activities for their age group.[18,19]

Adolescents with PIU engage in several Internet behaviors, with common forms being gambling, Internet-enabled sexual behavior (IESB), and online gaming. Several large-scale studies exist for problematic online gambling and suggest that online gamblers may be more likely to have PG than offline gamblers.[20] The Internet may provide access for adolescents and young adults,[21,22] as one study found that 25% of college students have wagered on the Internet.[23] It is difficult to determine the prevalence and extent of IESB, but Internet pornography grosses over $1 billion per year.[4] Online gaming may provide a social and interactive environment for adolescents, and adolescents and young adults may devote substantial time to massive multiplayer online games to the extent of neglecting important areas of life functioning.[4]

PREVALENCE

Although the prevalence estimates of PG and PIU are not precisely known, the disorders are believed to occur internationally and affect all ages, genders, and ethnic groups. It has been estimated that the prevalence of PG and serious problem gambling is two- to fourfold higher in youth aged 12 to 17 years than the prevalence in the adult population, with an additional 10% to 14% of adolescents considered "at risk" for developing PG later in life.[24,25] Studies have estimated adult prevalence of PG at 1% to 2% while estimating the adolescent PG rates at 3% to 8%.[26] The prevalence of gambling participation in teenagers may also be increasing over time, with some researchers noting increases from 45% to 66%[27–29] and others estimating even higher prevalences of juvenile gambling ranging up to 91% participation.[30,31] Some researchers contend these estimates are accurate,[26] and others suggest these rates may be inflated and that the trajectory of prevalence estimates over time are relatively stable.[32] Data in support of this notion that early estimates might be inflated come from recent studies of adults in which diagnostic assessments of PG were obtained rather than relying on screening instruments (which by design are developed to overidentify possible cases thus minimizing the risks of false negatives) to ascertain prevalence estimates. Several large, well-controlled studies using diagnostic assessments have estimated past-year PG to range from 0.1% to 0.3%, with lifetime estimates two- to threefold higher.[33–35] However, as subsyndromal levels of gambling have been associated with adverse measures of functioning in both adolescents and adults,[36,37] more research is needed to investigate the precise prevalence and clinical implications of syndromal and subsyndromal PG.

The prevalence of PIU in adolescents is also not precisely known and may be more difficult to determine than that for PG. Inconsistent assessment instruments, lack of formal diagnostic criteria, a focus primarily on young populations, and sampling of sections of the general population complicate conclusions that can be drawn regarding the prevalence and impact of PIU. Current assessment tools include the Diagnostic Questionnaire[5] and Internet Addiction Test,[38] instruments whose reliability and validity have been preliminarily tested, and many other instruments whose validity and reliability have yet to be empirically validated. These tools, while helpful in identifying individuals with PIU, may not replace a formal diagnostic clinical interview.[4,39] Large-scale offline community studies in Finland, Norway, and South Korea estimate a prevalence of PIU of 2% in adolescents,[4,40] and PIU is believed to represent a serious public health issue, particularly in regions of Asia including South Korea, Taiwan, and China.[41] Arguably the best current estimate of the prevalence of PIU comes from a study that used 4 positive indicators for Internet overuse as a screening tool for PIU. Aboujaoude and colleagues[42] found that in a population of individuals 18 years and older that 0.7% had 4 positive indicators, with 3.7% to 13.7% having 1 to 3 positive indicators. The study was interpreted to suggest that approximately 1% of the adult population may have narrow or "severe" PIU with another 4% to 14% possibly having problems with Internet overuse. The precise estimates in adolescents warrant direct examination, and given changes in Internet technologies and usage over time, longitudinal studies seem warranted.

FACTORS THAT MAY INFLUENCE PREVALENCE
Environmental Factors

The interaction of the environment with individual differences factors may influence the likelihood of developing PG or PIU. Some studies have suggested a link between the availability and accessibility of gambling and rates of gambling and PG.[18,43] Some investigators have proposed that there has been an increase in overall gambling rates in conjunction with increasing gambling availability.[44] In addition, new technological forms, for example, Internet gambling, allow for solitary and unsupervised gambling. Advertising campaigns for gambling may target youth directly or indirectly, encouraging gambling participation while using names and characters popular with adolescents.[18] Some have predicted that Internet gambling may increase tenfold in the near future.[45] The extent to which PIU, particularly among youth, may become more prevalent over time is difficult to predict, and direct investigation of PIU, in conjunction with factors that may be hypothesized to influence PIU, is indicated.

Social, Demographic, and Cultural Factors

Family and peer influences

Familial factors may significantly influence adolescent behavior.[13] There may be a widespread perception that gambling is acceptable and normal, and youths' initial experiences with gambling may often occur within their homes.[46] Parental and older sibling attitudes toward gambling may affect youth involvement, and adolescents with gambling problems are more likely to have parents who are perceived to gamble excessively, have other addictive behaviors, or participate in illegal activities.[30,47,48] Adolescents with parents who are ambivalent about youth gambling appear to have an approximately 50% greater probability of significant gambling problems.[43] In a recent Canadian national study, parents rated gambling least problematic among 13 potential adolescent behaviors (eg, alcohol, drug, and cigarette use, unprotected sex, and so forth).[49] Peer influence also warrants consideration. Up to 44% of adolescents report having gambled because of the influence of friends[50] and, as children age, a significant venue of choice for gambling may be in their homes with friends.[46] Social factors appear particularly relevant in adolescent gambling, perhaps even more so than other factors (eg, gambling to win money) that may be more salient for older age groups.[51] Gambling has been reported to give children the perception of feeling older and a way to show their skills to friends,[52] and there exists a strong social learning component involved in some gambling behaviors.[53] Overall, adolescents often view gambling as benign and less harmful than alcohol, drugs, and cigarettes,[54] and youth attitudes and behavior may predict patterns of gambling in adulthood.[45] Few data are available regarding family and peer influences on PIU, and future studies are needed to elucidate their influence on Internet behaviors.

Gender differences

Among youth, the ratio of males to females with PG is approximately 3:1 to 5:1.[24] Boys as compared with girls typically report higher gross wagers and increased risk-taking behavior, begin gambling earlier, on more games and more often, commit more time and money to gambling, and experience more gambling-related problems.[24,55] Some have proposed this pattern to result from parents encouraging boys to participate in gambling more than girls,[56] creating an environment in which gambling is a significant part of male culture.[57] However, gambling among girls is more closely linked to symptoms of depression than among boys,[37] perhaps because girls may tend to use gambling as a form of avoidance coping and an escape strategy more so than boys.[58] Among adults with gambling problems, men tend to have problems with "face-to-face" forms of gambling (poker, blackjack), substance abuse problems, and criminal behaviors, whereas women tend to develop problems with less personally interactive forms of gambling (bingo, electronic gambling machines) and are more likely to receive nongambling-related mental health services.[59]

As in PG, there is a male preponderance for PIU in adolescents. Boys as compared with girls tend to engage in computer activities associated with strong emotional-motivational states and are more likely to take part in the activities common in PIU including online games, cybersex, and gambling.[40,60] The gender-related differences in these behavioral syndromes suggest that there may exist different underlying motivations for participation that ultimately may require different prevention and treatment strategies.

Cultural differences

Cultural and ethnic backgrounds have been shown to influence gambling behaviors. A study in Minnesota high school students demonstrated that American Indians (30%) and Mexican Americans and African Americans (22%) gamble at greater weekly and daily rates than Asian and Caucasian Americans (4%–5%).[19] Additional studies have similarly found that Hispanic Americans, African Americans, and American Indian adolescents gamble at greater rates than Caucasian Americans.[61,62] Although existing studies have not directly examined cultural and ethnic differences in adolescents with respect to PIU, numerous studies and clinical reports have suggested that PIU may be a significant public health concern among specific Asian cultures.

Physiological and personality factors

There is evidence to suggest that individual physiological and personality characteristics may predispose some individuals to PG. Adolescents with PG have been found to have increased physiological resting states, greater sensation seeking, and greater arousability and excitability related to gambling.[1] Youth with PG also tend to dissociate more frequently while they participate in gambling behaviors.[28,30,63] Specific personality features suggest adolescent gamblers have been found to display more risk-taking behaviors[1,13] and score higher on measures of impulsivity,[46] extroversion, and state and trait anxiety.[64] Adolescents may also exhibit more self-blaming, guilt, anxiety, and emotional lability.[65] Gambling and/or PG among adolescents has also been shown to be associated with lower conformity and self-discipline scores[30] and increased frequency of attention deficit/hyperactivity disorder (ADHD), conduct-related problems,[48] antisocial behaviors, and alcohol and substance abuse.[48,66,67] Youth with PG also have maladaptive coping skills[1] that may be an important mediating factor, as adolescents may use gambling to help dissociate and escape from stressful events using money simply as a means to the end of continued playing.[30,58] Although less research has been performed on physiological and personality factors associated with adolescent PIU, the disorder has also been conceptualized within a stress-coping framework.[4,68]

AGE OF ONSET AND COURSE OF DISORDER

The average time of first gambling experience has been reported as 12 years old, an age considerably younger than the first use of alcohol, tobacco, or other drugs.[24] Adolescents with PG usually initiate gambling behaviors even earlier, at approximately 10 years old, compared with peers without problematic behaviors.[69] Initiation of gambling in youth has been associated with an increased likelihood of a substance use problem to begin during young adulthood.[66] Age of onset has been suggested to predict more severe problems later in life.[70]

Compared with adults, adolescents may progress more rapidly from social forms of gambling to PG, chase losses more consistently, and have erroneous perceptions when gambling.[53,71] Data indicate that early signs of impulsive behavior and ADHD are associated with excessive gambling involvement in adolescence and early adulthood.[72,73] These early signs of impulsive behavior and ADHD may also be associated with addictive behavioral syndromes such as PG and PIU in adolescence, and resultant adult behavior.

PIU has been reported in children as young as 6 years old.[4] It has been suggested that children and adolescents may be at increased risk for developing PIU, and anecdotal evidence suggests that the time of onset of PIU from first Internet use is often within the first 6 months, giving rise to the term "the newbie syndrome."[5] After an individual develops PIU, behaviors may lead to decreased offline social activities and increased depression and loneliness over the course of several years.[74] PIU may represent a chronic disorder with remissions and recurrences,[75] although systematic longitudinal studies to support this notion are lacking.

NEUROBIOLOGY
Adolescence and Impulsivity

Impulsivity is a construct with relevance to PG and multiple other psychiatric conditions.[2,76] Impulsivity may be conceptualized as a disturbance in reward motivation[77] and identified through risk taking.[76] Gambling involves ritualized risk taking and, therefore, impulsive individuals may be predisposed to gambling.[2] Impulsive individuals may fail to change risk-taking behaviors in the setting of past losses or assess risks appropriately, and thus individuals may demonstrate a lack of inhibition and a greater propensity to discount delayed rewards at an excessive rate.[2,78]

Adolescence, as a developmental stage, has often been associated with increased impulsivity.[2] One hypothesis regarding increased impulsivity during adolescence implicates the immaturity of the frontal cortical and subcortical monoamine systems during this developmental period.[2,65,79,80] Such immaturity may influence decision making to allow for an optimal learning drive during this developmental period, with dopamine and serotonin representing 2 contributing neurotransmitters. Dopamine discharge in the striatum may act to facilitate the action of a motivated drive in association with a reward benefit: (1) in the short term as a "go signal" for a motivated drive to result in behavior; and (2) in the long term to create neuroplastic changes underlying motivational memory and repertoire. Dopamine function within the nucleus accumbens may promote a range of motivated behaviors[81–83] with the short-term reward mechanism functioning such that events that are novel, salient, rewarding, or unpredictable are identified and given behavioral responses.[83–85] Neurodevelopmental changes within corticostriatal functioning thus may contribute to impulsivity and PG during adolescence.[2,83,85]

Prefrontal cortical networks have been proposed to control motivational drives. Serotonin systems, comprising serotonin tracts emanating from the raphe nuclei and synapsing into the prefrontal cortex, have been proposed to contribute importantly to this process.[2,80] Central markers for serotonin are decreased in individuals with impulse control disorders including PG,[86] and prefrontal cortex compromise is associated with disadvantageous decision making and engagement in seemingly impulsive behaviors.[87,88] In normal development, substantial changes occur in the prefrontal cortex during adolescence, and this may reflect a relatively diminished ability to exhibit self-control. The combination of changes within dopamine and serotonin systems and corticostriatal circuitry during adolescence may reflect a greater susceptibility to engage in impulse control disorders like PG and PIU,[2] although longitudinal biological investigations to directly investigate this hypothesis are warranted.

Unlike PG, there are limited biological data on PIU. The neurobiology may share similarities with those for substance abuse and impulse control disorders such as PG, although currently there is a lack of direct evidence. Some research has suggested that adolescents with PIU have higher impulsivity than controls,[89] but other studies have shown mixed results. It has been proposed that Internet use is a goal-directed behavior controlled by the ventral tegmental area projections to the nucleus accumbens that may become aberrantly active, leading to PIU.[4,90,91] One study using naltrexone, an opioid receptor antagonist, successfully treated IESB.[92] This finding suggests that medication may indirectly target dopamine function in the mesolimbic dopamine, thus being helpful for a broad range of impulse control disorders including PG and PIU.[93,94] Individuals with PIU who participate in excessive online gaming show increased emotional arousal and stronger cortical reactivity in response to computer game visual cues with increased urges to play, suggesting that gaming urges/cravings may share similar biological features with substance abuse craving.[95] Empirical investigations comparing these conditions are warranted to examine this hypothesis.

Comorbidities

Both PG and PIU are associated with multiple psychiatric conditions. There is a strong association between substance abuse and dependence and PG. The increased occurrence of alcohol and tobacco use in teenagers with PG suggests the 2 disorders may share a similar etiology.[96,97] Shared neural features have been found in association with cocaine cravings and gambling urges,[86] and a twin study with alcohol and PG suggest a common genetic vulnerability.[98] In addition to substance abuse, PG has also been found to be associated with psychotic disorders, internalizing disorders (forms of depression and anxiety), and personality disorders.[2,35,99–101] PG has been associated with suicidal ideation and attempts,[1] and behavioral problems including increased delinquent and criminal behavior, poor school performance, and disrupted family and peer relationships.[48]

Although less is currently known about the pathology of PIU, it is associated with co-occurring disorders, particularly depression.[4] A quarter of adolescents with PIU experience major depression,[102] and up to 70% of individuals with PIU have been diagnosed with bipolar I or II disorder at some point in their lives.[103] PIU may lead to isolation and depression, and the severity of depression may be correlated with the degree of Internet use. It is also hypothesized that the excessive depression may lead to PIU when Internet use is used as a coping strategy.[74] PIU has also been associated with ADHD. One study found that of 500 Korean students, 22.5% with PIU had ADHD, and it has been suggested that adult ADHD may be the best predictor of PIU among college students.[104,105] Obsessive-compulsive disorder (OCD) and other impulse control disorders have also been associated with PIU in small samples.[103] PIU has also been associated with heavy alcohol use in college students.[106] PIU may occur with social phobia and is believed to contribute to heavier Internet use, but this may not explain the compulsive pattern of use seen in PIU.[103] Unlike PG, psychotic disorders appear less commonly in PIU.

PREVENTION

Many prevention strategies for PG are based on approaches used in alcohol and substance abuse prevention, and use the concept of risk and protective factors and their resultant interaction. Risk factors for future gambling problems may include impulsivity, early age of initiation (before 12 years old), being male, prior substance misuse, low scores on measures of resiliency, and poor family and school connectedness.[30,58,70,107] These factors are associated with adolescent risk behavior in general and have been applied to PG. At this point, there is insufficient information to develop a full list of protective factors for PG, but family cohesion has been reported to be a protective factor.[54,108] A goal of prevention strategies involves limiting the effects of putative risk factors while enhancing resiliency through enhancing protective factors. In doing so, PG is approached through a harm-reduction and minimization strategy—typically not involving abstinence but rather promoting responsible gambling. Abstinence models prohibit youth from legally accessing regulated gambling activities, and while stricter enforcements and adherence may be required, it has already been found that many youths still access and participate in gambling even with prohibitive policies in place. For this reason, it seems reasonable to target informed use and use Beck's approach of "just say know" (1998) rather than a "just say no" approach. Canada's prevention efforts focused at the McGill University Center for Youth Problem Gambling and High Risk Behaviors has adopted and paved the way for a risk-protective factor model by including efforts to bring multimedia prevention programs to elementary students because reports of gambling begin early, often in children aged 9 and 10 years.[30,31] It is important to consider appropriate regulation and enforcement approaches to the prevention of youth gambling by advocating informed use.[109] For example, current adolescent opinion reflects that participating in the lottery is not gambling,[18] so one approach would focus on disseminating and communicating information and strategies that create more realistic understandings of and attitudes toward gambling.[110,111] Direct examination of the effectiveness of prevention strategies for adolescent gambling and PG is needed, as substance abuse prevention programs with seemingly logical tenets have not been found to be uniformly successful.[112]

At present little is known about the risk and protective factors in PIU, making the development of an effective prevention strategy difficult. A recent study found that depression and low family monitoring were discriminating factors for PIU in adolescents regardless of age or gender, with low connectedness to school, high family conflict, peers with habitual alcohol use, and rural living environments also associated with PIU.[113] These data suggest that parents might increase home monitoring of Internet use and aid youth in seeking treatment for depression to help prevent PIU.

TREATMENT

Evidenced-based treatments for PG have been reported, with advances over the past decade seen for both pharmacological and behavioral therapies for PG.[94,114] However, these approaches have largely been tested in adults with PG, and relatively few studies have systematically examined their efficacies and tolerabilities in youths.[115] Challenges related to lack of perceived gambling problems among youth identified via screening instruments as having such problems in conjunction with infrequent treatment seeking further complicate the treatment of adolescent PG.[116,117]

Data suggest that different types of adolescent gambling might require consideration in treatment development.[1,73,118] The pathways approach that defines behaviorally conditioned, emotionally vulnerable, and antisocial impulsive gamblers may have important implications for both the diagnosis and treatment of PG, and suggests that a dynamic and interactive strategy that takes into account the multifactorial nature of the disorder may be the most therapeutic.[1,65] Direct examination of this hypothesis in both adolescent and adult samples is warranted.

Both behavioral and pharmacological treatments for adult PG have shown initial positive results in controlled trials. Behavioral approaches including cognitive behavioral therapy, motivational interviewing, brief counseling, and imaginal desensitization have all shown initial positive results, as has attendance in self-help programs (specifically Gamblers Anonymous).[94,119] However, these approaches have largely not been systematically tested in youth populations. The transtheoretical model of intentional behavioral change has also been suggested to serve as a framework for treatment paradigm of adolescent PG.[27,120–122] Psychopharmacological approaches using serotonin reuptake inhibitors, mood stabilizers, opioid antagonists, and glutamatergic agents have shown efficacy and tolerability in controlled trials in adults with PG, albeit not uniformly with all classes.[94] Precise pharmacological recommendations for adolescents must wait until controlled treatment studies are performed.[115,123–125] As adolescents may not actively seek treatment, outreach programs (including telephone counseling and home-based treatment manuals) have been suggested.[121,122] Treatment approaches should consider addressing other co-occurring or underlying psychological problems that exist in addition to PG,[126] particularly as PG and other impulse control disorders may go unidentified in youth with psychiatric concerns. Although adolescence typically involves a relatively narrow range of ages (12–17 years), there is great variability in maturity, and different treatments should consider their appropriateness within a developmental framework.[65]

The lack of uniformly agreed on, formalized diagnostic criteria as well as valid and reliable assessment instruments for PIU makes designing and measuring treatment paradigms, and their efficacies and tolerabilities, difficult. Nonetheless, there exist a growing number of outpatient treatment services including those at the Computer Addiction Study Center at McLean Hospital of Harvard Medical School, the Illinois Institute for Addiction Recovery at Proctor Hospital, and a halfway house for adolescents with PIU in China. The goal of treatment for PIU in these programs is typically controlled use, not abstinence. Treatment for adolescents might include family-based interventions, skills for parents to improve communication, and increased monitoring of Internet use.[127] A study of cognitive behavioral therapy using a daily log in conjunction with software to restrict access showed improvement in symptoms but appeared poorly generalized.[8] Motivational interviewing using the transtheoretical model of behavioral change[128] and studies using both cognitive behavioral therapy and motivational interviewing showed improvements in quality of life and depression, but no significant changes in computer use behaviors.[92] Insight orient psychotherapy has also been suggested as a model for treatment. Internet support groups may also serve a role in the treatment of PIU. Online support groups provide wide accessibility and incorporate a medium that is familiar to these individuals. The extent to which these approaches might be helpful for youth with PIU warrants direct examination in controlled trials.

Psychopharmacology has been examined in some individuals with PIU. An open-label study in 19 patients given a serotonin reuptake inhibitor showed decreased time spent online, decreased impulsivity and compulsivity, and increased overall global function.[90] In addition, a case report demonstrated improvement in an online gambler with depression treated with a serotonin reuptake inhibitor,[129] and atypical antipsychotics, such as quetiapine, may represent augmentation strategies.[9] Naltrexone has also been successfully used to treat 3 of 4 men with PIU. Controlled trials are indicated to determine the extent to which these medications might be helpful, and direct examination with specific age groups is indicated to examine their efficacies and tolerabilities in a developmentally informed fashion.

PG and PIU share common negative consequences including disrupted interpersonal relationships, increased delinquent and criminal behavior, poor work and school performance, and greater social isolation.[30,130] Future directions in treatment-focused studies should further identify specific factors that motivate individuals with PG and PIU to engage excessively in gambling and Internet use, respectively. If these factors can be more precisely defined, clinical interventions may be designed to build resiliency such that individuals susceptible to PG and PIU may be better able to cope with adversity.

SUMMARY

PG and subsyndromal gambling have been shown to be associated with adverse measures of functioning in youth and older individuals. Although PIU may share similarities with PG regarding developmental impacts, few studies, particularly longitudinal ones, have been conducted to test this hypothesis. PG and PIU represent important and potentially growing public health issues that may go unrecognized by clinicians who focus on more "visible" behaviors such as drug and alcohol abuse. Parents, educators, clinicians, and public health officials should address PG and PIU in youth before they escalate. As various treatments for PG and PIU may not translate across developmental groups, direct examination of their efficacies and tolerabilities are warranted in youths. Similarly, although prevention strategies from other fields (eg, prevention of youth risk behaviors, including substance use and abuse) may be adopted and modified for PG and PIU, direct examination of their effectiveness is needed.

REFERENCES

1. Nower L, Derevensky JL, Gupta R. The relationship of impulsivity, sensation seeking, coping, and substance use in youth gamblers. Psychol Addict Behav 2004;18(1):49–55.
2. Chambers RA, Potenza MN. Neurodevelopment, impulsivity, and adolescent gambling. J Gambl Stud 2003;19(1):53–84.
3. Gupta R, Nower L, Derevensky J, et al. Problem gambling in adolescents: an examination of the pathways model. Report prepared for the Ontario Problem Gambling Research Center. Ontario, 2009.
4. Liu T, Potenza MN. Problematic internet use: clinical implications. CNS Spectr 2007;12(6):453–66.
5. Young KS. Psychology of computer use: XL. Addictive use of the internet: a case that breaks the stereotype. Psychol Rep 1996;79(3 Pt 1):899–902.
6. Shapira NA, Lessig MC, Goldsmith TD, et al. Problematic internet use: proposed classification and diagnostic criteria. Depress Anxiety 2003;17(4): 207–16.
7. Miller MC. Questions & answers. Is "internet addiction" a distinct mental disorder? Harv Ment Health Lett 2007;24(4):8.
8. Young KS. Cognitive behavior therapy with internet addicts: treatment outcomes and implications. Cyberpsychol Behav 2007;10(5):671–9.
9. Atmaca M. A case of problematic internet use successfully treated with an SSRI-antipsychotic combination. Prog Neuropsychopharmacol Biol Psychiatry 2007; 31(4):961–2.
10. Allison SE, von Wahlde L, Shockley T, et al. The development of the self in the era of the internet and role-playing fantasy games. Am J Psychiatry 2006; 163(3):381–5.
11. Griffiths M. Nicotine, tobacco and addiction. Nature 1996;384(6604):18.
12. Griffiths M. Psychology of computer use: XLIII. Some comments on 'addictive use of the internet' by Young. Psychol Rep 1997;80(1):81–2.
13. Abbott MW, Volberg RA, Ronnberg S. Comparing the New Zealand and Swedish national surveys of gambling and problem gambling. J Gambl Stud 2004;20(3):237–58.
14. Dowling N, Smith D, Thomas T. Electronic gaming machines: are they the 'crack-cocaine' of gambling? Addiction 2005;100(1):33–45.
15. Griffiths M. Gambling technologies: prospects for problem gambling. J Gambl Stud 1999;15(3):265–83.
16. Wood RT, Griffiths MD. Adolescent lottery and scratchcard players: do their attitudes influence their gambling behaviour? J Adolesc 2004;27(4): 467–75.
17. Welte JW, Barnes GM, Tidwell MC, et al. The association of form of gambling with problem gambling among American youth. Psychol Addict Behav 2009; 23(1):105–12.
18. Felsher JR, Derevensky JL, Gupta R. Lottery playing amongst youth: implications for prevention and social policy. J Gambl Stud 2004;20(2):127–53.

19. Stinchfield R. Gambling and correlates of gambling among Minnesota Public School students. J Gambl Stud 2000;16(2–3):153–73.

20. McBride J, Derevensky J. Internet gambling behaviour in a sample of online gamblers. Int J of Mental Health and Addiction 2009;7:149–67.

21. Labrie RA, Laplante DA, Nelson SE, et al. Assessing the playing field: a prospective longitudinal study of internet sports gambling behavior. J Gambl Stud 2007; 23(3):347–62.

22. Labrie RA, Kaplan SA, Laplante DA, et al. Inside the virtual casino: a prospective longitudinal study of actual internet casino gambling. Eur J Public Health 2008; 18(4):410–6.

23. Petry NM, Weinstock J. Internet gambling is common in college students and associated with poor mental health. Am J Addict 2007;16(5):325–30.

24. Jacobs DF. Youth gambling in North America: long-term trends and future prospects. In: Derevensky JL, Gupta R, editors. Gambling problems in youth: theoretical and applied perspectives. New York: Klewer Academic/Plenum Publishers; 2004. p. 1–24.

25. National Research Council. Pathological gambling: a critical review. Washington, DC: National Academy Press; 1999.

26. Derevensky JL, Gupta R, Winters K. Prevalence rates of youth gambling problems: are the current rates inflated? J Gambl Stud 2003;19(4):405–25.

27. DiClemente CC, Story M, Murray K. On a roll: the process of initiation and cessation of problem gambling among adolescents. J Gambl Stud 2000;16(2-3): 289–313.

28. Jacobs DF. Juvenile gambling in North America: an analysis of long term trends and future prospects. J Gambl Stud 2000;16(2-3):119–52.

29. Shaffer HJ, Hall MN. Updating and refining prevalence estimates of disordered gambling behaviour in the United States and Canada. Can J Public Health 2001; 92(3):168–72.

30. Gupta R, Derevensky JL. Adolescent gambling behavior: a prevalence study and examination of the correlates associated with problem gambling. J Gambl Stud 1998;14(4):319–45.

31. Derevensky JL, Gupta R. Prevalence estimates of adolescent gambling: a comparison of the SOGS-RA, DSM-IV-J, and the GA 20 questions. J Gambl Stud 2000;16(2–3):227–51.

32. Ladouceur R, Jacques C, Chevalier S, et al. Prevalence of pathological gambling in Quebec in 2002. Can J Psychiatry 2005;50(8):451–6.

33. Gerstein D, Hoffman J, Larison C, et al. Gambling impact and behavior study: National Opinion Research Center. Chicago: University of Chicago; 1999.

34. Kessler RC, Hwang I, LaBrie R, et al. DSM-IV pathological gambling in the National Comorbidity Survey Replication. Psychol Med 2008;38(9):1351–60.

35. Petry NM, Stinson FS, Grant BF. Comorbidity of DSM-IV pathological gambling and other psychiatric disorders: results from the National Epidemiologic Survey on Alcohol and Related Conditions. J Clin Psychiatry 2005;66(5):564–74.

36. Desai RA, Potenza MN. Gender differences in the associations between past-year gambling problems and psychiatric disorders. Soc Psychiatry Psychiatr Epidemiol 2008;43(3):173–83.

37. Desai RA, Maciejewski PK, Pantalon MV, et al. Gender differences in adolescent gambling. Ann Clin Psychiatry 2005;17(4):249–58.

38. Widyanto L, McMurran M. The psychometric properties of the internet addiction test. Cyberpsychol Behav 2004;7(4):443–50.

39. Beard KW. Internet addiction: a review of current assessment techniques and potential assessment questions. Cyberpsychol Behav 2005;8(1):7–14.

40. Johansson A, Gotestam KG. Internet addiction: characteristics of a questionnaire and prevalence in Norwegian youth (12–18 years). Scand J Psychol 2004;45(3):223–9.

41. Block JJ. Issues for DSM-V: internet addiction. Am J Psychiatry 2008;165(3):306–7.

42. Aboujaoude E, Koran LM, Gamel N, et al. Potential markers for problematic internet use: a telephone survey of 2,513 adults. CNS Spectr 2006;11(10):750–5.

43. Fisher S. Measuring the prevalence of sector-specific problem gambling: a study of casino patrons. J Gambl Stud 2000;16(1):25–51.

44. Korn DA, Shaffer HJ. Gambling and the health of the public: adopting a public health perspective. J Gambl Stud 1999;15(4):289–365.

45. Griffiths M, Wood RT. Risk factors in adolescence: the case of gambling, video-game playing, and the internet. J Gambl Stud 2000;16(2-3):199–225.

46. Gupta R, Derevensky J. Familial and social influences on juvenile gambling behavior. J Gambl Stud 1997;13(3):179–92.

47. Ladouceur R, Jacques C, Ferland F, et al. Parents' attitudes and knowledge regarding gambling among youths. J Gambl Stud 1998;14(1):83–90.

48. Hardoon KK, Gupta R, Derevensky JL. Psychosocial variables associated with adolescent gambling. Psychol Addict Behav 2004;18(2):170–9.

49. Derevensky J, Campbell C, Meerkamper E, et al. Parental attitudes towards youth gambling: results from a national Canadian study. Paper presented at the National Council on Problem Gambling Annual Conference. Indianapolis, Indiana, June, 2009.

50. Griffiths MD. Adolescent gambling: an observational pilot study. Percept Mot Skills 1990;70(3 Pt 2):1138.

51. Burge AN, Pietrzak RH, Petry NM. Pre/early adolescent onset of gambling and psychosocial problems in treatment-seeking pathological gamblers. J Gambl Stud 2006;22(3):263–74.

52. Fisher S. Gambling and pathological gambling in adolescents. J Gambl Stud 1993;9:277–88.

53. Hardoon KK, Derevensky JL. Social influences involved in children's gambling behavior. J Gambl Stud 2001;17(3):191–215.

54. Dickson LM, Derevensky JL, Gupta R. The prevention of gambling problems in youth: a conceptual framework. J Gambl Stud 2002;18(2):97–159.

55. Derevensky J, Gupta R, Della-Cioppa G. A developmental perspective of gambling behavior in children and adolescents. J Gambl Stud 1996;12:49–66.

56. Ladouceur R, Dube D, Bujold A. Prevalence of pathological gambling and related problems among college students in the Quebec metropolitan area. Can J Psychiatry 1994;39(5):289–93.

57. Huxley J, Carroll D. A survey of fruit machine gambling in adolescence. J Gambl Stud 1992;8:167–79.

58. Bergevin T, Gupta R, Derevensky J, et al. Adolescent gambling: understanding the role of stress and coping. J Gambl Stud July 12, 2006. [Epub ahead of print].

59. Potenza MN, Steinberg MA, McLaughlin SD, et al. Gender-related differences in the characteristics of problem gamblers using a gambling helpline. Am J Psychiatry 2001;158(9):1500–5.

60. Ko CH, Yen JY, Yen CF, et al. Screening for internet addiction: an empirical study on cut-off points for the Chen Internet Addiction Scale. Kaohsiung J Med Sci 2005;21(12):545–51.

61. Stinchfield R, Cassuto N, Winters K, et al. Prevalence of gambling among Minnesota public school students in 1992 and 1995. J Gambl Stud 1997;13(1):25–48.

62. Wallisch L. Gambling in Texas: 1992 Texas survey of adolescent gambling behavior. Austin (TX), 1993.

63. Powell J, Hardoon K, Derevensky JL, et al. Gambling and risk-taking behavior among university students. Subst Use Misuse 1999;34(8):1167–84.

64. Blaszczynski A, McConaughy N. The medical model of pathological gambling: Current shortcomings. Journal of Gambling Behavior 1989;5:42–52.

65. Gupta R, Derevensky JL. Adolescents with gambling problems: from research to treatment. J Gambl Stud 2000;16(2-3):315–42.

66. Lynch WJ, Maciejewski PK, Potenza MN. Psychiatric correlates of gambling in adolescents and young adults grouped by age at gambling onset. Arch Gen Psychiatry 2004;61(11):1116–22.

67. Winters KC, Anderson N. Gambling involvement and drug use among adolescents. J Gambl Stud 2000;16(2-3):175–98.

68. Ha JH, Kim SY, Bae SC, et al. Depression and Internet addiction in adolescents. Psychopathology 2007;40(6):424–30.

69. Wynne H, Smith G, Jacobs, D. Adolescent gambling and problem gambling in Alberta. Alberta (CA): Alberta Alcohol and Drug Abuse Commission (AADAC); 1996.

70. Winters KC, Stinchfield RD, Botzet A, et al. A prospective study of youth gambling behaviors. Psychol Addict Behav 2002;16(1):3–9.

71. Derevensky J, Gupta R, Dickson L. Prevention efforts toward reducing gambling problems. In: Derevensky J, Gupta R, editors. Gambling problems in youth: theoretical and applied perspectives. New York: Klewer Academic/Plenum Publishers; 2004. p. 211–30.

72. Pagani LS, Derevensky JL, Japel C. Predicting gambling behavior in sixth grade from kindergarten impulsivity: a tale of developmental continuity. Arch Pediatr Adolesc Med 2009;163(3):238–43.

73. Vitaro F, Wanner B, Ladouceur R, et al. Trajectories of gambling during adolescence. J Gambl Stud 2004;20(1):47–69.

74. Kraut R, Patterson M, Lundmark V, et al. Internet paradox. A social technology that reduces social involvement and psychological well-being? Am Psychol 1998;53(9):1017–31.

75. Ko CH, Yen JY, Yen CF, et al. Factors predictive for incidence and remission of internet addiction in young adolescents: a prospective study. Cyberpsychol Behav 2007;10(4):545–51.

76. Evenden J. Impulsivity: a discussion of clinical and experimental findings. J Psychopharmacol 1999;13(2):180–92.

77. Zuckerman M. P-impulsive sensation seeking and its behavioral, psychophysiological and biochemical correlates. Neuropsychobiology 1993;28(1–2):30–6.

78. Reynolds B. A review of delay-discounting research with humans: relations to drug use and gambling. Behav Pharmacol 2006;17(8):651–67.

79. Ernst M, Nelson EE, Jazbec S, et al. Amygdala and nucleus accumbens in responses to receipt and omission of gains in adults and adolescents. Neuroimage 2005;25(4):1279–91.

80. Casey BJ, Getz S, Galvan A. The adolescent brain. Dev Rev 2008;28(1):62–77.

81. Cardinal RN, Pennicott DR, Sugathapala CL, et al. Impulsive choice induced in rats by lesions of the nucleus accumbens core. Science 2001;292(5526):2499–501.

82. Pennartz CM, Groenewegen HJ, Lopes da Silva FH. The nucleus accumbens as a complex of functionally distinct neuronal ensembles: an integration of behavioural, electrophysiological and anatomical data. Prog Neurobiol 1994;42(6): 719–61.

83. Chambers RA, Bickel WK, Potenza MN. A scale-free systems theory of motivation and addiction. Neurosci Biobehav Rev 2007;31(7):1017–45.

84. Ferster CB. Concurrent schedules of reinforcement in the chimpanzee. Science 1957;125(3257):1090–1.

85. Waelti P, Dickinson A, Schultz W. Dopamine responses comply with basic assumptions of formal learning theory. Nature 2001;412(6842):43–8.

86. Potenza MN. The neurobiology of pathological gambling and drug addiction: an overview and new findings. Philos Trans R Soc Lond B Biol Sci 2008;363(1507):3181–9.

87. Bechara A. Neurobiology of decision-making: risk and reward. Semin Clin Neuropsychiatry 2001;6(3):205–16.

88. Bechara A, Damasio H, Damasio AR, et al. Different contributions of the human amygdala and ventromedial prefrontal cortex to decision-making. J Neurosci 1999;19(13):5473–81.

89. Cao F, Su L, Liu T, et al. The relationship between impulsivity and Internet addiction in a sample of Chinese adolescents. Eur Psychiatry 2007;22(7):466–71.

90. Dell'Osso B, Altamura AC, Allen A, et al. Epidemiologic and clinical updates on impulse control disorders: a critical review. Eur Arch Psychiatry Clin Neurosci 2006;256(8):464–75.

91. Liu CY, Kuo FY. A study of Internet addiction through the lens of the interpersonal theory. Cyberpsychol Behav 2007;10(6):799–804.

92. Orzack MH, Voluse AC, Wolf D, et al. An ongoing study of group treatment for men involved in problematic internet-enabled sexual behavior. Cyberpsychol Behav 2006;9(3):348–60.

93. Kim SW. Opioid antagonists in the treatment of impulse-control disorders. J Clin Psychiatry 1998;59(4):159–64.

94. Brewer JA, Grant JE, Potenza MN. The treatment of pathological gambling. Addict Disord Treat 2008;7:1–14.

95. Ko CH, Liu GC, Hsiao S, et al. Brain activities associated with gaming urge of online gaming addiction. J Psychiatr Res 2009;43(7):739–47.

96. Blanco C, Moreyra P, Nunes EV, et al. Pathological gambling: addiction or compulsion? Semin Clin Neuropsychiatry 2001;6(3):167–76.

97. Potenza MN. The neurobiology of pathological gambling. Semin Clin Neuropsychiatry 2001;6(3):217–26.

98. Slutske WS, Eisen S, True WR, et al. Common genetic vulnerability for pathological gambling and alcohol dependence in men. Arch Gen Psychiatry 2000; 57(7):666–73.

99. Potenza MN, Chambers RA. Schizophrenia and pathological gambling. Am J Psychiatry 2001;158(3):497–8.

100. Potenza MN, Xian H, Shah K, et al. Shared genetic contributions to pathological gambling and major depression in men. Arch Gen Psychiatry 2005;62(9): 1015–21.

101. Desai RA, Potenza MN. A cross-sectional study of problem and pathological gambling in patients with schizophrenia/schizoaffective disorder. J Clin Psychiatry 2009;70(9):1250–7.

102. Ha JH, Yoo HJ, Cho IH, et al. Psychiatric comorbidity assessed in Korean children and adolescents who screen positive for Internet addiction. J Clin Psychiatry 2006;67(5):821–6.

103. Shapira NA, Goldsmith TD, Keck PE, et al. Psychiatric features of individuals with problematic internet use. J Affect Disord 2000;57(1-3):267–72.

104. Yoo HJ, Cho SC, Ha J, et al. Attention deficit hyperactivity symptoms and internet addiction. Psychiatry Clin Neurosci 2004;58(5):487–94.

105. Yen JY, Yen CF, Chen CS, et al. The association between adult ADHD symptoms and internet addiction among college students: the gender difference. Cyberpsychol Behav 2009;12(2):187–91.

106. Yen JY, Ko CH, Yen CF, et al. The association between harmful alcohol use and Internet addiction among college students: comparison of personality. Psychiatry Clin Neurosci 2009;63(2):218–24.

107. Lussier I, Derevensky JL, Gupta R, et al. Youth gambling behaviors: an examination of the role of resilience. Psychol Addict Behav 2007;21(2):165–73.

108. Jessor R, Turbin MS, Costa FM. Protective factors in adolescent health behavior. J Pers Soc Psychol 1998;75(3):788–800.

109. Felsher J, Derevensky J, Gupta R. Parental influences and social modeling of youth lottery participation. J Community Appl Soc Psychol 2003;13:361–77.

110. Ferland F, Ladouceur R, Vitaro F. Prevention of problem gambling: modifying misconceptions and increasing knowledge. J Gambl Stud 2002;18(1):19–29.

111. Ferland F, Ladouceur R, Vitaro F. [Efficiency of a gambling prevention program for youths: results from the pilot study]. Encephale 2005;31(4 Pt 1):427–36 [in French].

112. Clayton RR, Cattarello AM, Johnstone BM. The effectiveness of drug abuse resistance education (project DARE): 5-year follow-up results. Prev Med 1996; 25(3):307–18.

113. Yen CF, Ko CH, Yen JY, et al. Multi-dimensional discriminative factors for Internet addiction among adolescents regarding gender and age. Psychiatry Clin Neurosci 2009;63(3):357–64.

114. Toneatto T, Ladoceur R. Treatment of pathological gambling: a critical review of the literature. Psychol Addict Behav 2003;17(4):284–92.

115. Grant JE, Potenza MN. Pharmacological treatment of adolescent pathological gambling. Int J Adol Med Health, in press.

116. Hardoon K, Derevensky JL, Gupta R. Empirical measures vs. perceived gambling severity among youth: why adolescent problem gamblers fail to seek treatment. Addict Behav 2003;28(5):933–46.

117. Cronce JM, Corbin WR, Steinberg MA, et al. Self-perception of gambling problems among adolescents identified as at-risk or problem gamblers. J Gambl Stud 2007;23(4):363–75.

118. Toneatto T, Millar G. Assessing and treating problem gambling: empirical status and promising trends. Can J Psychiatry 2004;49(8):517–25.

119. Grant JE, Donahue CB, Odlaug BL, et al. Imaginal desensitisation plus motivational interviewing for pathological gambling: randomised controlled trial. Br J Psychiatry 2009;195(3):266–7.

120. DiClemente CC, Schlundt D, Gemmell L. Readiness and stages of change in addiction treatment. Am J Addict 2004;13(2):103–19.

121. Hodgins DC, el-Guebaly N. Natural and treatment-assisted recovery from gambling problems: a comparison of resolved and active gamblers. Addiction 2000;95(5):777–89.

122. Hodgins DC, Currie SR, el-Guebaly N. Motivational enhancement and self-help treatments for problem gambling. J Consult Clin Psychol 2001;69(1): 50–7.

123. Grant JE, Potenza MN. Impulse control disorders: clinical characteristics and pharmacological management. Ann Clin Psychiatry 2004;16(1):27–34.

124. Grant JE, Potenza MN. Escitalopram treatment of pathological gambling with cooccurring anxiety: an open-label pilot study with double-blind discontinuation. Int Clin Psychopharmacol 2006;21(4):203–9.

125. Toneatto T, Brands B, Selby P. A randomized, double-blind, placebo-controlled trial of naltrexone in the treatment of concurrent alcohol use disorder and pathological gambling. Am J Addict 2009;18(3):219–25.

126. Grant JE, Williams KA, Potenza MN. Impulse-control disorders in adolescent psychiatric inpatients: co-occurring disorders and sex differences. J Clin Psychiatry 2007;68(10):1584–92.

127. Yen JY, Yen CF, Chen CC, et al. Family factors of internet addiction and substance use experience in Taiwanese adolescents. Cyberpsychol Behav 2007;10(3):323–9.

128. Prochaska JO, DiClemente CC, Velicer WF, et al. Criticisms and concerns of the transtheoretical model in light of recent research. Br J Addict 1992;87(6):825–8.

129. Sattar P, Ramaswamy S. Internet gaming addiction. Can J Psychiatry 2004; 49(12):869–70.

130. McBride J. Virtual interaction is still social interaction: how massively multiplayer online role-playing games and online gambling blur the distinction between normal and excessive internet use. Montreal (Canada): McGill University; 2009.

Problematic Use of Energy Drinks by Adolescents

Yifrah Kaminer, MD, MBA

KEYWORDS

- Adolescents • College students • Energy drinks
- Caffeine • Alcohol • High-risk behaviors

Since the introduction of the energy drink (ED) Red Bull in 1987 to Europe and in the 1990s to the United States, the popularity of EDs has increased, particularly with the youth population. In 2008, annual sales of EDs accounted for $3.2 billion in the United States and $7.8 billion worldwide.[1] To appeal to adolescents and young adults, many EDs carry names that have clear marketing reference to psychoactive drug use such as Cocaine and Blow, whereas others have names that glamorize antisocietal behavior like Pimp Juice and Venom. These beverages have been marketed as legal alternatives to gain status as cool beverages. An article with the catchy title A Can of Bull? represents a line of publications questioning the pivotal claim that EDs provide a source of physical and mental energy.[2] Given the popularity of EDs it is surprising that limited literature is available.

This article reviews the literature on EDs and examines their problematic use and the potential negative consequences that these drinks have on young people. Special emphasis is devoted to safety concerns regarding the combination of EDs with alcohol, whether as a commercially packaged beverage or as a mix tailored by the consumer.

THE COMPOSITION OF EDS

The 2 main ingredients in EDs are caffeine and sugar/carbohydrates. In addition, the natural products found in most EDs include several of the following: guarana, B complex vitamins, ginseng, amino acids (eg, taurine), gluconolactone, niacin, inositol, pantenol, and bitter orange. Bitter orange contains synephrine, a newly popular alternative to ephedrine. Ephedrine is the active ingredient in ephedra, once included in some diet and performance-enhancing drinks. The US Food and Drug Administration (FDA), banned ephedra in 2004 after it was linked to heart problems and approximately 80 heatstroke deaths among young athletes.[3] The main stimulating effects of

Department of Psychiatry & Pediatrics, Alcohol Research Center, University of Connecticut Health Center, 263 Farmington Avenue, Farmington, CT 06030-2103, USA
E-mail address: kaminer@uchc.edu

Child Adolesc Psychiatric Clin N Am 19 (2010) 643–650
doi:10.1016/j.chc.2010.03.015
1056-4993/10/$ – see front matter © 2010 Elsevier Inc. All rights reserved.

childpsych.theclinics.com

EDs have been attributed to caffeine as well as to the rush caused by the combination of caffeine and the high dosage of carbohydrates and sugar found in most beverages.

The content of caffeine in EDs varies from 116 mg in the leading brand Red Bull to 428 mg in Spike Shooter. In comparison, a cup of coffee contains 75 mg of caffeine and Coca-Cola Classic/Mountain Dew contains 23 mg. In addition, approximately 50 g of sugar/carbohydrates per serving are commonly present in EDs. All comparisons are in reference to a 340-g (12-oz) serving.

Several EDs do not contain carbohydrates and are therefore marketed as low-calorie energy beverages that charge the user at a cellular level. ACT Energy contains Stevia, a natural sweetener, and maca root, which has been promoted to improve cardiovascular function and act as an antidepressant. The beverage Cocaine not only contains 280 mg of caffeine but also includes a throat-numbing confidential ingredient added to justify its name.[4]

An important example of a low-calorie energy beverage is 5-Hour Energy, which controls 80% of the market of energy shots. The 59-mL (2-fluid oz) drink contains various B vitamins and amino acids. This ED is marketed as an energy blend with an antidepressant property due to phenylalanine[5] (http://5hourenergy.com/product. asp). This is now the most popular category of ED, with sales expected to double from 2008 to about $700 million. This power drink costs 20 times as much per ounce as Coca-Cola.[6]

THE EFFECTS OF EDS, AND TRUTH IN ADVERTISEMENT

It is claimed that EDs provide benefits to the user. The definition of a supplement refers to a substance that is taken to augment the diet. However, some supplements are drugs that exert an effect on a body system and might have physiologic side effects. Dietary supplements are treated as foods, as long as no drug claims are made for them.[7] When products are marketed for therapeutic use, the FDA regulates them. EDs can be viewed historically as an extension of the market for sports drinks (SDs). For example, Gatorade replenishes carbohydrates and electrolytes. Drinking SDs is superior to water because the added flavor stimulates the athlete to consume more fluids that are crucial after extensive physical effort. This consumption is especially important in young athletes more than 12 years of age who dehydrate more quickly and whose core temperature increases faster than in adults, thereby exposing them to increased risk for heat stroke.[8] SDs can be produced noncommercially by simply mixing sugar, salt, orange juice, lemon juice, and water.[9] EDs take the market a step further by adding stimulants.

There is no legal age limit to purchasing EDs. About 30% of 12 to 17 year olds admit to regular use of EDs. High school athletes frequently use supplements, vitamins, minerals, SDs, and EDs because of perceived short-term effects on sports performance.[10] Stimulants may be the most widely used supplement by high school athletes, including caffeine and guarana, which are commonly found in EDs. As the market grows, so do concerns of combining chemical stimulation with exercise. For more information on sport performance agents among high school athletes, which is beyond the scope of this article, please refer to a comprehensive review by Gregory and Fitch.[7]

According to a study among college students,[11] approximately one-third of those aged 18 to 24 years consume EDs. According to students' perceptions, the main reasons for consumption include coping with insufficient sleep (67%), increasing energy (65%), and increasing fun with alcohol at parties (54%). Most users consumed

1 drink to treat most situations; however, the use of 3 or more EDs with alcohol at parties was a common practice in half of ED users.

Alford and colleagues[12] reported that the effects of Red Bull significantly improved aerobic endurance and anaerobic performance on cycle ergometers compared with control drinks. Furthermore, significant improvements in mental performance included choice reaction time, concentration, and memory (immediate recall), which reflected increased subjective alertness. A placebo-controlled study concluded that effects on cognitive performance could not be predicted from the effects of glucose and caffeine in isolation. Data suggest some degree of short-term synergy between the cognition-modulating effects of glucose and caffeine.[13]

Caffeine, the main ingredient in EDs, has been reported to have stimulating effects; however, it is debatable whether these effects are usually the result of caffeine consumption among non–heavy drinkers or to the reversal of caffeine withdrawal among chronic users who have developed tolerance to caffeine. A recent study found no effect of overnight caffeine withdrawal on mood and performance. Caffeine challenges did have the predicted effect on alertness and vigilance, with the size of the effects increasing with caffeine dose in particular on non–heavy drinkers.[14]

Guarana has been a central component of EDs. This fruit of a domesticated rainforest vine is known for its caffeine content and became a soft drink in Brazil about a century ago. It has also been advertised as an aphrodisiac capable of boosting libido.

The amount of the natural products found in EDs is much less than the amounts expected to deliver therapeutic benefits or adverse events.[15]

EDS AND RISK-TAKING BEHAVIORS

Self-reported measures of risk-taking behaviors were positively associated with frequency of ED consumption, particularly among whites.[16] Risk-taking behaviors included tobacco smoking, marijuana and illicit prescription drug use, sexual risk taking, fighting, and seat-belt omission. It is plausible that a liking for EDs is a marker for high-risk behaviors.

It has been reported that a common genetic factor is associated with caffeine, nicotine, and alcohol abuse (see the article by Meyers and Dick elsewhere in this issue for further exploration of this topic).[17] Caffeine has been found to increase the reinforcing effects of nicotine and, because of increased caffeine metabolism among smokers, they consume more caffeine than nonsmokers.[18,19]

ADVERSE EFFECTS OF EDS ATTRIBUTED TO CAFFEINE

In addition to coffee, tea, and soft drinks, caffeine can be found in over-the-counter analgesics and cold remedies, antidrowsiness pills, and weight-loss aids. Chocolate and cocoa have much lower levels of caffeine. Average caffeine intake in the United States is 200 mg/d with up to 30% of Americans consuming 500 mg or more per day. According to the *Diagnostic and Statistical Manual of Mental Disorders* (Fourth Edition, Text Revision) (DSM-IV-TR),[20] caffeine-induced disorders include caffeine intoxication, caffeine-induced anxiety disorder, and caffeine-induced sleep disorder. Although some aspects of dependence have been reported, including tolerance and withdrawal, according to the DSM, the data are insufficient to determine abuse or dependence criteria. However, some reports indicate the potential for caffeine dependence in adolescents.[21,22]

A growing number of reports also show caffeine intoxication from EDs. Caffeine intoxication can be clinically significant. Diagnostic criteria include 5 or more of the following signs: restlessness, nervousness, excitement, insomnia, flushed face, diuresis, gastrointestinal disturbance, muscle twitching, rambling flow of thought and speech, tachycardia, cardiac arrhythmia, psychomotor agitation, and periods of inexhaustibility. Reissig and colleagues[23] note that the consumption of EDs may increase the risk for caffeine overdose for several reasons, including lack of adequate labeling of the amount of caffeine, lack of warning labels advising proper use, and lack of restrictions on the sale of EDs to children and adolescents.

Although individual responses to caffeine vary, the stimulating properties in EDs can increase heart rate and blood pressure, causing palpitations that may lead to emergency-room visits. EDs have also been reported to cause dehydration and insomnia.

Caffeine withdrawal is a research diagnosis in DSM-IV-TR, defined as "A phenomenon occurring after prolonged daily use of caffeine." It is diagnosed following the abrupt cessation of, or reduction in, the use of caffeine-containing products. The main symptom is a headache and 1 or more of the following symptoms: marked fatigue or drowsiness, marked anxiety or depression, and nausea or vomiting. These symptoms cause clinically significant distress or impairment in areas of functioning. Caffeine withdrawal has been identified in children[24,25] and adolescents,[21,22] and aggressive marketing of EDs to these populations may increase the incidence of caffeine-induced adverse effects.[23]

In a comprehensive review on caffeine as a pivotal ingredient in EDs, Reissig and colleagues[23] reported that EDs have been linked to seizures, acute mania, and stroke. A review by Clauson and colleagues[15] from 1980 to 2007 documented 4 case reports of caffeine-associated deaths, as well as 4 separate cases of seizures associated with EDs.

Among college students, weekly jolt and crash episodes were experienced by 29% (with a significant dose effect), headaches by 22%, and heart palpitations by 19% of ED users.[11] The combination of fluid loss from sweating and the diuretic properties of caffeine can also lead to dehydration, particularly among athletes and party goers.

A significant segment of adolescents in Western societies suffer from chronic sleep deprivation due to a maturational shift in the sleep-wakefulness cycle. EDs may be implicated in sleep deficits resulting in excessive daytime sleepiness. Caffeine consumption tended to be 76% higher by those who fall asleep during day time.[26]

It seems likely that problems with caffeine intoxication, dependence, and withdrawal will continue to grow with the increased popularity of EDs and the increase in consumption figures. Adolescents who are novice drinkers of caffeine are at greater risk for caffeine intoxication because they do not use caffeine daily, and also because EDs are served cold and therefore it is easier to consume large amounts of them compared with servings of hot coffee.

EDS AND ALCOHOL INTERACTION

The use of EDs with alcohol is an increasing public health concern. Alcoholic EDs (AEDs) are affordable, prepackaged beverages that commonly contain alcohol at concentrations up to 10%, caffeine, fruit juice, and other stimulants that are commercially available (eg, caffeinated beers such as Anheuser-Busch's B-to-the-E). AEDs are popular among club goers who also are being served AEDs mixed on the spot at the bar (eg, Red Bull and vodka). Approximately a quarter of 2 large samples of college students reported using EDs with alcohol during the last month.[11,27] College ED users consume alcohol more frequently than nonusers. These students got drunk twice as often as those who consumed alcohol only and were far more likely to be injured, require medical treatment, or ride with an intoxicated driver.[27] It was also reported that those who combine EDs and alcohol are more likely to be victims or perpetrators of aggressive sexual behavior. The effect remained even after controlling for the amount of alcohol consumed.[27]

Caffeine use with or after alcohol consumption has been erroneously and commonly perceived as a remedy to reverse the negative effects of alcohol intoxication, such as compromised motor coordination and visual reaction time. ED use simply masks alcohol effects leading to the wide-awake-and-drunk phenomenon, as demonstrated in a laboratory experiment with humans.[28] The ingestion of an ED did not alter the breath alcohol concentration.

A double-blind, placebo-controlled study in female participants showed that, compared with drinkers of EDs only, drinkers of EDs and alcohol at 6% by volume showed lower post-test performance on a global score of neuropsychological status. Specifically, deficits were found in visuospatial/constructional and language performance scores.[29] Therefore, the combined use of caffeine and alcohol may increase the rate of alcohol-related injury. Caffeine is a diuretic, and EDs and alcohol are dehydrating. Dehydration slows the metabolism of alcohol and might increase its toxicity.

Young drivers are more accident prone than adults, particularly after alcohol consumption, because of incomplete maturation of the prefrontal cortex (see the article by Rutherford and colleagues elsewhere in this issue for further exploration of this topic). The consumption of AEDs places them at an increased risk for alcohol-related consequences and having driving-associated deficits masked by the stimulating effects of the caffeine in the AED.[30,31]

The amino acid taurine is a common ingredient in EDs. Studies with laboratory animals showed pharmacologic interaction between alcohol and taurine affecting locomotor activity, dopamine release, and liver metabolism.[15,28] Endogenous taurine may be an important modulator of the effects of ethanol on the nervous system; however, there are no studies reported in humans. In addition, there are no data on the interaction of alcohol and other components of EDs.

LEGAL CONCERNS

Reissig and colleagues[23] noted that the FDA approved caffeine in soft drinks and limited the maximum content to 0.02%, or 71 mg per 355 mL (12 fluid oz); moreover, the FDA requires warning labels and information on the quantity of caffeine in over-the-counter stimulants. This requirement includes the recommendation of an age limit of 12 years. In contrast, there is a concerning inconsistency in FDA regulations because more than 130 EDs now exceed 0.02% of caffeine but are not marketed with warnings or information on the amount of caffeine in the product.[23]

The National Association of Attorneys General (NAAG) has requested that the FDA use its authority under the Food, Drug and Cosmetics Act to remove caffeinated alcoholic beverages from the market place unless the manufacturers empirically demonstrate their safety.[32] The law places the burden of proof on the safety of beverages on the manufacturers and forbids false advertising that may create a misleading impression.[31] Some commercially prepackaged drinks were withdrawn from the market as a result of state and federal legal action. In addition, caffeine and other additives were removed from flavored malt beverages. However, other AEDs are still available and the consumer may simply mix EDs and alcohol at will.[30,31]

The FDA responded by announcing its plan to study concerns regarding the safety of caffeinated alcoholic beverages (ie, intoxicating EDs). There are estimates of consumption rates of 18% for college-age students.[33]

RECENT DEVELOPMENT IN THE ED MARKET

There is a dynamic market for EDs that is continually expanding. This trend was illustrated by a report on CBS radio 880 in New York, in early spring of 2010, that chewable EDs will be available shortly in the form of beef jerky.

The enormous success of energy shots such as the 5-Hour Energy has forced big beverage makers to develop similar products. Dr Pepper began marketing an 85-g (3-oz) version of its Venom ED, called Venom Bite. Coca-Cola and Red Bull also introduced a shot drink.[6]

A new line of mood-altering beverages with a cannabis-oriented marketing campaign (eg, weed in a bottle) known as Anti EDs has recently appeared in the American market.[1,34] These drinks are marketed as an alternative to alcohol or to caffeine-laced EDs by producing calming and relaxing effects without losing focus and concentration. These sugary drinks are laced with folk-medicine sedatives, such as chamomile, valerian root, the south pacific kava root, rose hips (a source of vitamin C and antioxidants derived from rose plants), and the hormone melatonin (used to treat insomnia and jet lag). New drinks carry names such as Mary Jane's Relaxing Soda, Slow Cow, Ex Chill and VIB (ie, vacation in a soda). There are neither age restrictions on the sale of kava-based products nor any known negative effects associated with their consumption; most probably because of the lack of research. Wahlgren[1] cites health information from WebMD that side effects of valerian root may include headache, upset stomach, abnormal heartbeat, and insomnia. Melatonin may cause lower body temperature and affect blood flow. It remains to be seen whether this new lifestyle trend will have the success of EDs.

It has been reported that online drug use information is associated with increasing general curiosity about drugs and intent to use drugs.[35] Therefore, it is likely that as the word on these new beverages spreads by mouth and Internet, more youth will experiment and perhaps continue to use Anti EDs.

SUMMARY AND CONCLUSIONS

The consumption of EDs does not seem to carry adverse effects that are any different from drinking similar amounts of other caffeinated beverages. However, frequent consumption of EDs may serve as a useful screening indicator to identify students at risk for substance use and other problem behaviors.

Communities, state, and federal governments should educate, monitor, and collect data on consumption and adverse effects, and look for legal actions to control the potential harm by excessive use of EDs and of any consumption of AEDs. Special emphasis on prevention-intervention is necessary to protect the impressionable minds of adolescents who are exposed to manipulating advertisements that encourage the consumption of EDs and AEDs. (For a detailed recommendation on legal action please refer to a review by Simon and Mosher.[31])

The qualitative and quantitative effects resulting from excessive and chronic consumption of EDs, as well as from potential interactions with medications and the dynamic innovation and availability of new street drugs, are not fully known. For example, anecdotal information has been provided regarding a combination of EDs and Adderall, a prescription drug for attention deficit disorder that is popular on college campuses. Adderall improves focus and the EDs maintain wakefulness.[6] The label on the drink Endo-Rush carries a warning against its consumption by individuals less than 18 years of age, and those with depression, high blood pressure, or who are pregnant. Therefore, the potential for adverse effects from ED/AED use and drug interaction should always be considered until more empirical data are available.[36] This precaution may be particularly important in youths with psychiatric disorders (see the article by Bukstein and Horner elsewhere in this issue for further exploration of this topic).[37,38]

The debate about taxing sugar-sweetened beverages to combat youth obesity[39] may serve as a platform to consider taxing EDs, particularly for youth. Such an approach might improve prevention of adverse effects by forcing the manufacturers of these drinks to place warning labels and provide age limit and consumption guidelines.

REFERENCES

1. Wahlgren E. Adios, Red Bull? Anti-energy drinks seek to soothe frazzled Americans. Available at: http://www.dailyfinance.com/story/company-news/anti-energy-drinks. Accessed October 7, 2009.
2. Heidmann M, Urquhart G. A can of bull? Do energy drinks really provide a source of energy?. Available at: http://www.sciencecases.org/energy_drinks/retrieved. Accessed January 10, 2010.
3. Severson K. Energy drinks are fueling concerns. Available at: http://www.nytimes.com/2006/06/19/health/healthspecial/19drinks. Accessed February 20, 2010.
4. Sowery M. The ultimate energy drink: cocaine? Available at: http://abcnews.go.com/health/story. Accessed September 18, 2006.
5. Available at: http://5hourenergy.com/product.asp. Accessed February 20, 2010.
6. Neuman W. Energy shots stimulate power drink sales. Available at: http://www.nytimes.com/2009/07/11/business/11energy. Accessed February 20, 2010.
7. Gregory AJM, Fitch RW. Sports medicine: performance enhancing drugs. Pediatr Clin North Am 2007;54:797–806.
8. Decher NR, Casa DJ, Yeargin SW. Hydration status: knowledge and behavior in youths at summer sports camps. Int J Sports Physiol Perform 2008;3(3):262–78.
9. Clark N. Sports nutrition guidebook. 4th edition. Champaign (IL): Human Kinetics; 2009.
10. O'Dea JA. Consumption of nutritional supplements among adolescents: usage and perceived benefits. Health Educ Res 2003;18(1):98–107.
11. Malinauskas BM, Aeby VG, Overton RF, et al. A survey of energy drink consumption patterns among college students. Nutr J 2007;31(6):35.
12. Alford C, Cox H, Wescott R. The effects of Red Bull energy drink on human performance and mood. Amino Acids 2001;21(2):139–50.
13. Scholey AB, Kennedy DO. Cognitive and physiological effects of an energy drink: an evaluation of the whole drink and of glucose, caffeine and herbal fractions. Psychopharmacology 2004;176(3-4):320–30.
14. Hewlett P, Smith A. Effects of repeated doses of caffeine on performance and alertness: new data and secondary analyses. Hum Psychopharmacol 2007;22(6):339–50.
15. Clauson KA, Shields KM, McQueen CE. Safety issues associated with commercially available energy drinks. J Am Pharm Assoc 2008;48(3):e55–63.
16. Miller KE. Energy drinks, race, and problem behaviors among college students. J Adolesc Health 2008;43(5):490–7.
17. Kendler KS, Myers J, Prescott CS. Specificity of genetic and environmental risk factors for symptoms of cannabis, cocaine, alcohol, caffeine and nicotine dependence. Arch Gen Psychiatry 2007;64:1313–20.
18. Swanson JA, Lee JW, Hopp JW. Caffeine and nicotine: a review of their joint use and possible interactive effects in tobacco withdrawal. Addict Behav 1994;19:229–56.

19. Parsons WD, Neims AH. Effect of smoking on caffeine clearance. Clin Pharm 1978;24:40–5.
20. American Psychiatric Association. Diagnostic and statistical manual of mental disorders. Text Revision (DSM-IV-TR). 4th edition. Washington, DC: APPI; 2000.
21. Bernstein GA, Carroll ME, Thuras PD, et al. Caffeine dependence in teenagers. Drug Alcohol Depend 2002;66:1–6.
22. Oberstar JV, Bernstein GA, Thuras PD. Caffeine use and dependence in adolescents: one-year follow-up. J Child Adolesc Psychopharmacol 2002;12:127–35.
23. Reissig CJ, Strain EC, Griffiths RR. Caffeinated energy drinks: a growing problem. Drug Alcohol Depend 2009;99:1–10.
24. Bernstein GA, Carroll ME, Dean NW, et al. Caffeine withdrawal in normal school-age children. J Am Acad Child Adolesc Psychiatry 1998;37:858–65.
25. Goldstein E, Wallace ME. Caffeine dependence in school children? Exp Clin Psychopharmacol 1997;5:388–92.
26. Calamaro CJ, Mason TB, Ratcliffe SJ. Adolescents living the 24/7 lifestyle: effects of caffeine and technology on sleep duration and daytime functioning. Pediatrics 2009;123(6):e1005–10.
27. O'Brien MC, McCoy TP, Rhodes SD, et al. Caffeinated cocktails: energy drink consumption, high-risk drinking, and alcohol related consequences among college students. Acad Emerg Med 2008;15(5):453–60.
28. Ferreira SE, De Mello MT, Pompela S, et al. Effects of energy drink ingestion on alcohol intoxication. Alcohol Clin Exp Res 2006;30:598–605.
29. Curry K, Stasio MJ. The effects of energy drinks alone and with alcohol on neuropsychological functioning. Hum Psychopharmacol 2009;24(6):473–81.
30. Marczinski CA, Fillmore MT. Clubgoers and their trendy cocktails: implications of mixing caffeine into alcohol on information processing and subjective reports of intoxication. Exp Clin Psychopharmacol 2006;14:450–8.
31. Simon M, Mosher J. Alcohol, energy drinks, and youth: a dangerous mix. A report by the Marin Institute. San Rafael (CA): Marin Institute; 2007.
32. Arria A, O'Brien MC, Goldberger B, et al. Safety of alcoholic energy drinks to be reviewed by FDA. Available at: Bcatone@tresearch.org. November 13, 2009.
33. Gardiner H. F.D.A. says it may ban alcoholic drinks with caffeine. Available at: http://nytimes.com/2009/11/14/health/policy/14fda.
34. Hirsch J. Kava anti energy drinks takes root in the southland. Los Angeles Times. January 10, 2010.
35. Belenko S, Dugosh KL, Lynch K, et al. Online illegal drug use information: an exploratory analysis of drug related website viewing by adolescents. J Health Commun 2009;14(7):612–30.
36. Kaminer Y, Goldberg P, Connor D. Psychotropic medications and substances of abuse interactions in youth. Subst Abus 2010;31:53–7.
37. Kaminer Y, Bukstein O, editors. Adolescent substance abuse: dual diagnosis and high risk behaviors. New York: Routledge/Taylor & Francis; 2008.
38. Kaminer Y, Winters K, editors. Clinical manual of adolescent substance abuse treatment. Washington DC: American Psychiatric Publishing Inc; 2010.
39. Brownell KD, Farley T, Willett WC, et al. The public health and economic benefits of taxing sugar-sweetened beverages. N Engl J Med 2009;261(16):1599–605.

Index

Note: Page numbers of article titles are in **boldface** type.

A

Acamprosate, for alcohol abuse in adolescents, 593
Adaptive treatment, after substance abuse management in adolescents, 583–585
Adolescence, early, described, 493
Adolescent(s)
    decision making by, neurobiology of, 480–482
    energy drink use by, **643–650.** See also *Energy drinks.*
    impulsivity of, 631
    SUDs in. See Substance use disorders (SUDs), among adolescents; *specific agents and* Substance use/abuse, in adolescents.
Adult(s), substance use/abuse in, vs. adolescent substance use/abuse, 578
Advertisement(s), truth in, energy drinks–related, 644–645
Age of onset, of pathological gambling and problematic Internet use, 630
Alcohol expectancies, as risk factor for adolescent alcohol abuse, 497–498
Alcohol use/abuse
    energy drinks and, in adolescents, 646–647
    in adolescents, 466, 495–498
        demographic factors, 457
        development of, **493–504**
        deviance prone model, 498–499
        epidemiology trends in, 456–457
        protective factors, 457
        rates of, 456
        risk factors, 456, 495–498
            alcohol expectancies, 497–498
            cognitive functioning, 497
            conduct problems, 496–497
            family history of alcoholism, 495
            peer relations, 498
            social relations, 498
            temperamental traits, 495–496
        treatment of, 593–594, 597, 601
        variations in, 494–495
        vulnerability factors, **493–504**
Alcoholism, family history of, as risk factor for adolescent alcohol abuse, 495
Amphetamine(s), in adolescents, epidemiology trends in, 460
Anti-craving agents, in SUDs management in adolescents, 592–597
Assessment reactivity, in adolescent substance abuse management, **577–590**
    baseline measures in, 578–580
    behavioral change in, mechanisms of, 580–581

Child Adolesc Psychiatric Clin N Am 19 (2010) 651–660
doi:10.1016/S1056-4993(10)00051-9
1056-4993/10/$ – see front matter © 2010 Elsevier Inc. All rights reserved.

childpsych.theclinics.com

Moving?

Make sure your subscription moves with you!

To notify us of your new address, find your **Clinics Account Number** (located on your mailing label above your name), and contact customer service at:

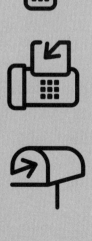

Email: journalscustomerservice-usa@elsevier.com

800-654-2452 (subscribers in the U.S. & Canada)
314-447-8871 (subscribers outside of the U.S. & Canada)

Fax number: 314-447-8029

Elsevier Health Sciences Division
Subscription Customer Service
3251 Riverport Lane
Maryland Heights, MO 63043

*To ensure uninterrupted delivery of your subscription, please notify us at least 4 weeks in advance of move.